ACUTE RENAL FAILURE

Clinical and Experimental

ADVANCES IN EXPERIMENTAL MEDICINE AND BIOLOGY

Recent Volumes in this Series

Volume 205
NEW MOLECULAR AND CELLULAR ASPECTS OF REPRODUCTION
Edited by Dharam S. Dhindsa and Om P. Bahl

Volume 206
ESSENTIAL NUTRIENTS IN CARCINOGENESIS
Edited by Lionel A. Poirier, Paul M. Newberne, and Michael W. Pariza

Volume 207
THE MOLECULAR AND CELLULAR BIOLOGY OF FERTILIZATION
Edited by Jerry L. Hedrick

Volume 208
PHOSPHATE AND MINERAL HOMEOSTASIS
Edited by Shaul G. Massry, Michel Olmer, and Eberhard Ritz

Volume 209
AMYOTROPHIC LATERAL SCLEROSIS
Therapeutic, Psychological, and Research Aspects
Edited by V. Cosi, Ann C. Kato, W. Parlette, P. Pinelli, and M. Poloni

Volume 210
LIPOPROTEINS AND ATHEROSCLEROSIS
Edited by C. L. Malmendier and P. Alaupovic

Volume 211
BIOPHYSICS OF THE PANCREATIC β-CELL
Edited by Illani Arwater, Eduardo Rojas, and Bernat Soria

Volume 212
ACUTE RENAL FAILURE: Clinical and Experimental
Edited by Alberto Amerio, Pasquale Coratelli, Vito M. Campese, and Shaul G. Massry

Volume 213
MECHANISMS OF LYMPHOCYTE ACTIVATION AND IMMUNE REGULATION
Edited by Sudhir Gupta, William E. Paul, and Anthony S. Fauci

---

ACUTE RENAL FAILURE

Clinical and Experimental

Edited by

Alberto Amerio
and Pasquale Coratelli

University of Bari
Bari, Italy

and

Vito M. Campese
and Shaul G. Massry

University of Southern California
Los Angeles, California

PLENUM PRESS • NEW YORK AND LONDON

Library of Congress Cataloging in Publication Data

Bari Seminar in Nephrology on Acute Renal Failure (1986: Bari, Italy)
Acute renal failure.

(Advances in experimental medicine and biology; v. 212)
"Proceedings of the Second Bari Seminar in Nephrology, on Acute Renal Failure, held April 3-5, 1986, in Bari Italy"—T.p. verso.
Includes bibliographies and index.
1. Renal insufficiency, Acute—Congresses. I. Amerio, A. II. Title. III. Series.
[DNLM: 1. Kidney Failure, Acute—congresses. W1 AD559 v. 212/WJ 342 B252a 1986]
RC918.R4B37 1986 616.6′14 87-7714

DOI 10.1007/978-1-4684-8240-9

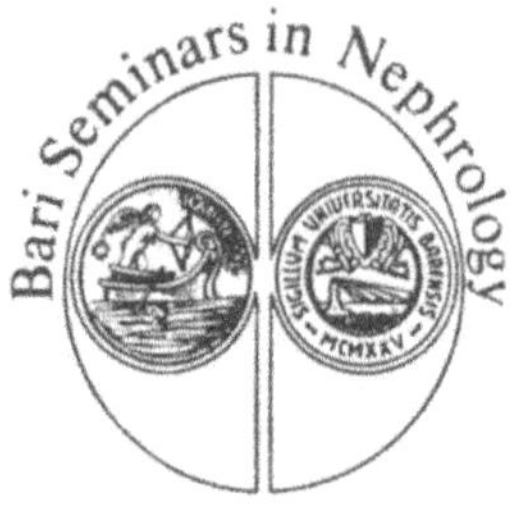

Proceedings of the Second Bari Seminar in Nephrology, on Acute Renal Failure, held April 3-5, 1986, in Bari Italy

TO OUR WIVES

Pia Amerio
Liliana Coratelli
Stefania Campese
Meira Massry

AND OUR CHILDREN

PREFACE

We are pleased to present to our readers the proceedings of the Second Bari Seminars in Nephrology. The topic of theses proceedings deals with clinical and experimental aspects of acute renal failure.

The Bari Seminars in Nephrology were initiated in 1984 and will be held every two years. It is attended by a large number of international clinical scientists in the disciplines of nephrology and related fields.

The next Bari Seminars in Nephrology will take place during April 20-24 in 1988 and the theme of the gathering will be Drugs, Systemic Diseases and the Kidney. We are indebted for the generous financial support of the Centro Nazionale delle Richerche, Italy.

Alberto Amerio
Pasquale Coratelli
Vito M. Campese
Shaul G. Massry

CONTENTS

I. PATHOPHYSIOLOGY AND STRUCTURAL CHANGES OF ACUTE RENAL FAILURE

PATHOPHYSIOLOGY AND STRUCTURAL CHANGES OF ACUTE RENAL FAILURE

PATHOGENESIS OF ACUTE RENAL FAILURE

Michel Burnier and Robert W. Schrier

Department of Medicine
University of Colorado School of Medicine
Denver, CO

INTRODUCTION

Several theories have been proposed to explain the reduced glomerular filtration rate (GFR) occurring in acute renal failure (ARF). Initially, mechanisms related primarily to disturbances of the tubules were advanced and later, others suggested that abnormalities of the renal circulation contributed to the impairment in GFR. It is now clear that the pathogenesis of ARF is multifactorial involving both tubular and vascular events. However, the relative contribution of these tubular and vascular factors varies considerably depending on the model of ARF. Furthermore, it appears that the mechanisms responsible for the initiation of the decrease in GFR differ from those required for its maintenance.

More recently, the cellular abnormalities developing during an ischemic or a toxic renal injury have been examined in more detail and have led to a better understanding of the pathogenesis of ARF. The purpose of the present review is 1) to discuss the vascular and tubular theories proposed to explain the decrease in GFR in ARF and 2) to describe the biochemical changes occurring at the cellular level following an acute renal injury. Since renal ischemia has been one of our major topics of interest during the past several years, this review will emphasize mostly the pathogenesis of ischemic ARF.

VASCULAR THEORY

Clinical and experimental studies have suggested that the initiation phase of most varieties of ARF involves renal ischemia due to renal vasoconstriction and resultant decrease in renal blood flow (RBF). According to these studies the decrease in GFR may result from a decrease in renal perfusion pressure or preglomerular vasoconstriction. A significant decrease in RBF has been demonstrated using different techniques such as Xenon washout, para-aminohippurate clearance, angiography, or microsphere distribution both in patients with established ARF and in various animal models of ARF including glycerol, mercuric or uranyl-induced ARF (1).

The mechanisms responsible for the renal vasoconstriction and the resultant decrease in RBF during ARF are still not precisely defined. Since ARF frequently occurs in clinical settings where adrenergic activity is increased, such as shock or surgery, adrenergic mechanisms have been suggested to cause the renal vasoconstriction of ARF. In experimental situations, renal denervation and administration of phenoxybenzamine after the injection of glycerol have been shown to afford significant protection from glycerol-induced ARF in the rat (2). However, the occurrence of ARF in transplanted, non-innervated kidneys and the failure of phenoxybenzamine to increase RBF and improve ARF in humans are used as arguments against a significant role for adrenergic mechanism (3). Others have focused on the role of prostaglandins and a failure of the kidney to synthetize and release prostaglandins when renal vasoconstriction occurs has been proposed as a possible mechanism during the initiation phase of ARF (4,5). The administration of prostaglandins during hypotensive shock, however, failed to improve renal function (6).

Flores et al proposed that the ischemic injury to the renal vasculature leads to swelling of the endothelial cells causing a reduction of the diameter of renal arterioles and an increase resistance to blood flow (7). Although this hypothesis was attractive, it has been weakened by several observations. First, studies have shown that RBF recovers progressively following an injury and does not deteriorate further as one would expect if Flores' theory was correct. In addition, morphologic studies of the cellular abnormalities developing during ARF indicate that cell swelling involves mainly the tubules rather than the endothelial cells.

Stimulation of the renin-angiotensin system also has been demonstrated in clinical and experimental ARF and a pathogenic role for activation of the renin-angiotensin system in ARF has been proposed (8-10). Thurau and co-workers first suggested that the impaired tubular solute reabsorption developing during the early phase of ARF leads to an increase in sodium chloride delivery to the macula densa which then activates a tubuloglomerular feedback system whereby increased renin-angiotensin activity constricts afferent arterioles (11). However, the failure to observe any changes in the course of ARF with administration of either saralasin, a specific antagonist of angiotensin II, or inhibitors of the angiotensin converting enzyme would suggest that mechanisms other than angiotensin II stimulation are involved in initiating renal vasoconstriction (12).

ARF frequently occurs in the setting of activation of the coagulation system and therefore a role for intravascular coagulation to diminish RBF has been suggested. Although in one clinical study, patients with intravascular coagulation had a high incidence of ARF, histological evidence argued against a participation of the coagulopathy in the decreased RBF (13). Taken together, these observations support the idea that the origin of renal vasoconstriction in ARF is multifactorial, involving probably the renin-angiotensin system, the sympathetic nervous system, and maybe the coagulation system and endothelial cell swelling.

Among the other possible mechanisms contributing to the fall in GFR in ARF, a decrease in glomerular permeability has been suggested. Using transmission electron microscopy, glomerular abnormalities have been demonstrated in the norepinephrine model of ARF. Twenty-four hours after a 2 hour norepinephrine infusion into the renal artery, Cox et al have described the fusion of epithelial processes in the glomeruli (14). Because the endothelial fenestrae may represent a site of water and solute transport, the authors speculated that these changes may induce a defect in glomerular permeability. Glomerular abnormalities have also been found in the glycerol and uranyl nitrate models of ARF (15,16). In addition, in the latter model, micropuncture studies of the surface glomeruli have shown a reduction in total glomerular permeability (17). However, the authors did not determine whether the decrease in glomerular permeability was due to a decrease in filtering surface or a decrease in hydraulic permeability. Thus, the significance of these glomerular changes in the pathogenesis of ARF still needs to be defined. Although some decrease in glomerular permeability has been measured in a few models of ARF, it generally was not of a sufficient degree to explain the severe reduction in GFR. Furthermore, the abnormalities in glomerular morphology could not be confirmed in a reversible model of ARF when norepinephrine was infused for only 40 minutes, suggesting that the glomerular changes are dependent on the severity of the injury (15).

In summary, there is considerable evidence from the literature to support the vascular theory of the pathogenesis during the initiation phase of ARF. However, during the maintenance phase of ARF, ARF persists despite the normalization of RBF. Indeed, if RBF is increased during ARF with the administration of vasoactive agents such as intrarenal dopamine, little if any improvement in GFR occurs. This interesting observation suggests that the maintenance phase of ARF has different characteristics than the initiating phase and supports a role for a tubular component in the pathogenesis of ARF.

TUBULAR THEORY

Tubular obstruction by intraluminal debris and backleak of glomerular filtrate across the injured tubules into the peritubular capillaries are the two main components of the tubular theory. The presence of proximal tubule dilatation and intraluminal casts and debris has been documented both in clinical and experimental forms of ARF and has led to the hypothesis that tubular obstruction is an important factor in the pathogenesis of ARF. Using micropuncture studies, high intratubular pressures have been measured in the norepinephrine and renal artery clamping models of ischemic ARF (19,20) and in ARF induced by mercuric chloride (11), uranyl nitrate (11), hyperuricosuria (21), and methemoglobin (11). Morphologic studies by Venkatachalam et al have also provided some interesting insights into the mechanisms of tubular obstruction (22). Following 25 minutes of renal ischemia, S3 segments of the proximal tubules were severely damaged and often desquamated into the tubular lumen whereas the S1 and S2 segments were only moderately damaged (22). Tubular obstruction can also be caused by the presence of intratubular casts. In human ischemic ARF, studies in the 1950's demonstrated that the distal nephron appeared occluded by urinary casts of the hyaline, granular and pigmented varieties (23). The role of tubular obstruction in the decrease in GFR is supported also by the fact that mannitol or furosemide which inhibit tubular reabsorption and increase tubular pressure protect against ischemic ARF (20,24).

As tubular integrity is disrupted, conditions are created which will allow glomerular filtrate to leak back through the injured tubules into the peritubular capillaries. Evidence for tubular backleak was first supported by microinjection studies using ^{3}H or ^{14}C labeled inulin which showed that the recovery of labeled inulin in the urine was significantly decreased in injured kidneys (16,25). More recently, Myers et al used the fractional clearance of dextran/inulin to demonstrate the presence of tubular backleak (26). Because dextran molecules are larger than inulin molecules, a fractional clearance greater than one would suggest backleak of inulin. With this method Myers et al have shown that about 40% of the filtered inulin was lost by tubular backleak in patients presenting with

ARF following cardiac surgery (26). However, as with changes in glomerular permeabilities, the significance of tubular backleak in some models of ARF is still questioned. For example, no evidence of backleak could be found in reversible models of norepinephrine-induced ARF (20). In addition, it appears that the degree of tubular backleak during ischemic ARF is dependent on the duration of the ischemic insult and the duration of recovery.

In summary, there is evidence to support a role for tubular obstruction and backleak of glomerular filtrate in clinical and experimental ARF. However, it appears that in most forms of ARF, both vascular and tubular factors contribute to the pathogenesis of ARF, with the vascular component being probably more important during the initiation phase of ARF and the tubular component contributing essentially to the maintenance of ARF.

CELLULAR ASPECTS OF THE PATHOGENESIS OF ARF

The study of the pathogenesis of cell injury has provided considerable new information regarding the pathogenesis of tissue injury particularly in the heart and liver. Although the cellular abnormalities occurring during ischemic or nephrotoxic ARF have been investigated for many years, progress in understanding the pathogenesis of cell injury in ARF has been complicated by the morphologic heterogeneity of the kidney and by the different susceptibilities of the nephron segments to injury. Because ischemia is by far the most common cause of ARF, our attention has been focused during the past several years on the mechanisms of ischemic renal cell injury. In vivo studies in ischemic hearts and kidneys have suggested that two steps are involved in the development of ischemic cell injury. First, cellular metabolic changes develop during the period of ischemia which involve a decrease in energy metabolism as the primary event. Then, upon reperfusion, new conditions appear (oxygen and calcium delivery and correction of acidosis) which may actually enhance cellular injury.

CELLULAR INJURY DEVELOPING DURING ISCHEMIA

As soon as ischemia occurs, cellular adenosine triphosphate (ATP) concentrations quickly decline (27) and in presence of very low cellular ATP levels, intracellular electrolyte homeostasis is lost. Mason et al have shown that following renal ischemia, intracellular sodium and chloride concentrations increase whereas cellular potassium, phosphate and magnesium decrease (28). In addition, a shift from aerobic to anaerobic metabolism is observed due to the lack of oxygen and intracellular acidosis develops. Finally, free calcium concentration may increase due to a loss of calcium from intracellular storage sites such as mitochondria or endoplasmic reticulum. Mitochondria isolated from ischemic tissues have been studied extensively and depression of mitochondrial respiration following ischemia is well documented (29,30). In the presence of mitochondrial dysfunction, the capacity of the mitochondria to buffer any increase in cytosolic calcium will be reduced leading to an increase in cytosolic calcium concentration. In addition, calcium may leak from the mitochondria into the cytosol and further increase cytosolic calcium. Intracellular calcium could also increase because the ATP-mediated calcium efflux is decreased or because of the passive calcium influx down a calcium concentration gradient. However, Snowdowne et al could not find any decrease in calcium efflux in cultured kidney cells subjected to 60 minutes of anoxia (31). In the contrary, calcium efflux increased proportionally to the increase in cytosolic-free calcium. Moreover, studies from our laboratory in isolated proximal tubules have shown that in the presence of acidosis calcium influx was not increased following anoxia (32). This latter observation would suggest that any increase in intracellular calcium observed during ischemia when acidosis is present is not due to an increase calcium influx but rather represents a redistribution of intracellular calcium. An hypothetical schema of the progression of cellular events leading to the increase cytosolic calcium during ischemia is presented in Figure 1.

The main consequence of these intracellular changes, in the context of the pathogenesis of ARF, is the development of cell swelling during ischemia, because the increase in intracellular sodium will induce an osmotic flow of water into the cells. Cell swelling may participate in the fall in GFR in many ways. As discussed previously, swelling of the endothelial cells could reduce post-ischemic reperfusion and prolong the period of ischemia. Tubular swelling also may allow the glomerular filtrate to leak back through the more permeable tubular membranes. In addition, if ischemia is prolonged, cell swelling could lead to cell necrosis and possibly cause tubular obstruction by desquamation of the necrotic tubules into the lumen.

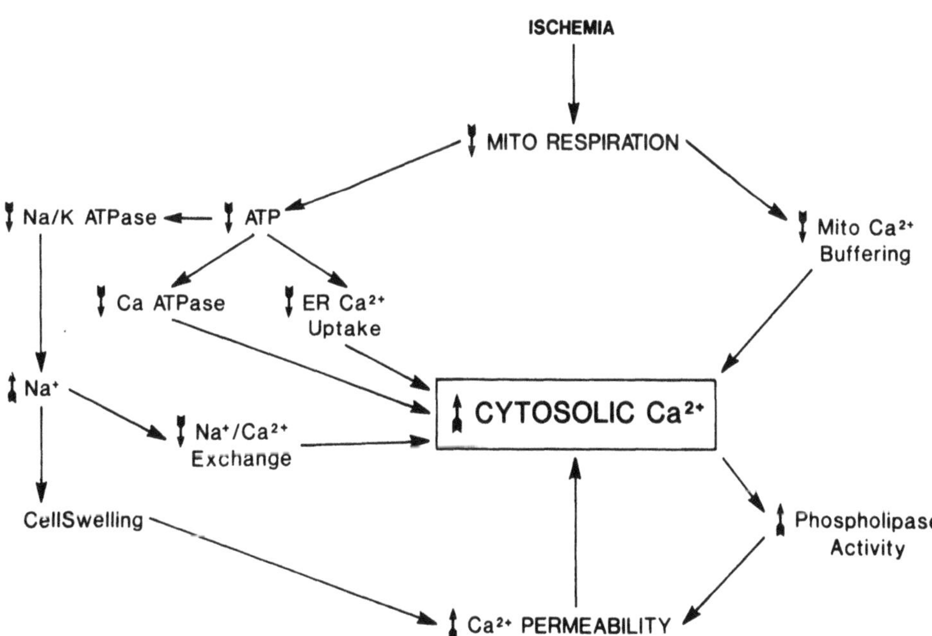

Figure 1. Cellular events leading to increase cytosolic calcium during ischemia and reflow. (With permission from R. W. Schrier, P. E. Arnold, V. J. Van Putten, T. J. Burke, Pathophysiology of cell ischemia, in Diseases of the Kidney, R. W. Schrier, C. W. Gottschalk eds., Little Brown, Boston, in press.)

CELLULAR INJURY OCCURRING DURING REPERFUSION

During reperfusion, oxygen and metabolic substrates delivery is restored and one would expect that these changes are beneficial to the cells. In fact, it does not appear to be the case, at least following ischemia, since an increase in cell injury has been observed upon return of blood flow to both ischemic kidney and heart (33,34). Three factors may contribute to the increase cell injury during reperfusion: 1) increase oxygen delivery, 2) increase ionized calcium delivery, and 3) correction of cellular acidosis.

Oxygen

In healthy tissues, the enzyme xanthine dehydrogenease allows xanthine to be metabolized into uric acid with reduction of NAD into NADH. During ischemia, it has been shown that xanthine dehydrogenase is converted into xanthine oxydase and it has been postulated that the increase in intracellular calcium activates a protease capable of inducing the conversion (35). In the heart, the oxidase content doubles within 10 minutes whereas in the kidneys the same increase is observed after about 30 minutes. Xanthine oxidase can use molecular oxygen instead of NAD to metabolize xanthine and this results in the production of oxygen-free radicals. The formation of oxygen-free radicals will lead to peroxidation of unsaturated fatty acids and ultimately to membrane damage.

Although conversion of xanthine dehydrogenase to xanthine oxydase occurs during ischemia, the formation of free radicals has been shown to develop strictly during reperfusion when adequate oxygen supply is restored. After 60 minutes of renal ischemia, Paller et al could not find any increase in lipid peroxide formation (36). However, a significant increase in lipid peroxide was observed after 15 minutes of reperfusion (36).

The main consequence of the formation of free radicals is the deterioration of both the plasma membrane and the intracellular membranes resulting ultimately in the destruction of the cell. The important role of free radicals in the pathogenesis of cell injury is supported also by the morphologic and functional protection afforded by the xanthine oxidase inhibitor, allopurinol, and free radical scavengers such as superoxide dismutase or catalase (37,38).

Calcium

Reperfusion is also accompanied by an increase ionized calcium delivery to the cells which may contribute to enhance cell injury. Several mechanisms might be involved in the increase intracellular calcium during reperfusion. Initially, as membrane damage occurs, permeability to extracellular calcium will increase and a massive, passive calcium influx will occur down the concentration gradient. As a result, calcium load to the cytosol will be increased and may actually aggravate the membrane damage by activation of phospholipases. As discussed above, it has been suggested that intracellular calcium increases during ischemia mainly because of organelles dysfunction. Recent studies in our laboratory have shown in the rat that mitochondrial function was severely depressed prior to reflow but recovered to near normal levels within 3 hours of reflow (39,40). Subsequently, however, a progressive decline in mitochondrial function was observed which correlated with an increase in mitochondrial calcium content. Simultaneously, the capacity of the mitochondria to buffer any increase in extra-mitochondrial calcium was significantly reduced (27). Thus, although mitochondria are able to buffer an increase in cytosolic calcium during the early post-ischemic phase, mitochondrial calcium overload will ultimately lead to mitochondrial dysfunction allowing cytosolic calcium to increase.

The pathogenic role of alteration in cellular calcium homeostasis is supported by studies in the heart and liver suggesting that increase cellular calcium can convert a reversible membrane injury into an irreversible lesion (40,41). Recently, the detrimental role of calcium in the development of ischemic cell injury has been confirmed in the kidney both in vivo and in vitro.

The intrarenal administration of verapamil or nifedipine in dogs with norepinephrine-induced ARF was associated with significant functional protection as assessed by a better recovery of inulin clearance during reperfusion (42). In addition, verapamil prevented the increase in mitochondrial calcium content observed after 24 hours of reflow in untreated animals and prevented the decrease in State 3 mitochondrial respiration (oxidative phosphorylation). A similar effect of verapamil has been observed in vivo in ischemic ARF in the rat (43). Furthermore, using the isolated perfused rat kidney, Shapiro et al have shown that verapamil was beneficial both in a model of warm and in a model of cold ischemia (44).

Because the extracellular medium can easily be manipulated in in vitro conditions such as cell culture or tubules suspensions, these techniques appear ideal to study the role of extracellular calcium in the development of ischemic cell injury. Wilson et al have shown in cultured tubular cells that cell viability significantly increased following 45 minutes of anoxia if the tubules were incubated in calcium-free medium for the first 2 hours of reoxygenation (45) and in the same circumstances calcium channel blockers also improved cell viability (46). Moreover, when verapamil is added to a suspension of proximal tubules subjected to 30 minutes of anoxia, a decrease in ^{45}Ca influx and particularly the membrane bound calcium occurs. These effects of verapamil on calcium influx were associated with cellular protection against the development of ischemic injury (47).

Acidosis

The contribution of acidosis to organ dysfunction remains unclear but it appears from recent studies that the role of acidosis may vary when one considers the functional versus the biochemical aspect of cell injury. Studies addressing the effect of acidosis on the recovery of renal function in renal preservation did not show any beneficial effect of acidosis (48). At the cellular level, however, acidosis has been shown to protect isolated proximal tubules against an ischemic injury (32,49,50). This apparent discrepancy could be explained by the effect of intracellular pH on cellular metabolism. Because many enzymatic reactions occur at a pH optimum greater than 7.0, intracellular acidosis may reduce cellular activity thus compromising cellular functions such as tubular reabsorption or secretion or blood vessel contraction. The resultant decrease in energy expenditure associated with the decreased metabolic activity may actually protect against cell injury. Indeed, studies by Brezis et al in the isolated perfused rat kidney have suggested that the morphologic protection afforded by various agents against ischemic injury was related to a decrease in energy expenditure due to a decrease in transport activities (51).

As with reoxygenation, pH may become an important factor in the development of cell injury when acidosis is corrected during reperfusion.

For example, on correction of intracellular acidosis, optimal pH for enzymatic reactions will be reached and an increase in phospholipases activity might lead to membrane damage. In addition, studies from our laboratory in isolated proximal tubules subjected to 30 minutes of anoxia have shown that the presence of extracellular acidosis prevented the increase in ^{45}Ca uptake observed in anoxic tubules maintained in an extracellular pH of 7.4 (32). This observation suggests that massive calcium influx into injured cells does not occur when acidosis is present but rather it occurs when acidosis is corrected, e.g. during reperfusion.

Recent studies in human neutrophils have suggested that intracellular pH modulates the generation of superoxide radicals (52). Although this possibility has not been addressed in renal or vascular cells, it could represent another mechanism whereby correction of intracellular pH may be detrimental to the cells.

CONCLUSION

The understanding of the pathogenesis of ARF has progressed considerably within the last several years and the progress has been due, at least in part, because of the availability of new techniques and preparations such as cultured cells and isolated tubule suspensions. These new approaches have provided interesting insights into several major aspects of renal cell injury and have allowed the separate study of the vascular and the tubular events classically described in ARF. While this review has focused on the new information relating to the pathogenesis of ischemic ARF, equally important observations have been reported recently regarding the cellular response to nephrotoxic agents.

ACKNOWLEDGEMENTS

Dr. Michel Burnier is a recipient of a grant from the Swiss Foundation for Medicine and Biology supported by the Swiss Academy of Medical Sciences.

REFERENCES

1. M. S. Paller and R. J. Anderson, Use of vasoactive agents in the therapy of acute renal failure, in: Acute Renal Failure, B. M. Brenner and J. M. Lazarus, eds., W. B. Saunders, Philadelphia (1983).
2. D. McLean and A. E. Thompson, Effect of phenoxybenzamine on glycerol-induced acute renal failure in the rat, Fed. Proc. 29:1313 (1970).
3. A. E. Thompson and H. Y. M. Fung, Adrenergic and cholinergic mechanisms in acute renal failure in the dog and in man, Proc. Conf. Acute Renal Failure, DHEW Publication, Washington, DC, p. 293 (1974).
4. L. G. Fine, Acquired prostaglandin E_2 (medullin) deficiency as the cause of oliguria in acute tubular necrosis: A hypothesis, Israel J. Med. Sci. 6:346 (1970).
5. F. C. Reubi, The pathogenesis of anuria following shock, Kidney Int. 5:106 (1974).
6. V. E. Torres, J. C. Romero, C. G. Strong, D. M. Wilson and V. R. Walker, Renal prostaglandin E during acute renal failure, Prostaglandins 8:353 (1974).
7. J. Flores, D. R. DiBona, C. H. Beck and A. Leaf, The role of cell swelling in ischemic renal damage and the protective effect of

hypertonic solute, J. Clin. Invest. 51:118 (1972).
8. W. E. Mitch and W. G. Walker, Plasma renin and angiotensin II in acute renal failure, Lancet 1:328 (1977).
9. G. F. DiBona and L. L. Sawin, The renin-angiotensin system in acute renal failure in the rat, Lab. Invest. 25:528 (1971).
10. P. G. Mathews, T. O. Morgan and C. I. Johnston, The renin-angiotensin system in acute renal failure in rats, Clin. Sci. Mol. Med. 47:79-88 (19).
11. J. Mason, C. Olbricht, T. Takabatake and K. Thurau, The early phase of experimental acute renal failure. I. Intratubular pressure and obstruction, Pfluegers Arch. 37:155 (1977).
12. J. D. Powell-Jackson, J. MacGregor, J. J. Brown, A. F. Lever and I. S. Robertson, The effect of angiotensin II antisera and synthetic inhibitors of the renin-angiotensin system on glycerol-induced acute renal failure in the rat, in: Proceedings of the Contress on Acute Renal Failure, E. A. Friedman and H. E. Eliahou eds., Department of Health, Education and Welfare, Washington, DC, Publication No. 74-608, pp. 281 (1973).
13. M. J. Mant and E. G. King, Severe acute disseminated intravascular coagulation, Am. J. Med. 67:557 (1979).
14. J. W. Cox, R. W. Baehler, H. Sharma, T. O'Dorisio, R. W. Osgood, J. H. Stein and T. F. Ferris, Studies on the mechanism of oliguria in a model of unilateral acute renal failure, J. Clin. Invest. 53:1546 (1974).
15. T. Suzuki and F. K. Mostoffi, Electron microscopy studies of acute tubular necrosis: Early changes in the glomeruli of rat kidney after subcutaneous injection of glycerin, Lab. Invest. 23:8 (1970).
16. J. H. Stein, J. Gottschalk, R. W. Osgood and T. F. Ferris, Pathophysiology of a nephrotoxic model of acute renal failure, Kidney Int. 8:27 (1975).
17. R. C. Blantz, The mechanism of acute renal failure after uranyl nitrate, J. Clin. Invest. 55:621 (1975).
18. R. E. Cronin, A. deTorrente, P. D. Miller, R. E. Bulger, T. J. Burke and R. W. Schrier, Pathogenic mechanisms in early norepinephrine induced acute renal failure: Functional and histological correlates of protection, Kidney Int. 14:155 (1978).
19. W. J. Arendhorst, W. F. Finn and C. W. Gottschalk, Micropuncture study of acute renal failure following temporary renal ischemia in the rat, Kidney Int. 10:S100 (1976).
20. T. J. Burke, R. E. Cronin, K. L. Duchin, L. N. Peterson and R. W. Schrier, Ischemia and tubule obstruction during acute renal failure in dogs: Mannitol in protection, Am. J. Physiol. 238:F305 (1980).
21. J. D. Conger and T. J. Burke, Pathogenesis and prevention of acute urate nephropathy, J. Clin. Invest. 58:681 (1976).
22. M. A. Venkatachalam, D. B. Bernard, J. F. Donohoe and N. G. Levinsky, Ischemic damage and repair in the rat proximal tubule: Differences among the S1, S2 and S3 segments, Kidney Int. 14:31 (1978).
23. C. Brun and D. Munck, Lesions of the kidney in acute renal failure following shock, Lancet 1:603 (1957).
24. A. deTorrente, P. D. Miller, R. E. Cronin, P. E. Paulsen, A. L. Erickson and R. W. Schrier, Effects of furosemide and acetylcholine in norepinephrine-induced acute renal failure, Am. J. Physiol. 235:F131 (1978).
25. G. A. Tanner, K. L. Sloan and S. Sophasan, Effects of renal artery occlusion on kidney function in the rat, Kidney Int. 4:377 (1973).
26. B. D. Myers, B. J. Carrie, R. R. Yee, M. Hilberman and A. B. Michaels, Pathophysiology of hemodynamically mediated acute renal failure in man, Kidney Int. 18:495 (1980).
27. P. E. Arnold, V. J. Van Putten, D. Lumlertgul, T. J. Burke and R. W. Schrier, Adenine nucleotide metabolism and mitochondrial Ca

transport following renal ischemia, Am. J. Physiol. 250:F357 (1986).
28. J. Mason, F. Beck, A. Dorge, R. Rick and K. Thurau, Intracellular electrolyte composition following renal ischemia, Kidney Int. 20:61 (1981).
29. P. E. Arnold, D. Lumlertgul, T. J. Burke and R. W. Schrier, In vitro versus in vivo mitochondrial calcium loading in ischemic acute renal failure, Am. J. Physiol. 248:F845 (1985).
30. T. Takano, S. P. Soltoff, S. Murdaugh and L. J. Mandel, Intracellular respiratory dysfunction and cell injury in short-term anoxia of rabbit renal proximal tubules, J. Clin. Invest. 76:2377 (1985).
31. K. W. Snowdowne, C. G. Freudenrich and A. B. Borle, The effects of anoxia on cytosolic free calcium, calcium fluxes, and cellular ATP levels in cultured kidney cells, J. Biol. Chem. 260:11619 (1985).
32. M. Burnier, P. Shanley, T. J. Burke and R. W. Schrier, Effect of extracellular acidosis on enhanced Ca influx in anoxic renal proximal tubules (PT) (abstract), Kidney Int. 29:299 (1986).
33. N. S. Frega, D. R. DiBona, B. Guertler and A. Leaf, Ischemic renal injury, Kidney Int. 10:517 (1976).
34. R. A. Kloner, C. E. Ganote, D. Whalen and R. B. Jennings, Effect of transient period of ischemia on myocardial cells. II. Fine structure during the first few minutes of reflow, Am. J. Pathol. 74:399 (1979).
35. J. M. McCord, Oxygen-derived free radicals in post-ischemic tissue injury, N. Engl. J. Med. 312:159 (1985).
36. M. S. Paller, J. R. Hoidal and T. F. Ferris, Oxygen-free radicals in ischemic acute renal failure in the rat, J. Clin. Invest. 74:1156 (1984).
37. J. R. Stewart, W. H. Blackwell, S. L. Crute, V. Loughlin, M. L. Hess and L. J. Greenfield, Prevention of myocardial ischemia/reperfusion injury with oxygen free radicals scavengers, Surg. Forum 33:317 (1982).
38. L. H. Toledo-Pereyra, R. L. Simmons and J. S. Najarian, Effect of allopurinol on the preservation of ischemic kidneys perfused with plasma or plasma substitutes, Ann. Surg. 180:780 (1974).
39. D. R. Wilson, P. E., Arnold, T. J. Burke and R. W. Schrier, Mitochondrial calcium accumulation and mitochondrial respiration in ischemic acute renal failure in the rat, Kidney Int. 25:519 (1984).
40. J. L. Farber, The role of calcium in cell death, Life Sci. 29:1289 (1981).
41. W. G. Nayler, P. A. Poole-Wilson and A. Williams, Hypoxia and calcium, J. Mol. Cell. Cardiol. 11:683 (1979).
42. T. J. Burke, P. E. Arnold, J. A. Gordon, R. E. Bulger, D. C. Dobyan and R. W. Schrier, Protective effect of intrarenal calcium membrane blockers before or after renal ischemia. Functional, morphological and mitochondrial studies, J. Clin. Invest. 74:1830 (1984).
43. D. Goldfarb, A. Iaina, I. Serbon, S. Gavendo, S. Koupler and H. E. Eliahou, Protective effect of verapamil in ischemic acute renal failure in the rat, Proc. Soc. Exp. Biol. Med. 172:389 (1983).
44. J. I. Shapiro, C. Cheung, A. Itabashi, L. Chan and R. W. Schrier, The effect of verapamil on renal function after warm and cold ischemia in the isolated perfused kidney, Transplantation 40:596 (1985).
45. P. D. Wilson and R. W. Schrier, Nephron segments and calcium as determinants of ischemic cell death in primary renal cell cultures, Kidney Int. (in press).
46. U. Schwertschlag, R. W. Schrier and P. D. Wilson, Beneficial effects of calcium channel blockers and calmodulin binding drugs on in vitro renal cell anoxia, J. Pharmacol. Exp. Ther. (in press).
47. M. Burnier, V. Van Putten, P. D. Wilson, T. J. Burke, and R. W. Schrier, Beneficial effects of verapamil (V) and nifedipine (N) on

Ca influx and cell viability in anoxic renal cortical proximal tubules (CPT) (abstract), Mineral Electrolyte Metab. 11:390 (1985).
48. P. J. Bore, L. Chan, P. A. Sehr, K. R. Thulborn, B. D. Ross and G. K. Radda, The importance of pH in renal preservation, Transplant. Proc. 13:707 (1981).
49. J. M. Weinberg, Oxygen deprivation-induced injury to isolated rabbit kidney tubules, J. Clin. Invest. 76:1193 (1985).
50. J. V. Bonventre and J. Y. Cheung, Effects of metabolic acidosis on viability of cells exposed to anoxia, Am. J. Physiol. 249:C149 (1985).
51. M. Brezis, S. Rosen, P. Silva and F. H. Epstein, Renal ischemia: A new perspective, Kidney Int. 26:375 (1984).
52. L. Simchowitz, Intracellular pH modulates the generation of superoxide radicals by human neutrophils, J. Clin. Invest. 76:1079 (1985).

STRUCTURAL-FUNCTIONAL CORRELATES IN ACUTE RENAL FAILURE

Garabed Eknoyan, Dennis C. Dobyan*, and Ruth E. Bulger*

Baylor College of Medicine and *The University of Texas
Health Science Center at Houston
Houston, Texas

INTRODUCTION

The acute renal failure syndrome (ARF) may result from a variety of causes. This discussion will focus on one of the major subtypes of this entity, specifically that of acute tubular necrosis (ATN) which by definition includes those forms of acute renal failure in which tubular injury of acute onset is the primary basis for renal failure, and excludes other causes of ARF, such as those due to glomerular, vascular and interstitial lesions. ATN is by far the most common cause of ARF, and accounts for some 40% of cases encountered clinically.

The appropriateness of the term "acute tubular necrosis" to describe a form of ARF has been controversial, and the contention that tubular damage determines renal failure has been challenged. However, over the past two decades, experimental studies of ischemic and nephrotoxic models of ARF have established the primacy of tubular injury and characterized it by a progression of well defined events in which the structural integrity of the renal tubule is frequently compromised. Actually, it is the application of transmission and scanning electron microscopy which provided experimental pathologists with the potent tools necessary to characterize the structural changes that follow insult (1-8). Figures 1 through 4 illustrate the sequential changes that are observed by scanning electron microscopy following one prototype model of ARF induced by mercuric chloride injection in the rat. The same general pattern has been described in other models of ARF. It has been shown that the initial nephrotoxic insult affects the cells lining the proximal tubule (Figure 1) which will then exhibit varying degrees of sublethal injury which, if allowed to persist, can ultimately culminate in cellular necrosis (Figure 2). The rate at which the cells progress from potentially reversible injury to irreversible necrosis is dependent on the type and magnitude of the insult, and on the underlying metabolic state of the cell which can alter its susceptibility to the injurious stimulus. When cell necrosis occurs it results in sloughing of the injured cells or cellular debris into the tubular lumen with subsequent denudation of the tubular basement membrane and cast formation in the distal nephron (Figures 3 and 4). The earlier controversy as to whether morphological injury of epithelial cells accounts for the development of ARF in the clinical setting seems to be resolving with more careful studies where cell injury is quantitated and reviewed critically (9).

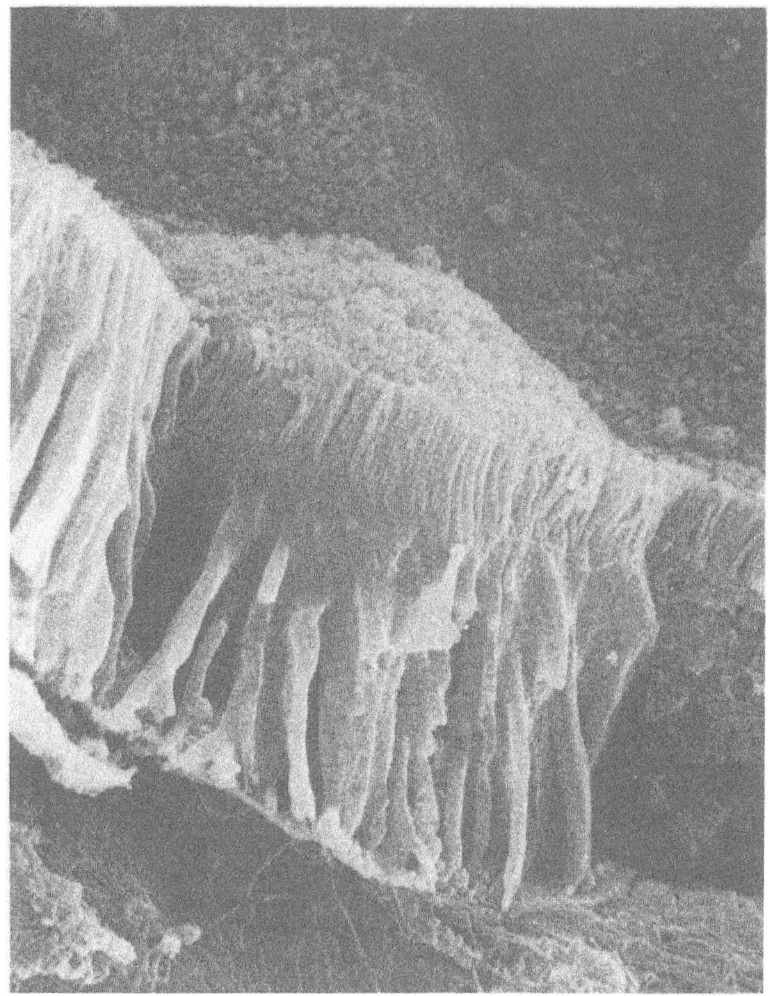

Figure 1. Scanning electron micrograph of the normal proximal tubule of a rat. Note the smooth velvety appearance of the villi.

Prompted by these initial studies which provided a descriptive sequence of events over the past decade, rigorous attempts have been made to correlate the structural changes seen in experimental models of ARF with concomitant measurements of renal function. In order to arrive at meaningful correlations of structural and functional changes it is important to adhere to the basic principles shown in Table I.

TABLE I. CONSIDERATIONS IN ESTABLISHING STRUCTURE-FUNCTION CORRELATES

1. Determine renal function at the same time that the morphologic studies are undertaken.
2. Optimize tissue preservation by in-vivo vascular perfusion.
3. Determine severity and extent of tissue injury by preset criteria.
4. Evaluate different regions of the kidney.
5. Evaluate several areas, within each region, at random.

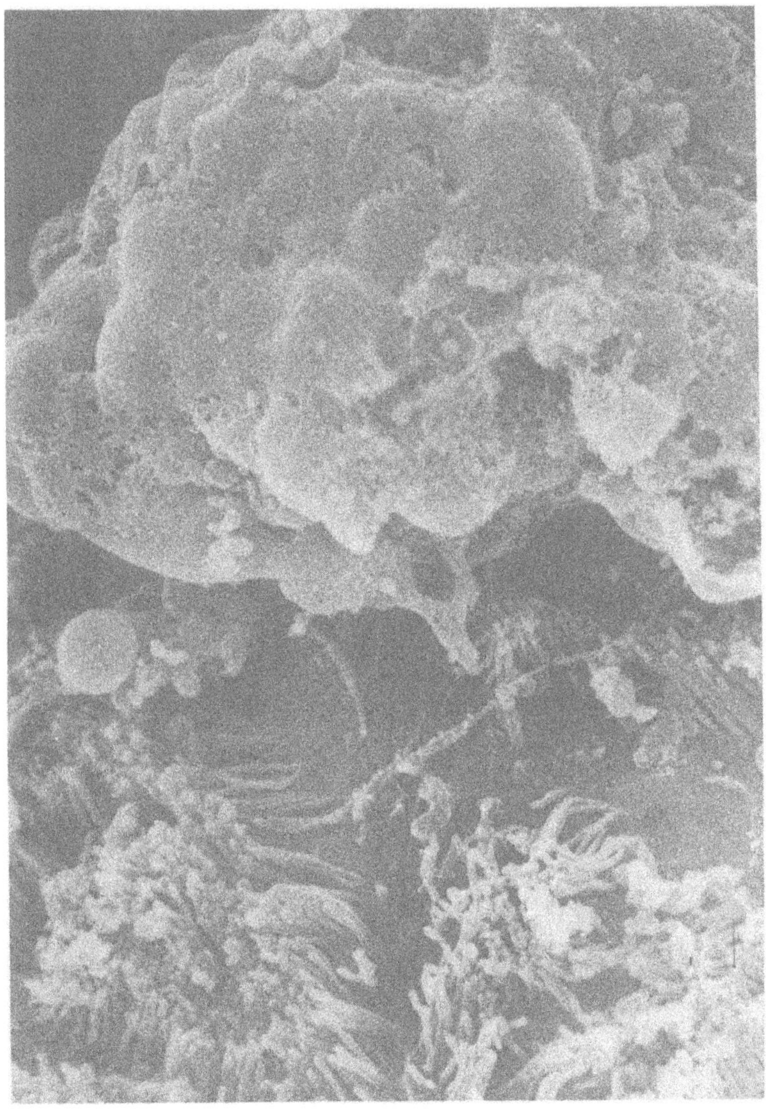

Figure 2. Scanning electron micrograph of the proximal tubule of a rat less than 24 hours after exposure to mercuric chloride. The cell in the upper part of the figure is necrotic. The cells in the lower part of the figure are injured and have lost the normal velvety appearance of the microvilli.

CORRELATION OF RENAL FUNCTION AND STRUCTURAL CHANGES IN THE PROXIMAL TUBULE IN NEPHROTOXIC MODELS OF A.R.F.

As an example of the feasibility of quantitative examination of tubular and glomerular alterations we will summarize the data from several sets of studies completed in our laboratories (10-12). The first of these was an effort to determine whether there is a correlation between the morphologic and functional changes that occur in a nephrotoxic model of acute renal failure in rats, induced by the subcutaneous administration of mercuric chloride at a dose of 2 mg/kg body weight. In this study, renal function was determined from the clearance of inulin (GFR) and the frac-

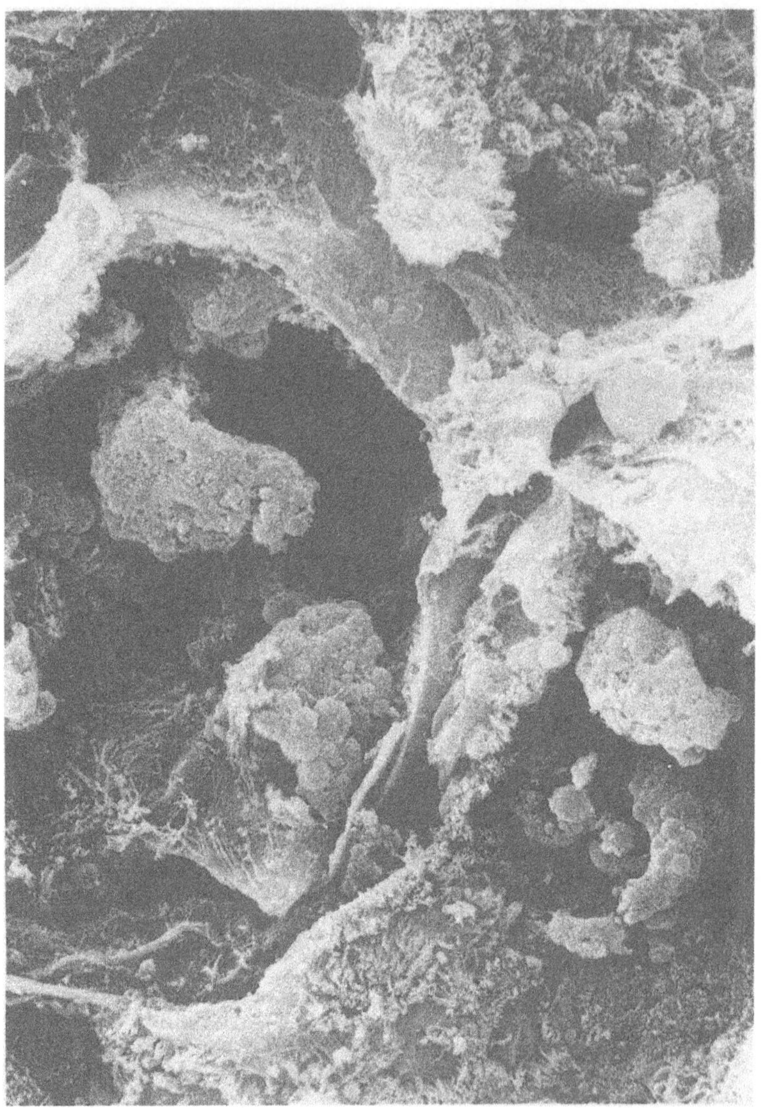

Figure 3. Scanning electron micrograph of the proximal tubule of a rat more than 24 hours after exposure to mercuric chloride. Compared to Figure 2, most of the cells now are necrotic and sloughing. Note the denuded areas of basement membrane.

tional excretion of sodium (F_ENa) measured immediately prior to the in-situ fixation of the kidney by vascular perfusion. In each kidney, five separate areas from the outer cortex, the inner cortex and the outer zone of the medulla were analyzed. A total of 144 cells in each of the areas examined were categorized and the proximal tubular cells were classified as normal, injured or necrotic. The data from each specific region was then combined to yield a single value per region per animal.

When the GFR was plotted against the percent of necrotic cells there was a significant linear relationship between the percent of necrotic cells in the pars recta of the proximal tubule and in the inner cortical region, with a correlation coefficient of 0.767. This was also the case when the

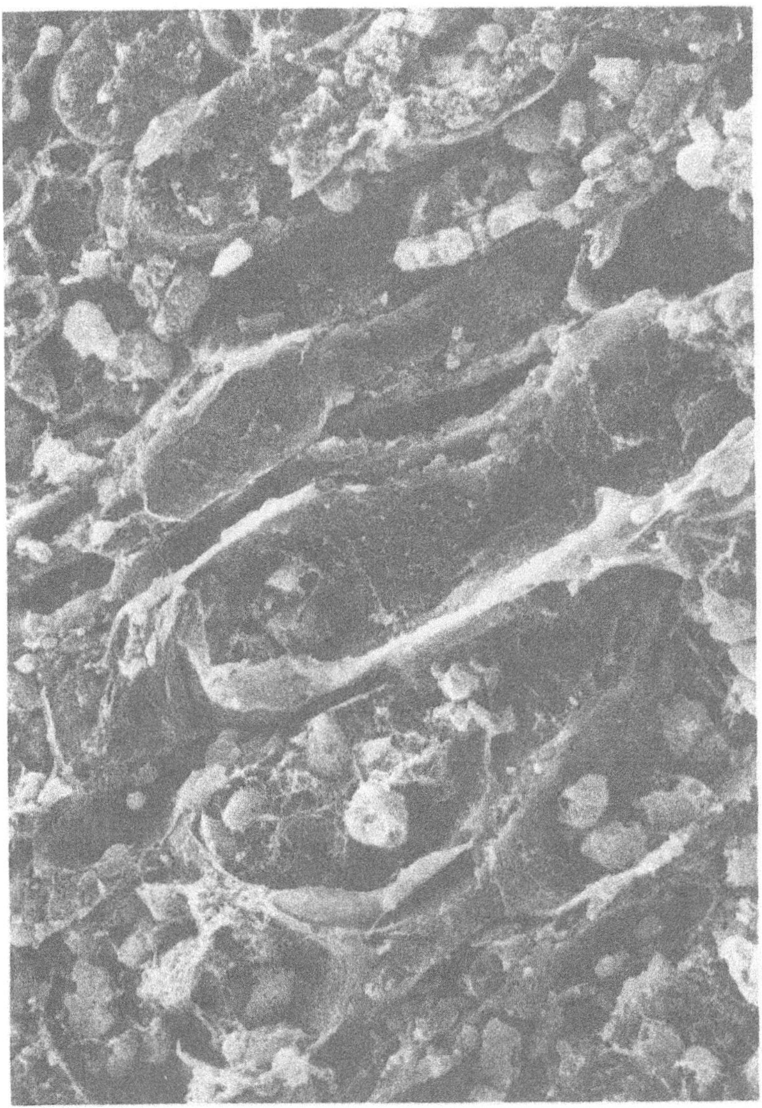

Figure 4. Scanning electron micrograph of the proximal tubule of a rat after ischemic injury induced by norepinephrine infusion. Extensive cell necrosis and sloughing is evident with the consequent exposure of denuded segments of the basement membrane.

GFR was plotted as a function of the percent of the necrotic cells in the pars recta in the outer stripe of the medulla. There was also a significant ($p < 0.01$) linear increase in the fractional excretion of sodium with the increase in percent of necrotic cells, with a correlation coefficient of 0.475. While these observations may not be totally unexpected, they illustrate one type of quantitative correlation that can be established between the functional and morphologic changes in acute renal failure. Similar correlations between the serum creatinine and that of the number of casts, accumulation of leukocytes in the vasa recta, interstitial inflammation, tubular necrosis and tubular dilatation have also been noted in glycerol and gentamicin-induced acute renal failure (9, 13, 14). While the data presented focuses on the changes in the proximal tubule, over the past few years, Brezis and his associates (15), using a model of isolated kidney, have demonstrated preferential lesions in the ascending thick limb of Henle's loop in a variety of experimental situations.

CORRELATION OF RENAL FUNCTION AND STRUCTURAL CHANGES IN THE GLOMERULUS

Interest in endothelial changes in acute renal failure has been prompted by the quest for a structural basis to explain the decrease in balance between hydrostatic and controlled osmotic forces governing the transcapillary filtration of fluid; applied to the ultrafiltration of plasma in the glomerular capillaries gives the now well popularized formula for single nephron glomerular filtration rate (16):

$$SNGFR = K_f[(P_{GC}-P_T) - (\pi_{GC}-\pi_T)]$$

Where K_f is the ultrafiltration coefficient, P_{GC} and P_T are the mean glomerular capillary and proximal tubular hydrostatic pressures; and π_{GC} and π_T the glomerular capillary and proximal tubular colloid osmotic pressures. Of note in this formula is K_f which stands for ultrafiltration coefficient. The demonstration of a decline in ultrafiltration coefficient determined from direct measurements of transcapillary hydrostatic pressure and oncotic pressure in different experimental models of acute renal failure (17-20), has provided a functional explanation for the drop in GFR in acute renal failure. Since the ultrafiltration coefficient is the product of hydraulic or water permeability or "k", and the available surface area for ultrafiltration or "S", attention has been focused on this latter value (21). The hydraulic permeability of fenestrated capillaries are several orders of magnitude higher that that of non-fenestrated capillaries, suggesting that the fenestrated glomerular capillaries are functional channels of convective transport (22, 23). Interest has, therefore, focused on the role of fenestrae in the decrease in GFR, and evidence has been presented that fenestral size and density are altered in different models of acute renal failure (24, 25).

Prior to embarking on a study of the endothelial changes that might occur in acute renal failure, we felt it important to determine the normal endothelial cell morphology and to define the variations that might exist under control conditions. Using a freeze-cracking technique which exposes the endothelial surface for examination by scanning electron microscopy, we conducted a detailed morphometric study of the endothelium (26). In this study, low magnification scanning electron micrographs were taken of four individual cortical and juxtamedullary glomeruli per kidney for mapping of the capillary loops. All those capillaries whose endothelial surfaces were exposed were then photographed at a high magnification, and fifteen micrographs from each animal were chosen at random for morphometric analysis of the capillary mechanism.

As can be seen in Figure 5, the attenuated endothelial surface is divided into compartments by non-fenestrated cytoplasmic crests and ridges radiating from the nucleated non-fenestrated portion of the endothelium. As part of the study, Xerox copies were made of the fifteen randomly chosen micrographs from each animal used for endothelial pore size measurement. Of these copies, the endothelial structures were color coded as ridges, attenuated fenestrated areas, and non-fenestrated areas. The figures were then cut out and weighed to determine the percent component of each type of structure. The fenestrated areas constituted 56% of the surface area, whereas the ridges occupied about 32.5% of the surface, while the remaining 11.5% was occupied by non-fenestrated areas (12, 26).

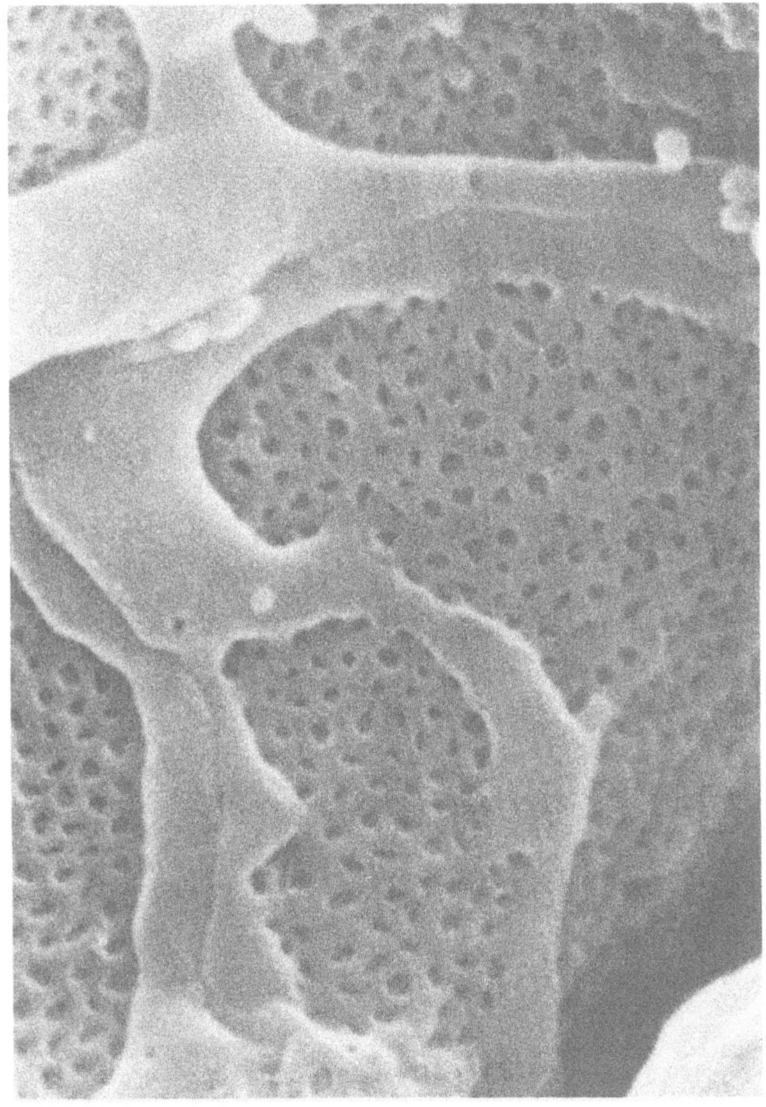

Figure 5. Scanning electron micrograph of the endothelial cell surface of a glomerular capillary from the kidney of a normal rat. The fenestrated areas are separated by cytoplasmic ridges. Note the variation in the size and shape of the fenestrae.

Closer examination of the fenestrated areas (Figure 5), reveals that whereas some of the pores are roughly circular, the bulk of the fenestrae are conspicuously variable in shape, being at best, oval or ellipsoidal in most, and more irregular in others, some of which have distinct angular components. Three-dimensional representations of the glomerulus that have been developed and used in the various texts show the glomerular capillary fenestrations as perfect circles, and the diameter of the pores as given as an expression of pore size, with given values ranging from 500-1000 A° (27, 28). Therefore, a fallacy that needs to be corrected is that the pores are not circles and a more correct or physiological expression of their size would be that of their area. When pore area was measured, the

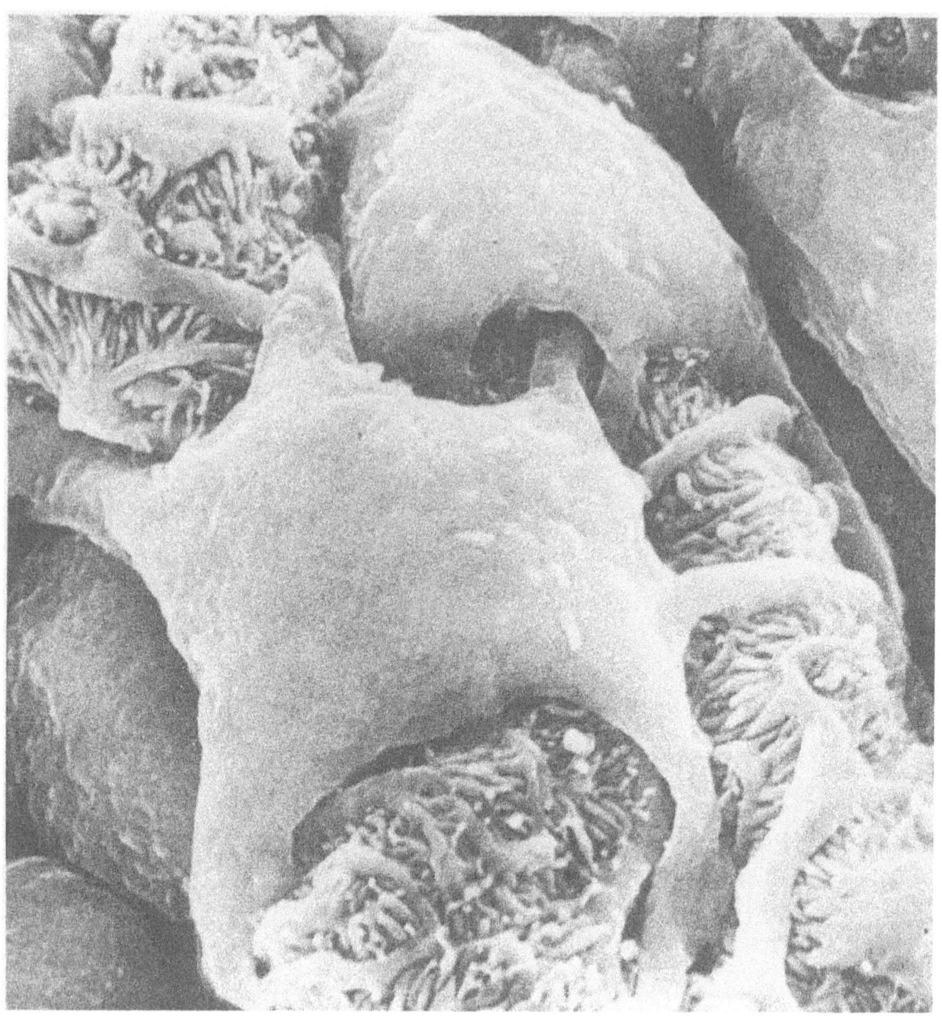

Figure 6. Scanning electron micrograph of the epithelial surface of a glomerular capillary from the kidney of a normal rat. Note the interdigitating pedicels or foot processes forming the filtration slits.

variations noted visually were substantiated. Pores varied in size, ranging from 815 to 2100 nm^2, with an average value of 1560 nm^2. The pore size in the fenestrated areas adjacent to the ridges and non-fenestrated endothelium were smaller, averaging 1200 nm^2, occurred less frequently, and occupied less of the available surface area (Figure 5). The aggregate area occupied by pores in the fenestrated area of the endothelium was about 12.5%, and the number of pores per μm^2 of fenestrated area of the endothelium was about 90. Here again, there was considerable variation with the values for the latter ranging from 53 to 118 pores per μm^2, and the former 6.6% to 18%.

Obviously, unless this kind of careful analysis is made in any study of endothelial morphometry, the results are bound to be altered upward or downward depending on how many of the variable pores are included in the final evaluation. When we applied this kind of meticulous study to the examination of experimental models of acute renal failure induced by mercuric chloride or gentamicin in rats, we could not detect a difference in endothelial characteristics from that of normal (12).

Another aspect of the glomerulus that can affect GFR is the visceral epithelial surface. The main cell body of the visceral epithelial cells is somewhat removed from the glomerular capillary wall and is separated from the underlying glomerular basement membrane by a layer of abundant cytoplasmic projections. Primary processes emanating from the main cell body radiate and branch into secondary and tertiary processes which terminate in club-shaped foot processes or pedicels, that lie immediately over the glomerular capillary wall (Figure 6). These pedicels interdigitate with pedicels from adjacent epithelial cells to form an intricate system of slits that are part of the glomerular filtration barrier (21). Here again, some of the early descriptive studies of the epithelial surface in experimental models of acute renal failure noted significant changes (2, 4, 29). However, when subjected to quantitative analysis, it became evident that although detectable changes can be ascertained by scanning electron microscopy, these are evident only very early after ischemic insult and tend to diminish quickly after a very short period of time, and are more evident in models that develop severe post-ischemic acute renal failure (30, 31). Most investigators have been able to detect only minimal changes in epithelial cell, reflecting the transient nature of the phenomena and have concluded that the glomerular podocyte changes are not a primary pathophysiological mechanism that could cause the decreased glomerular filtitration rate in ARF (31).

CONCLUSIONS

The structural changes in ATN and attendant functional changes can be summarized as being: 1) tubular injury resulting in abnormal permeability that could account for the polyuria and increased fractional excretion of sodium, and intratubular cell necrosis and sloughing resulting in tubular obstruction that could account for oliguria and anuria; 2) glomerular changes which are manifested by minimal or transient structural changes but significant functional changes that could account for the decreased SNGFR; and 3) vascular changes which involve the afferent arteriole and could contribute to the decreased SNGFR, and the vasa recta which could account for the injury to the thick ascending limb of the loop of Henle. There is convincing evidence that all these factors, to varying degrees, contribute to the impairment of renal function in ARF. However, the bulk of the evidence indicates that tubular damage constitutes the primary defect.

Finally, it must be noted that the process of tubular damage is reversible, with tubular regeneration and recovery following in the footsteps of injury (11). This recovery process may extend over weeks or months, during which tubular function remains abnormal manifesting itself principally as an inability to concentrate the urine maximally with resultant polyuria and nocturia that is noted clinically after an episode of ATN.

REFERENCES

1. Bulger, R. E., Cronin, R. E. and Dobyan, D. C.: Glomerular architectural changes after a two-hour infusion of norepinephrine. AMER. J. ANAT. 159: 379-384, 1980.
2. Cox, J. W., Baehler, R. W., Sharma, T., O'Dousio, R. W., Osgood, J. H., Stein, J. H. and Ferris, T. F.: Studies on the mechanism of oliguria in a model of unilateral acute renal failure. J. CLIN. INVEST. 53: 1564-1578, 1974.

3. Cronin, R. E., DeTorrente, A., Miller, P. D., Bulger, R. E., Burke, T. J. and Schrier, R. E.: Pathogenic mechanisms in early norepinephrine-induced acute renal failure: Functional and histological correlates of protection. KIDNEY INT. 14: 114-125, 1978.
4. Dach, J. L. and Kurtzman, N. A.: A scanning electron microscopic study of the glycerol model of acute renal failure. LAB. INVEST. 34: 406-414, 1976.
5. Ganote, C. E., Reimer, K. A. and Jennings, R. B.: Acute and mercuric chloride nephrotoxicity: An electron microscopic and metabolic study. LAB. INVEST. 31: 633-647, 1974.
6. Ideura, T., Solez, K. and Heptinstall, R. H.: The effect of clonidine on tubular obstruction in postischemic acute renal failure in the rabbit demonstrated by microradiography and microdissection. AMER. J. PATHOL. 98: 123-129, 1980.
7. Siegel, F. L. and Bulger, R. E.: Scanning and transmission electron microscopy of mercuric chloride-induced acute tubular necrosis in the rat. VIRCHOWS ARCH. (Cell Pathol) 18: 243-262, 1975.
8. Suzuki, R. and Mostofi, F. K.: Electron microscopic studies of acute tubular necrosis. Early changes in the glomeruli of rat kidney after subcutaneous injection of glycerin. LAB. INVEST. 23: 8-14, 1970.
9. Solez, K., Morel-Maroger, L. and Sraer, J. D.: The morphology of "acute tubular necrosis" in man: Analysis of 57 renal biopsies and a comparison with the glycerol model. MEDICINE 58: 362, 1979.
10. Eknoyan, G., Bulger, R. E. and Dobyan, D. C.: Mercuric chloride-induced acute renal failure in the rat. Correlation of functional and morphologic changes and their modification by clonidine. LAB. INVEST. 46: 613-620, 1982.
11. Eknoyan, G., Dobyan, D. C., Senekjian, H. O. and Bulger, R. E.: Protective effect of oral clonidine in the prophylaxis and therapy of mercuric chloride-induced acute renal failure in the rat. J. LAB. CLIN. MED. 192: 699-713, 1983.
12. Bulger, R. E., Eknoyan, G., Purcell, D. J. II and Dobyan, D. C.: Endothelial characteristics of glomerular capillaries in normal and mercuric chloride-induced acute renal failure in the rat. J. CLIN. INVEST. 72: 128-141, 1983.
13. Solez, K., D'Agostini, R. J., Stowowy, L., Freedman, M. T., Scott, W. W. Jr., Siegelman, S. S. and Heptinstall, R. H.: Beneficial effect of propranolol in a histologically appropriate model of postischemic acute renal failure. AMER. J. PATHOL. 88: 163, 1977.
14. Kourilsky, O., Solez, K., Morel-Maroger, L., Whelton, A., Dohoux, P. and Sraer, J. D.: The pathology of acute renal failure due to interstitial nephritis in man with comments on the role of interstitial inflammation and sex in gentamicin nephrotoxicity. MEDICINE 61: 258, 1982.
15. Brezis, M., Rosen, S., Silva, P. and Epstein, F.: Renal ischemia: A new perspective. KIDNEY INT. 26: 375-383, 1984.
16. Deen, W. M., Troy, J. L., Robertson, C. R. and Brenner, B. M.: Dynamics of glomerular ultrafiltration in the rat. IV. Determination of the ultrafiltration coefficient. J. CLIN. INVEST. 52: 1500-1508, 1973.

17. Blantz, R. C.: The mechanism of acute renal failure after uranyl nitrate. J. CLIN. INVEST. 55: 621-635, 1975.
18. Baylis, C., Rennke, H. R. and Brenner, B. M.: Mechanisms of the defect in glomerular ultrafiltration associated with gentamicin administration. KIDNEY INT. 12: 344-353, 1977.
19. Schor, N., Ichikawa, I., Rennke, H. G., Troy, J. L. and Brenner, B. M.: Pathophysiology of altered glomerular function in aminoglycoside-treated rats. KIDNEY INT. 19: 288-296, 1981.
20. Williams, R. H., Thomas, C. E., Mavar, L. G. and Evan A. P.: Hemodynamic and single nephron function during the maintenance phase of ischemic acute renal failure in the dog. KIDNEY INT. 19: 503-515, 1981.
21. Venkatchalam, M. A. and Rennke, H. G.: The structural and molecular basis of glomerular filtration. CIRC. RES. 43: 337-347, 1978.
22. Renkin, E. M. and Gilmore, J. P.: Glomerular filtration. In: HANDBOOK OF PHYSIOLOGY, Section 8, Renal Physiology; edited by: Orloff, J. and Berliner, R. W., Washington, D. C., 1973.
23. Landis, E. M. and Pappenheimer, J. R.: Exchange of substances through the capillary walls. In: HANDBOOK OF PHYSIOLOGY, Section 2, Circulation, Vol. II; edited by: Hamilton, D. F. and Down, P., Washington, D. C., American Physiological Society, 1963, pp. 961-1034.
24. Avashti, P. S., Evan, A. P. and Hay, D.: Glomerular endothelial cells in uranyl nitrate-induced acute renal failure in rats. J. CLIN. INVEST. 65: 121-127, 1980.
25. Avashti, P. S., Evan, A. P., Huser, J. W. and Luft, F. C.: Effect of gentamicin on glomerular ultrastructure. J. LAB. CLIN. MED. 98: 444-454, 1981.
26. Eknoyan, G., Bulger, R. E., Purcell, D. J. II and Dobyan, D. C.: Ultrastructural functional-anatomic correlations in acute renal failures and normal variations in endothelial morphology. In: ACUTE RENAL FAILURE: Correlations Between Morphology and Function; edited by: Solez, K. and Whelton, A., New York, Marcel Dekker, Inc., 1984, pp. 105-117.
27. Latta, H.: Ultrastructure of the glomerulus and juxtaglomerular apparatus. In: HANDBOOK OF PHYSIOLOGY, Section 8, Renal Physiology; edited by: Orloff, J. and Berliner, R. W., Washington, D. C., American Physiology Society, 1973, pp. 1-29.
28. Rhodin, J. A. G.: The diaphragm of capillary endothelial fenestrations. J. ULTRASTRUCT. RES. 6: 171-185, 1962.
29. Barnes, J. L., Osgood, R. W., Reineck, H. J. and Stein, J. H.: Glomerular alterations in an ischemic model of acute renal failure. LAB. INVEST. 45: 378, 1981.
30. Dobyan, D. C., Nagle, R. B. and Bulger, R. E.: Acute tubular necrosis in the rat kidney following sustained hypotension. Physiologic and morphologic observations. LAB. INVEST. 37: 411, 1977.
31. Racusen, L. C. and Solez, K.: Podocyte changes in post-ischemic ARF. In: ACUTE RENAL FAILURE: Correlations Between Morphology and Function; edited by: Solez, K. and Whelton, A., New York, Marcel Dekker Inc., 1984, pp. 134-145.

LONG TERM CLINICAL AND MORPHOLOGICAL EVALUATION OF ACUTE RENAL FAILURE

V. Bonomini, A. Vangelista, G. Frasca, S. Stefoni, M.P. Scolari, and G. Feliciangeli

Institute of Nephrology, St. Orsola University Hospital Bologna, Italy

INTRODUCTION

Acute Renal Failure(ARF)is a severe clinical event characterized by a sudden reduction in renal function.This apparently well defined condition may be the result of different etiological and pathogenetic mechanims which largely determine the type of renal lesions and influence the immediate outcome and long-term prognosis.

Clinical results have greatly improved since the introduction of artificial substitutive procedures in the therapeutic management of patients with ARF enabling most of them to survive until renal function recovery is regained,or even in the absence of renal function recovery.Patient prognosis and kidney prognosis,in fact,do not necessarily tally nowadays(1) owing to the availability of various kinds of renal substitution therapy.

The undoubtedly great improvement in clinical results,however,mostly refers to the immediate patient survival rates.Little is known until today about the long-term results,especially as far as the behaviour of renal function according to the type of renal lesions responsible for ARF is concerned.As far as we know,in fact,no previous papers have dealt in detail with the correlation between basic renal biopsy findings and renal survival,especially long-term renal survival.Isolated reports on kidney prognosis do exist in the literature,but describe either one type of renal lesions alone(2-4)or inadequate case material in terms of quantity and time(5,6).Chief among the various factors which may account for this inadequacy is the difficulty of marshalling such different data in differing conditions and keeping a regular check on the patient once the acute episode is over.In an attempt to throw some light on long-term clinico-functional correlations,we have reviewed our cases of ARF in order to establish:a)the importance,if any,of prognostic factors on immediate patient outcome;b)the correlation between renal morphological findings and the degree of renal function recovery after 1 year;c)the correlation between basic morphological findings and the appearance of chronic renal failure after 5 years.

This study is an updated review of our experience in the field drawing on over 20 years of clinical and renal biopsy findings.

MATERIAL AND METHODS

The overall case material observed from 1962 until the end of 1985 comprises 1794 patients with ARF.Among these patients 827 required admission to our intensive care unit.Renal biopsy has been performed in 640 of them.In order to evaluate the prognostic importance of various factors on patients' immediate outcome a careful investigation have been made on: 1)presence of extrarenal complications,2)timing of substitutive therapy, and 3)the nature of renal lesions at the time of acute episode.In an attempt to investigate the importance of the last parameter on short-term and long-term renal function,the case material has been deliberately restricted to 238 patients out of the 640 submitted to renal biopsy,since they alone fulfilled the following criteria for inclusion:1)at least 5-year follow-up,2)at least two renal biopsies performed,3)clinical and functional investigations carried out at least once a year during the study.

RESULTS

Patient Prognosis

The analysis of the various factors which may influence the immediate outcome of patients with ARF demonstrated that the presence of extrarenal complications and the choice of therapeutic strategy are of the utmost importance for patient survival.Among the 827 patients admitted to the intensive care unit,in fact,mortality rate was 7.4% in uncomplicated patients, and 53.7% in patients with extrarenal complications.The more frequent causes of death were:hemorrage(above all digestive and cerebral),infection, cardiac failure,severe hypertension,and severe acid-base imbalance.

Table I. Mortality Rate According to Renal Lesions

Diagnosis	Patients	Mortality Rate(%)
ATN	472	32.4
AGN	215	21.8
AIN	49	16.3
AVN	53	45.2
Others	38	52.6

ATN:acute tubular necrosis;AGN:acute glomerulonephritis;AIN:acute interstitial nephritis;AVN:acute vascular nephropathy.

Table I shows the mortality rate according to the clinico-pathological diagnosis of renal lesions.In ARF due to acute tubular necrosis, patients with surgical or obstetrical problems and severe traumatic lesions had the worse prognosis as compared to patients with toxic acute tubular necrosis. Among patients with acute vascular nephropathy,cortical necrosis secondary to obstetrical causes(septic abortion,placenta disruption),thrombotic microangiopathy,and malignant hypertension were associated with the highest mortality rates.

The use of prophylactic dialysis (i.e. used with BUN < 200 mg/dl;serum creatinine < 8 mg/dl;before the onset of clinical signs of acute uremia) significantly improved the survival rate,enabling a better control of acute uremic symptoms,and reducing the number of severe clinical complications. Mortality rate,in fact,was 42.1% in patients treated with late dialysis,23.3% when prophylactic dialysis was employed.

Renal Prognosis

1-year Follow-up. Table II shows the recovery rate in renal function 1 year after the acute episode.Renal function was most severely affected in patients with ARF due to vascular and glomerular lesions.No functional recovery occurred in 50% of patients with acute vascular nephropathy.Better results were found in patients with acute tubular necrosis and acute interstitial nephritis;among the former 78 cases(62.4%) recovered normal renal function;39(31.2%) showed a partial recovery,while only in 8 cases(6.4%) no functional recovery was documented.In acute interstitial nephritis due to hypersensitivity reaction or bacterial infection,10(76.9%) of the 13 patients examined showed a normal renal function after 1 year.In ARF due to glomerular lesions(table III),extracapillary proliferative glomerulonephritis was associated with the poorest prognosis.In no patient was normal renal function observed,while 57.7% of cases showed absence of functional recovery. More favorable results were documented when ARF was associated with endocapillary proliferative lesions,diffuse proliferative lupus nephritis,and Schönlein-Henoch syndrome.

Table II. Renal Function After 1 Year from the Acute Episode

Diagnosis	Cases n	Complete recovery		Partial recovery		No recovery	
		n	%	n	%	n	%
ATN	125	78	62.4	39	31.2	8	6.4
AGN	84	33	39.3	31	36.9	20	23.8
AIN	13	10	76.9	3	23.1	-	-
AVN	16	2	12.5	6	37.5	8	50.0
	238	123	51.7	79	33.2	36	15.1

Table III. Renal Function After 1 Year from the Acute Episode in ARF due to Glomerular Lesions

Glomerular lesion	Cases n	Complete recovery n	Complete recovery %	Partial recovery n	Partial recovery %	No recovery n	No recovery %
Extracapillary proliferative	23	-	-	11	42.3	15	57.7
Endocapillary proliferative	29	20	68.9	9	31.1	-	-
Membrano-proliferative	6	2	33.3	4	66.6	-	-
Diffuse Lupus nephritis	8	6	75.0	2	25.0	-	-
Schönlein-Henoch	4	3	75.0	1	25.0	-	-
Others	11	3	27.6	4	36.4	4	36.4
	84	34	40.5	31	37.0	19	22.6

5-year Follow-up. Table IV shows the results after 5 years.About 43% of the cases had normal renal function,30.2% chronic renal insufficiency, and 30.7% chronic uremia.However the distribution of these data varied remarkably according to the nature of the original renal lesions.62.6% of patients with acute vascular nephropathy reached terminal renal failure and were submitted to regular dialysis or transplantation.Among the patients with ARF due to acute tubular necrosis or acute interstitial nephritis,normal renal function was observed in 56.8% and 61.5% respectively.In ARF of glomerular origin(table V) extracapillary proliferative lesions were associated with a progression towards chronic uremia in most cases after 5 years(84.6%).Poor long-term prognosis was also observed in the presence of membranoproliferative lesions associated with acute nephritic syndrome and renal failure:of the 6 patients studied,none had a normal function after 5 years from the acute episode .In diffuse proliferative lupus nephritis,the long-term results indicate a progression of renal lesions in about

Table IV. Renal Function After 5 Years From the Acute Episode

Diagnosis	Cases n	GFR > 80 n	GFR > 80 %	GFR > 15 n	GFR > 15 %	GFR < 15 n	GFR < 15 %
ATN	125	71	56.8	40	32.0	14	11.2
AGN	84	23	27.4	23	27.4	38	45.2
AIN	13	8	61.5	4	30.8	1	7.7
AVN	16	1	6.2	5	31.2	10	62.6
	238	103	43.3	72	30.2	73	30.7

Table V. Renal Function After 5 Years From the Acute Episode in ARF due to Glomerular Lesions

Glomerular lesion	Cases n	GFR > 80 n	GFR > 80 %	GFR > 15 n	GFR > 15 %	GFR < 15 n	GFR < 15 %
Extracapillary proliferative	26	-	-	4	15.4	22	84.6
Endocapillary proliferative	29	18	62.0	8	27.6	3	10.4
Membrano-proliferative	6	-	-	3	50.0	3	50.0
Diffuse Lupus nephritis	8	3	37.5	3	37.5	2	25.0
Schönlein-Henoch	4	3	75.0	1	25.0	-	-
Others	11	1	9.1	3	27.3	7	63.6
	84	25	29.8	22	26.2	37	44.0

60% of cases:only in 3 out of 8 patients was renal function normal after 5 years.A more favorable prognosis was shown in ARF due to diffuse endocapillary glomerulonephritis or Schönlein-Henoch syndrome:only 10.4% of patients from the first group had chronic uremia, while 1 patient out of 4 with Schönlein-Henoch syndrome showed a reduction of renal function after 5 years.

DISCUSSION

The improvement in technology during the last years has been associated with an improvement in survival in renal failure.Survival figures of 70-80% in severe ARF would have been simply incredible only a few years ago.This occurs provided that the patient is admitted to a center with proven experience and adequate facilities.

Patient prognosis and kidney prognosis do not necessarily tally nowadays.Rational therapy is of importance for immediate patient survival.This holds for example in tubulointerstitial ARF due to drugs:according to whether the lesion is toxic or immunological,a different approach is obviously required(hemodialysis alone or hemodialysis combined with steroids). Another example concerns ARF due to glomerular and vascular injuries,where various therapeutic measures(steroids,immunosuppressive drugs,plasma exchange,anticoagulants,etc.) should be employed,combined with hemodialysis, according to renal biopsy findings.Even admitting that certain forms of ARF result in more severe prognosis for both the patient and the kidney, (thrombotic microangiopathy,malignant hypertension,Goodpasture's syndrome),it is more likely that extrarenal factors play the major role in patient outcome.The mortality rate is higher when severe extrarenal complications supervene in the clinical course of ARF,with a 53.7% mortality rate in complicated patients,and a 7.4% mortality in uncomplicated cases. Another factor of importance for patient prognosis is the use of early dialysis.The mortality rate is lower,extrarenal complications are less frequent and the clinical course is better when dialysis is employed before the onset of clinical signs of uremia,with plasma creatinine less than 8 mg/dl and blood urea less than 200 mg/dl(7).

When Should Renal Biopsy Be Performed ? The value of renal biopsy in patients with ARF due to intrinsic renal damage is generally accepted today.The importance of early morphological diagnosis(8,9),the connections between morphological results and clinical data (5,10)and the reliability of renal biopsy for assessing treatment(4,8,9,11) have been already outlined.In general ARF due to intrinsic renal damage is regarded as a condition where renal biopsy is necessary for a more correct clinical comprehension.Contrary to previous observations(9,12) our experience suggests that renal biopsy does not carry higher morbidity in ARF than in other conditions(13).Therefore,if there are no specific contraindications,it should be undertaken in nearly all cases,especially in patients with rapid onset and/or persistence of severe oliguria.

In ARF renal biopsy provides a more appropriate diagnosis.Glomeruli, vessels,tubuli and interstitium may be variably affected,even in the presence of similar clinical pictures.The same etiology may produce different lesions,while,conversely,the same lesion may result from different causes. The reasons for this nephrological dilemma are still obscure today. However,the value of early morphological diagnosis for provision of appropriate treatment goes without saying.

ARF is one of the clinical conditions where the main features of responsible lesions(localization,nature,degree,etc.) can best be appreciated by renal biopsy.Early morphological diagnosis enables:1)early treatment, before renal lesions become irreversible;2)early substitutive therapy before the appearance of severe extrarenal complications,which play an important role for patient survival;3)avoidance of useless and/or dangerous therapeutic measures.

In conclusion:The functional and morphological results reported in this paper are an improvement on those reported only a few years ago(1). Immediate and long-term prognosis,however,will further improve in the future if appropriate treatment based on morphological findings starts earlier.Unfortunately this is impossible in many cases since either the diagnosis is made too late,or the patient is admitted too late to the proper nephrological center.The alleged risks of renal biopsy are overstated;its advantages(for diagnosis,further treatment and prognosis)are still insufficiently appreciated.

REFERENCES

1. V.Bonomini,A.Vangelista,G.M.Frascà,Value of renal biopsy for long-term prognosis in acute renal failure,in:"Acute Renal Failure",D.Seybold and U.Gessler,ed,Karger,Basel(1981)
2. V.Bonomini,V.Mioli,A.Albertazzi,A.Vangelista,Osservazioni clinico-funzionali-nefrobioptiche sugli esiti a distanza della insufficienza renale acuta su base prevalentemente glomerulare,Min.Nefrol.17:27 (1970)

3. A. Segonds,N.Louradour,J.M.Suc,C.Orfila,Postpartum hemolytic uremic syndrome:a study of three cases with a review of the literature,Clin. Nephrol. 12:229 (1979)
4. L.Morel-Maroger,A.Kanfer,K.Solez,J.D.Sraer,G.Richet,Prognostic importance of vascular lesions in acute renal failure with microangiopathic hemolytic anemia:clinico-pathological study in 20 adults,Kidney Int. 15:548 (1979)
5. P.Duhoux,O.Kourilsky,A.Kanfer,J.D.Sraer,L.Morel-Maroger,G.Richet,Les insuffisances renales aigües necessitant un traitment etiopathogenique. Utilité de la biopsie renale precoce,in:"Seminaires d'Uro-Nephrologie", Küss and Legrain ed,Masson,Paris(1981)
6. V.Bonomini,P.Zucchelli,V.Mioli,The significance of renal biopsy for the prognosis of patients with acute renal failure treated by hemodialysis, Proc.EDTA:371 (1966)
7. V.Bonomini,L.Baldrati,M.P.Scolari,S.Stefoni,A.Vangelista,Acute renal failure:10 year experience,in"Acute Renal Failure",H.E.Eliahou ed,Libbey, London (1982)
8. P.Kincaid-Smith,Severe acute oliguric renal failure in glomerular and vascular disease,in:"The Kidney",P.Kincaid-Smith,Blackwell,Oxford (1975)
9. D.M.Wilson,D.R.Turner,J.S.Cameron,C.S.Ogg,C.B.Brown,C.Chantler,Value of renal biopsy in acute intrinsic renal failure,Br.Med.J.:459(1976)
10. G.Ganeval,F.Daniel,F.Lhoste,P.Bouchard,Problemes diagnostiques et therapeutiques au cours de l'insuffusance renal aigue,in:Actualites Nephrologiques,Hamburger,Crosnier,Funck-Brentano ed,Flammarion,Paris (1976)
11. G.Richet,J.D.Sraer,O.Kourilsky,A.Kanfer,F.Mignon,J.Withworth,L.Morel-Maroger,La ponction biopsie renale dans les insuffusances renales aigues, Ann.Int.Med.,129:445 (1978)
12. J.A.Diaz-Boxo,J.V.Donadio,Complications of percutaneous renal biopsy:an analysis of 1000 consecutive biopsies,Clin.Nephrol.,4:223 (1975)
13. A.Vangelista,V.Bonomini,Indagine nefrobioptica nell'IRA:impiego estensivo o limitato?,in:Nefrologia,Dialisi,Trapianto 1983,A.Albertazzi ed, Wichtig,Milano(1983)

THE ROLE OF RENAL BIOPSY IN ACUTE RENAL FAILURE

Giuseppe D'Amico and Giuliano Colasanti

Division of Nephrology, S. Carlo Hospital, Milan (Italy)

There is agreement among the nephrologists that renal biopsy is of value for selected patients with acute uremia. It may be indicated for making or confirming a clinical diagnosis, to assess prognosis or to provide a basis for treatment.

However, there are consistent differences in the criteria for the selection of those patients who might benefit from the diagnostic procedure and in how frequently it really should be applied. The different attitudes toward the use of biopsy in renal disease in general are probably responsible for this disagreement, and may explain why the percentage of biopsied patients in the total number of patients with intrinsic acute renal failure (ARF) ranged between 12% and 92% in the different series reported in the literature (Table I). Undoubtedly, those renal pathologists who use biopsy often for patients with ARF will admit that one aim of this unrestricted use, and probably the most important, is research, to enlarge their knowledge about the morphological features of different clinical situations to the advantage of all future patients with similar clinical picture, rather than better treatment of the patient who is being biopsied. We think that the biopsying of all the 91 consecutive patients with ARF observed at the University of Tampere in Finland (Mustonen et al,1984) can be justified only on the basis of evaluating the usefulness of this procedure in an unselected series of patients with ARF.It is difficult to decide to what extent such a policy should be widely accepted. Unfortunately, everyone thinks he is the right person to make a definite contribution to scientific progress through unrestricted use of the renal biopsy.

What are the indications for renal biopsy in patients with ARF, if for any given patient the benefit to be derived from the procedure is to exceed the risks of renal biopsy, especially in patients with uremia (Diaz-Buxo and Donadio,1975)? A prevalence of severe complications as high as 2.2% and 2.1% was reported in patients with ARF by the nephrologists of the Hopital Tenon (Duhoux et al,1981) and of the Hopital Necker (Ganeval et al,1976) in Paris, although Vangelista and

Bonomini (1983) did not have a high rate of complications in their series.

Although the respective frequencies of the renal lesions responsible for intrinsic acute renal failure are difficult to state precisely because of differences in patient populations and in the diagnostic attitudes in the different nephrological centers, we can estimate that acute tubular necrosis (ATN) accounts for approximately 70-80% of cases, glomerular and vascular diseases for 5-10% each,and acute interstitial nephritis (AIN) for another 3-5%. Hence, in the great majority of patients ATN is responsible for the syndrome with sudden reduction in renal function, usually associated with anuria or oliguria, commonly called "acute renal failure". Its incidence becomes even greater than 80%, if cases without oliguria are taken into consideration.

In our opinion, patients suspected of having reversible ATN, if they have typical well-defined clinical and laboratory signs, do not require tissue diagnosis. Renal biopsy will add little to the diagnosis and management. In fact, the extent of tubular cell necrosis does not correlate with the duration of renal failure (Solez et al,1979), and it is very unusual in this group of patients for the histological diagnosis not to confirm the diagnosis made on clinical grounds 10% of cases, according to Mustonen et al (1984), especially when ischemic or pigment-associated renal damage is evident.

As Table I illustrates, all nephrological groups who restrict use of renal biopsies report histological diagnosis of ATN in no more than 30% of patients, a definitely low percentage considering the frequency of this disease as a cause of ARF.

Clinical diagnosis may be less accurate when nephrotoxic damage from some specific drugs is documented, since the alternative possibility of an immunologically-mediated AIN can not always be excluded on clinical grounds. It is well known that systemic signs of an allergic reaction often do not accompany the renal lesion in drug-induced AIN. This diagnosis has been confirmed histologically in 5-10% of all biopsied patients (Table I) and very frequently the clinical features in these patients had not suggested the disease [(63% cases according to Vangelista and Bonomini (1983) and 44% according to Duhoux et al (1981)]. Therefore, there is an indication for taking a biopsy from patients for whom one of the drugs (the list is unfortunately becoming longer every year) capable of giving an hyper-sensitivity reaction, systemic or circumscribed to the renal interstitium, is suspected to be the cause of ARF. Currently, we perform biopsies in these patients, because we are interested in the morphological study of the interstitial infiltrates with monoclonal antibodies and are convinced that the more accurate histological diagnosis which this study permits will help us to establish a more correct treatment. In fact, steroid administration is probably helpful when there is histological evidence of AIN. However, in our experience the prognosis is good in patients with this disease even without giving steroids, provided the causative drug is immediately stopped.

Table I. Prevalence of various types of morphological lesions in some large series of ARF

	Mustonen et al. 1984	Vangelista and Bonomini, 1983	Duhoux et al. 1981	Wilson et al. 1976	Ganeval et al. 1976	Personal Experience, 1986
No. of biopsied pts (% of pts with ARF)	91 92%	594 36%	178 20%	84 13%	93 12%	106 25%
ACUTE TUBULAR NECROSIS	56*	39	30	17	29	24
ACUTE INTERSTITIAL NEPHRITIS	4	12	9	11	5	10
MYELOMA KIDNEY	3	-	4	2	2	10
RAPIDLY PROGRESSIVE GN (with or without vasculitis)	32	38	26	52	34	33
ACUTE VASCULAR DISEASE (except vasculitis)	-	10	28	18	20	27

* % of biopsied patients

To summarize, whenever the history and clinical features strongly suggest a diagnosis of ATN, all measures are put into practice to eliminate the nephrotoxic insult, to correct the hemodynamic abnormalities, to reconstitute fluid and electrolytes balance and to substitute renal function with dialysis if necessary. In these circumstances, renal biopsy should be considered only when oligo-anuria is prolonged (more than 10 days), or when acute cortical necrosis, which is very uncommon (Table I), is suspected. However,we are convinced of the usefulness of performing this procedure as soon as possible for all patients in whom the cause of ARF is not clinically evident, or for whom AIN or a glomerular or vascular disease is suspected. In a good number of such patients, although a diagnosis of AIN, or glomerulonephritis, or thrombotic microangiopathy could have been proposed on clinical grounds (consistent proteinuria,moderate hemolytic anemia and/or thrombocytopenia, history of use of drugs capable of inducing AIN), renal biopsy will reveal the existence of ATN, leading to the stopping or discarding of useless and potentially harmful drugs (Table II).

As is shown in Table I, glomerular disease is found in a high percentage of biopsied patients (as high as 50%). In most of these patients extracapillary GN with cellular crescents in the majority of glomeruli is found, and in more than 1/3 of them the focal nature of the necrotizing crescentic GN, associated with completely negative IF, suggests or confirms renal vasculitis even when there are no definite lesions of the renal arterioles. Histological diagnosis appears to be particularly helpful for guiding treatment and establishing the prognosis, since in the last 10 years therapeutic procedures have become available that consistenly change the prognosis for all types of extracapillary GN, whether due to anti-GBM antibodies, to immune complexes, or to vasculitis. These include concomitant use of steroid therapy (starting with 3 i.v. high dose pulses of methylprednisolone), cyclophosphamide and plasma exchange (Sinico et al,1983). It is common experience that the efficacy of such treatment depends largely on its early institution, possibly before uremia requiring dialysis has developed. Therefore, renal biopsy should be performed as soon as possible when there is clinical suspicion of this, to obtain a morphological validation before prescribing drugs and procedures which are complicated to manage and potentially dangerous.

Finally, what should be done when vascular diseases such as thrombotic microangiopathy (hemolytic-uremic syndrome) or malignant nephroangiosclerosis are suspected on clinical grounds to be responsible for ARF? There is little doubt about the potential utility of renal biopsy in such circumstances, especially if the differential diagnosis between these two diseases, which is not always easy without histology, will influence the decision to start heparin and/or plasma exchange. However, if there is thrombocytopenia, coagulation defects and/or severe arterial hypertension the risks of complications after a renal biopsy are markedly increased. The most severe complications, requiring nephrectomy, reported by the two experienced nephrological groups from Paris (Duhoux et al,1981; Ganeval et al,1976) occurred in patients with such vascular diseases. In spite of these risks, we think that the advantages of biopsy justify its use. Obviously, one must wait long enough to carefully control hypertension and to permit a rise in platelet count, before one can proceed to biopsy with sufficient safety.

Table II. Prevalence of histological diagnosis of ATN in patients suspected on clinical ground to be affected by other types of ARF

	% found to be affected by ATN at biopsy		
SUGGESTED CLINICAL DIAGNOSIS	Duhox et al. 1981	Vangelista and Bonomini, 1983	Mustonen et al. 1984
GLOMERULAR DISEASE	24%	21%	26%
VASCULAR DISEASE	5%	23%	-
ACUTE INTERSTITIAL NEPHRITIS	55%	48%	-

We prefer sometimes,in these circumstances,to use surgical biopsy instead of percutaneous biopsy,even though severe complications may occur even with the former procedure.

In conclusion, the criteria we use for deciding to take biopsies from patients with intrinsic ARF are as follows:

1) ATN is suspected, but there is no obvious cause for it (exposure to toxins, hypotension, sepsis, etc).

2) A drug is suspected to be the cause of ARF, but it is difficult to differentiate on clinical grounds between ATN and immunologically-mediated AIN.

3) There are renal and/or extrarenal signs that suggest a diagnosis of acute primary or secondary glomerular disease or of systemic vasculitis, or of some other vascular disease, such as thrombotic microangiopathy or malignant nephroangiosclerosis.

4) ATN is suspected, but anuria lasts more than 10-15 days, and cortical necrosis or one of the diseases indicated in point 3 must be excluded.

REFERENCES

Diaz-Buxo, J.A. and Donadio, J.A., 1975, Complications of percutaneous renal biopsy: an analysis of 1000 consecutive biopsies, Clin Nephrol 4:223.

Duhoux, P., Kourilsky, O., Kanfer, A., Sraer, J.D., Morel-Maroger, L. and Richet, G., 1981, Les insuffisances renales aigues necessitant un traitment ethiopathogenigue, in:"Seminaires d'Uro-Nephrologie", R. Kuss and M. Legrain ed., Masson, Paris

Ganeval, D., Daniel F., Lhoste, F. and Bouchard, P.,1976, Problemes diagnostique et therapeutïque au cours de l'insuffisance renale aigue,in: Actualités Nephrologique de l'Hopital Necker",J. Hamburger, J. Crosnier and J.L. Funck-Brentano ed., Flammarion, Paris.

Mustonen, J.,Pasternack, A., Helin, H., Pystynen, S. and Tuominen,T., 1984, Renal biopsy in acute renal failure, Am J Nephrol 4:27.

Sinico, R.A.,Fornasieri, A.,Fiorini, G., Paracchini, M.L.,Pagella, G., Ferrario, F., Gibelli, G. and D'Amico, G., 1983, Plasma exchange in glomerulonephritis associated with systemic lupus erythematosus and essential mixed cryoglobulinemia, Int J Art Organs 6: 21.

Solez, K., Morel-Maroger L. and Sraer, J.D., 1979, The morphology of "Acute Tubular Necrosis" in man: Analysis of 57 Renal Biopsies and a Comparison with the Glycérol model, Medicine 58:362

Vangelista, A., Bonomini, V., 1983, Indagine nefrobioptica nell'IRA: impiego estensivo o limitato?, in "Nefrologia, Dialisi e Trapianto", D. Brancaccio ed., Wichtig, Milan.

Wilson, D.M., Turner, D.R., Cameron, J.S., Ogg, C.S., Brown C.B. and Chantler, C., 1976, Value of renal biopsy in acute intrinsic renal failure, Br Med J 2: 459

CATABOLISM IN ACUTE RENAL FAILURE:

IMPORTANCE OF GLUCOCORTICOIDS AND LYSOSOMAL ENZYMES

August Heidland[1], Roland M. Schaefer[1], Joachim Weipert[1], Ekkehart Heidbreder[1], Markus Teschner[1], Gernot Peter[2], and Walter H. Horl[3]

Departments of [1]Medicine and [2]Dermatology
University of Wurzburg, FRG
Department of [3]Medicine, University of Freiburg
Freiburg, FRG

Renal failure has been previously shown to be a catabolic event[1-6]. There is growing evidence for a certain role of proteolytic enzymes in the catabolism of acute uremia[7-13]. Thus, frank proteolytic activity has been demonstrated in ultrafiltrated plasma fractions, in the urine and bronchoalveolar-lavage (BAL) fluid[14-15]. The type of proteinases involved, is up to now not totally defined. There are some data, which indicate a participation of broad spectrum serine proteinases in the BAL-fluid and in the plasma of ureter-ligated rats[16].

Furthermore, enhanced plasma concentrations of elastase in complex with α_1-proteinase inhibitor were found in various forms of acute renal failure such as traumatic, septic and drug-induced forms[16-20]. On the other hand, there are findings that other proteinases, besides leukocyte elastase, contribute to the proteolytic activity found in ARF.

Schaefer et al.[21] showed that the proteolytic activity, found in the plasma of ARF patients, was distinct from polymorphonuclear (PMN) elastase. In addition, Hörl et al. recently described a metalloproteinase both in plasma fractions and in the urine of patients suffering from ARF[22]. Enhanced proteolytic activity has not only been detected in the plasma and urine of such patients, but also in skeletal muscle. Especially, an alkaline myofibrillar proteinase could be related to various catabolic conditions[23].

As a consequence of activated muscle proteolysis degradation of muscle proteins and increased release of amino acids might occur[4-6]. The enhanced proteolytic activity of plasma is associated with an increase of plasma levels of non-TCA precipitable proteins (split products)[10]. Furthermore, low plasma levels of key components of the coagulation-, fibrinolytic-, complement-, and of the kallikrein-kinin system, are described in acutely uremic rats and in patients suffering from ARF[24]. These findings might be, at least partly, the result of increased specific as well as unspecific protein degradation.

During bacterial and viral infections, numerous proteolytic processes might be involved[25-27]. Especially, pseudomonas bacteria display a high content of serine-proteinase activity[28]. Own investigations with 7 strains of pseudomonas, obtained from patients with pseudomonas-septicemia, showed a dramatic digestion of elastin (2 %) in vitro (Fig. 1). In addition to the direct release of proteinases, bacterial infection causes PMN leukocyte activation with subsequent degranulation[29-31]. During infectious or inflammatory conditions monocytes and macrophages secret a circulating peptide or a class of peptides which have been related to interleukin-1[32]. Its proteolysis-stimulating effect on skeletal muscle is mediated by protaglandin E_2 and therefore completely suppressible by indomethacin[33].

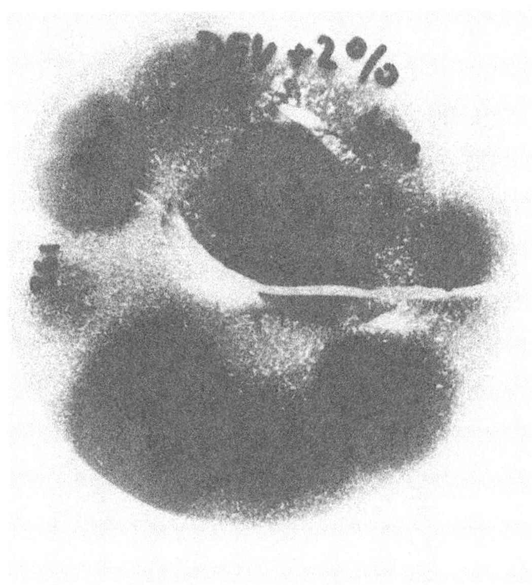

Fig. 1: Demonstration of elastolytic activity in several human-pathogenetic strains of pseudomonas bacteria by digestion of elastin (2%).

Various hormonal factors, which display a potiental stimulating effect on proteolysis, might also contribute to the enhanced catabolism of ARF. These include glucagon and glucocorticoids, as well as insulin resistance[34-37]. Furthermore, there is some evidence[38] for a catabolic effect of parathyroid hormone (PTH). High levels of corticosterone, the main glucocorticoid in the rat, have been found after bilateral nephrectomy (BN)[39]. In patients suffering from trauma induced ARF, plasma cortisol levels are markedly enhanced (Fig. 2). The catabolic effect of glucocorticoids results from both decreased synthesis and enhanced protein degradation of skeletal muscle[40-48].

Finally, metabolic acidosis, a consistent finding of uremia, seems to be a potent stimulator of muscle protein breakdown[49]. May et al. were able to demonstrate that this effect is mediated by glucocorticoids[50].

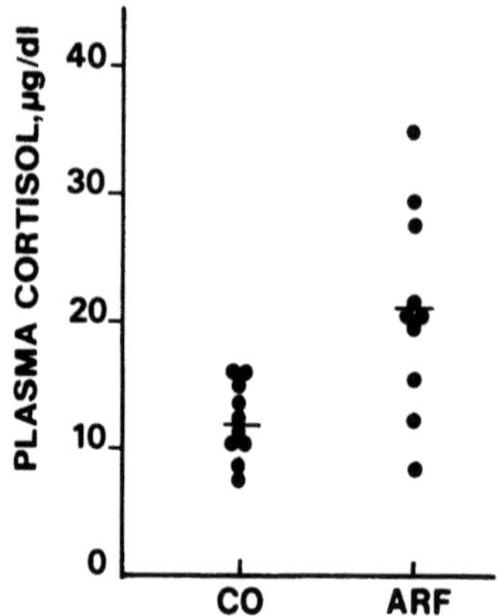

Fig. 2: Plasma levels of cortisol, obtained from 10 ARF patients and 10 age- and sex matched, healthy controls. Blood was collected between 8°° and 9°° am. Despite a considerable scatter, the difference between both groups reached significance (Mann-Whitney test, $p<0.05$).

THERAPEUTIC TRIALS IN THE CATABOLISM OF UREMIA

Glucocorticoids

As early as 1949, Bondy et al.[51] were able to show that adrenalectomy (ADX) decreased BUN in acutely uremic rats. In order to further evaluate the role of glucocorticoids in the catabolism of uremia, we recently investigated the effect of ADX in BN rats on urea-N appearance and on plasma levels of 3-methylhistidine[52]. 3-Methylhistidine has been found to be a suitable indicator of myofibrillar protein degradation, since it is present within actin and myosin and is released from muscle by degradation of myofibrillar proteins. There is no reutilization or oxidation once it is released from skeletal muscle[53-56]. Fourty-eight hours after BN/ADX, rats showed significantly reduced BUN levels and a curtailment of urea-N appearance (Fig. 3).

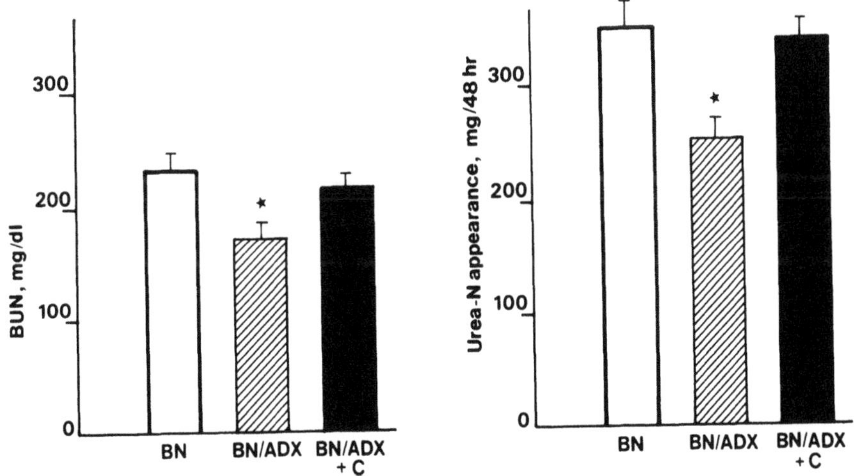

Fig. 3: Effect of ADX on BUN levels and urea-N appearance 48 hours after induction of uremia. Corticosterone (C) was administered in a dose of 5mg/kg/day subcutaneously. For statistical analysis, the Student's t test was applied. Data are given as mean values ± SEM, obtained from 9 animals. *$p<0.01$, for BN/ADX vs. BN or BN/ADX+C.

As a sign of decreased muscle protein degradation, plasma levels of 3-methylhistidine were also lowered compared to BN rats (Fig. 4). After the substitution of corticosterone in BN/ADX animals these benefical biochemical effects were readily reversed (Fig. 4). It is of note that in BN/ADX animals, blood levels of ionized calcium were significantly increased. Administration of corticosterone readily reversed this phenomenon.

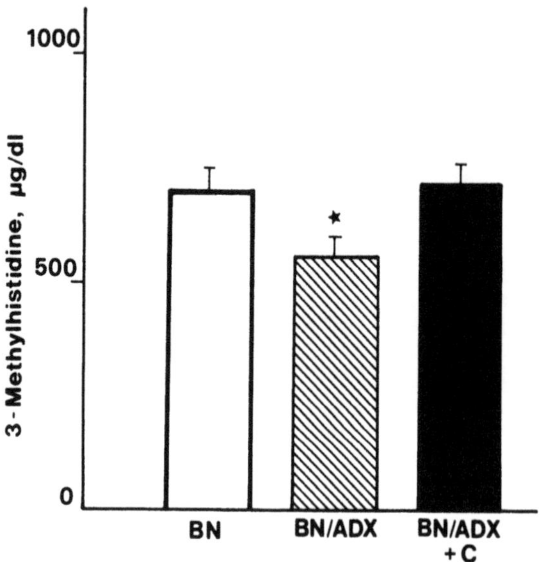

Fig. 4: Effect of ADX on serum levels of 3-methylhistidine 48 hours after induction of uremia. For details, see legend to Fig. 3.

These data clearly indicate that glucocorticoids play a major role in the enhanced muscle protein degradation of acute uremia. Moreover the increased urea-N appearance suggests that amino acids, released from skeletal muscle, are used for gluconeogenesis in the liver with a consecutive rise of hepatic ureogenesis.

Finally, the high levels of ionized calcium in the BN/ADX animals led us to assume that glucocorticoids might be involved in the PTH-resistance of the bone in uremia[57]. Unfortunately, the administration of inhibitors of the synthesis of glucocorticoids (aminoglutethimide and metyrapone) did not reduce urea-N appearance and 3-methylhistidine levels in acutely uremic rats. In the future, peripheral antagonists of glucocorticoids might gain some importance in the treatment of catabolic conditions, induced by an excess of these hormones.

Prostaglandin-synthetase inhibitors

The potential involvement of prostaglandins in protein breakdown[58] under physiologic and pathological conditions, led us to investigate the effect of indomethacin on muscle protein degradation in acutely uremic animals. However, the administration of indomethacin (6 mg/kg/24 hr) did not affect the concentration of BUN and 3-methylhistidine. These results are in agreement with data from Laidlaw et al.[59] who also could not observe an effect of indomethacin on 3-methylhistidine release in the perfused hemicorpus of acutely uremic rats, despite profound lowering of prostaglandin E_2 production. In general, these data suggest that prostaglandins do not play a major role in the degradation of muscle proteins in acute uremia, quite in contrast to experimental septicemia.

Proteinase inhibitors

Leupeptin is a low-molecular weight proteinase inhibitor, produced by streptomyces species[60], whose activity is predominantly directed (85%) against lysosomal enzymes, in particular thiol-proteinases, and partly (15 %) against non-lysosomal proteinases, including Ca-activated proteinases[61].

In order to study the effect of lysosomal proteinases on uremic catabolism, we administered leupeptin to acutely uremic rats and measured BUN as well as urea-N appearance.

The experiments were performed in 2 groups of BN rats. One group received leupeptin (180 mg/kg/24hr) in 3 hour intervals up to 24 hours after nephrectomy, whereas control BN rats received only the vehicle (0.9% NaCl). The leupeptin treated uremic animals displayed a significant decrease of BUN and urea-N appearance compared to untreated BN rats (Fig. 5).

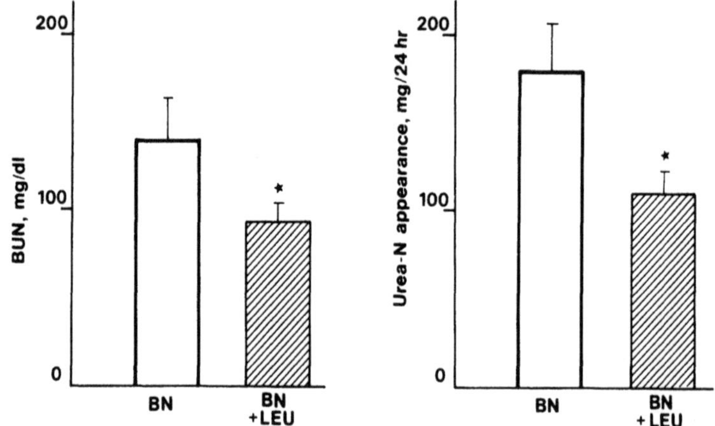

Fig. 5: Effect of leupeptin (LEU) on BUN levels and urea-N appearance 24 hours after induction of uremia. Data are given as mean values ± SEM, obtained from 10 animals. For statistical analysis, the Student's t test was used. *$p < 0.01$, for BN vs. BN+LEU.

However, leupeptin did not prevent the decrease in plasma levels of plasminogen and C_3-complement, which occurs during acute uremia in the rat. Infact, there was a paradoxical decrease of these key components of plasma proteolytic enzyme systems. Thus, in the uremic rat leupeptin exerts both proteolytic and anti-proteolytic actions.

CONCLUSIONS

Numerous factors contribute to the enhanced catabolism in acute uremia. Besides glucocorticoids, metabolic acidosis and systemic infectious or inflammatory conditions, there is ample evidence for the participation of proteolytic enzymes, namely serine-, metallo-, and cystein proteinases. Enhanced proteolytic degradation could be, as consequence of uremic intoxication, the result of both, enhanced activity of proteinases and/or increased susceptibility of protein substrates to proteolytic digestion. Therefore, the treatment with anti-proteolytic compounds might represent the therapeutical key for the management of catabolic patients suffering from ARF.

REFERENCES

1. J. D. Kopple, Metabolic and endocrine abnormalities: C. nitrogen metabolism, <u>in</u>: "Clinical Aspects of Uremia and Dialysis", S. G. Massry, ed., Charles C. Thomas, Springfield (1976).
2. J. D. Kopple, M. Jones, S. Fukuda, M. E. Swendseid, Amino acid and protein metabolism in renal failure, <u>Am. J. Clin. Nutr</u>. 31: 1532 (1978).
3. C. Giordano, N. G. DeSanto, R. Senatore, Effects of catabolic stress in acute and chronic renal failure, <u>Am. J. Clin. Nutr</u> 31: 1561 (1978).

4. W.E. Mitch, Amino acid release from the hindquarter and urea appearance in acute uremia, Am. J. Physiol. 241: E415 (1981).

5. W.E. Mitch, A.S. Clark, Muscle protein turnover in uremia, Kidney Int. 24 (suppl 16): 2 (1983).

6. R.M. Flügel-Link, I.B. Salusky, M.R. Jones, J.D. Kopple, Protein and amino acid metabolism in posterior hemicorpus of acutely uremic rats, Am. J. Physiol. 244: E615 (1983).

7. G. Richet, H. Villiers, R. Ardaillou, Activite tripeptidasique du plasma au cours de l'insuffisance renale: contribution a l'etude du catabolisme protidique, Revue Fr. Etud. Clin. Biol. 2: 808 (1957).

8. G. Richet, R. Ardaillou, L'activite tripeptidasique du plasma au cours des affections severes: contribution a l'etude de l'hypercatabolisme protidique, Presse Med. 30: 1229 (1959).

9. W.H. Hörl, A. Heidland, Enhanced proteolytic activity - cause of protein catabolism in acute renal failure, Am. J. Clin. Nutr. 33: 1423 (1980).

10. W.H. Hörl, J. Stepinski, C. Gantert, M. Hörl, A. Heidland, Evidence for the participation of proteinases on protein catabolism during hypercatabolic renal failure, Klin. Wochenschr. 59: 751 (1981).

11. W.H. Hörl, J. Stepinski, A. Heidland, Further evidence for the participation of proteases in protein catabolism during hypercatabolic renal failure, in: "Acute renal failure", H.E. Eliahou, ed., J. Libbey, London (1982).

12. W.H. Hörl, J. Stepinski, R.M. Schäfer, C. Wanner, A. Heidland, Role of proteases in hypercatabolic patients with renal failure, Kidney Int. 24 (suppl 16): 37 (1983).

13. W.H. Hörl, R.M. Schäfer, K. Scheidhauer, M. Jochum, A. Heidland, Proteolytic activity in patients with hypercatabolic renal failure, Adv. Exp. Biol. Med. 167: 405 (1984).

14. C. Wanner, P. Schollmeyer, W.H. Hörl, Urinary proteinase activity in patients with multiple traumatic injuries and sepsis, J. Lab. Clin. Med. in press (1986).

15. A. Heidland, H. Heine, J. Haunschild, J. Weipert, E. Heidbreder, W.H. Hörl, Uremic pneumonitis: Evidence for participation of proteolytic enzymes, Contrib. Nephrol. 41: 352 (1984).

16. W.H. Hörl, M. Jochum, A. Heidland, H. Fritz, Release of granulocyte proteinases during hemodialysis, Am. J. Nephrol. 3: 213 (1983).

17. W.H. Hörl, A. Heidland, Evidence of the participation of granulocyte proteinases on intradialytic catabolism, Clin. Nephrol. 21: 314 (1984).

18. A. Heidland, W.H. Hörl, N. Heller, H. Heine, S. Neumann, E. Heidbreder, Proteolytic enzymes and catabolism: Enhanced release of granulocyte proteinases in uremic intoxication and during hemodialysis, Kidney Int. 24 (suppl 16): 27 (1983).

19. A. Heidland, J. Weipert, R.M. Schäfer, E. Heidbreder, G. Peter, W.H. Hörl, Proteases and other catabolic factors in renal failure, Kidney Int. (suppl) in press (1986).

20. A. Heidland, W.H. Hörl, N. Heller, H. Heine, S. Neumann, R.M. Schaefer, E. Heidbreder, Granulocyte lysosomal factors and plasma elastase in uremia: A potential factor of catabolism, Klin. Wochenschr. 62: 218 (1984).

21. R.M. Schaefer, A. Heidland, W.H. Hörl, Role of leukocyte proteinases and proteinase inhibitors in the catabolism of acute renal failure, Kidney Int. (suppl) in press (1986).

22. W.H. Hörl, C. Wanner, F. Thaiss, P. Schollmeyer, Detection of a metalloproteinase in patients with acute and chronic renal failure, Am. J. Nephrol. 6: 6 (1986).

23. R.M. Schaefer, A. Heidland, W.H. Hörl, The effect of adrenalectomy on protein degradation in acutely uremic rats, Kidney Int. 29: 309 (1986).

24. A. Heidland, W.H. Hörl, Contribution of proteases to hyper. catabolism in acute renal failure, in: "Nephrology", R.R. Robinson, ed., Springer, New York, Berlin, Heidelberg, Tokyo (1984).

25. J.Y. Tai, A.A. Kortt, T.Y. Liu, S.D. Elliot, Primary structure of streptococcal proteinase. III. Isolation of cyanogen bromide peptides: completes covalent structure of the polypeptide chain, J. Biol. Chem. 251: 1955 (1976).

26. A.L. Goldberg, J.F. Dice, Intracellular protein degradation in mammalian and bacterial cells: part I, Annu. Rev. Biochem. 43: 835 (1974).

27. A. L. Goldberg, A.C. St. John, Intracellular protein degradation in mammalian and bacterial cells: part II, Annu. Rev. Biochem. 45: 747 (1976).

28. K. Morihara, H. Tsuzuki, Production of protease and elastase by Pseudomonas aeruginosa strains isolated from patients, Infect. Immunitiy 15: 679 (1977).

29. K. Havemann, M. Gramse, Physiology and pathophysiology of neutral proteinases of human granulocytes, Adv. Exp. Med. Biol. 167: 1 (1984).

30. R. Egbring, W. Schmidt, G. Fuchs, K. Havemann, Demonstration of granulocyte proteases in plasma of patients with acute leukemia and septicemia with coagulation defects, Blood 49: 219 (1977).

31. M. Jochum, K.H. Duswald, S. Neumann, J. Witte, H. Fritz, Proteinases and their inhibitors in septicemia: Basic concepts and clinical implications, Adv. Exp. Med. Biol. 167: 391 (1984).

32. V. Baracos, H.P. Rodemann, C.A. Dinarello, A.L. Goldberg, Stimulation of muscle protein degradation and prostaglandin E_2 release by leukocytic pyrogen (interleukin-1), N. Engl. J. Med. 308: 553 (1983).

33. R.L. Raff, D. Secrist, Inhibitors of prostaglandin synthesis or cathepsin B prevent muscle wasting due to sepsis in the rat, J. Clin. Invest. 73: 1483 (1984).

34. G.L. Bilbrey, G.R. Faloona, M.G. White, J.P. Knochel:

Hyperglucagonemia of renal failure. J. Clin. Invest. 53: 841 (1974).

35. C.E. Mondon, C.B. Dolkas, G.M. Reaven, P. Alto, M. Field, The site of insulin resistance in acute uremia, J. Am. Diabetes Assoc. 27: 571 (1978).

36. D. Smith, R.A. DeFronzo, Insulin resistance in uremia mediated by post-binding defects, Kidney Int. 22: 54 (1982).

37. W.C. Arnold, M.A. Holliday, Tissue resistance to insulin stimulation of amino acid uptake in acutely uremic rats, Kidney Int. 16: 124 (1979).

38. J.D. Kopple, B. Cianciaruso, S.G. Massry, Does parathyroid hormone cause protein wasting?, Contrib. Nephrol. 20: 138 (1980).

39. H. Wernze, Changes of plasma renin substrate in physiological and pathophysiological states, in: "Radioimmunoassay: Renin, Angiotensin", D.K. Krause, W. Hummerich, K.Poulsen, ed., Georg Thieme, Stuttgart (1978).

40. H.G. Rose, M.C. Robertson, T.B. Schwartz, Hormonal and metabolic influences on intracellular peptidase activity, Am. J. Physiol. 197: 1063 (1959).

41. I.G. Wool, E.I. Weinshelbaum, Incorporation of C^{14}-amino acids into protein of isolated diaphragms: role of the adrenal steroids, Am. J. Physiol. 197: 1089 (1959).

42. A.L. Goldberg, Protein turnover in skeletal muscle. II. Effect of denervation and cortisone on protein catabolism in skeletal muscle, J. Biol. Chem. 244: 3223 (1969).

43. A.L. Goldberg, M. Tischler, G. DeMartino, G. Griffin, Hormonal regulation of protein degradation and synthesis in skeletal muscle, Fed. Proc. 39: 31 (1980).

44. S.R. Rannels, L.S. Jefferson, Effects of glucocorticoids on muscle protein turnover in perfused rat hemicorpus, Am. J. Physiol. 238: E564 (1980).

45. F.M. Thomas, A.J. Murray, L.M. Jones, Interactive effects of insulin and corticosterone on myofibrillar protein turnover in rats as determined by N-methylhistidine excretion, Biochem. J. 220: 469 (1984).

46. F.M. Thomas, H.N. Munro, V.R. Young, Effect of glucocorticoid administration and the rate of muscle protein breakdown in vivo in rats, as measured by urinary excretion of N-methylhistidine, Biochem. J. 178: 139 (1979).

47. S.R. Rannels, D.E. Rannels, A.E. Pegg, L.S. Jefferson, Glucocorticoid effect on peptide-chain initiation in skeletal muscle and heart, Am. J. Physiol. 235: E134 (1978).

48. P.S. Simmons, J.M. Miles, J.E. Gerich, M.W. Haymond, Increased proteolysis - an effect of increases in plasma cortisol within the physiologic range, J. Clin. Invest. 73: 412 (1984).

49. N.J. Papadoyannakis, C.J. Stefanidis, M. McGeown, The effect of the correction of metabolic acidosis on nitrogen and potassium balance of patients with chronic renal failure, Am. J. Clin. Nutr. 40: 623 (1984).

50. R.C. May, R.A. Kelly, E. Mitch, Metabolic acidosis stimulates protein degradation in rat muscle by a glucocorticoid-dependent mechanism, J. Clin. Invest. 77: 614 (1986).

51. P.K. Bondy, F.L. Engel, B. Farrar, The metabolism of amino acids and protein in the adrenalectomized-nephrectomized rat, Endocrinology 44: 476 (1949).

52. J. Weipert, G. Peter, R.M. Schaefer, E. Heidbreder, A. Heidland, Reduction of urea nitrogen appearance and skeletal muscle degradation by adrenalectomy in binephrectomized rats, Nephron, submitted for publication (1986).

53. V.R. Young, S.D. Alexis, B.S. Baliga, H.N. Munro, Metabolism of administered 3-methylhistidine, J. Biol. Chem. 247: 3592 (1972).

54. L.C. Ward, P.J. Buttery, N-methylhistidine: An index of the true rate of myofibrillar degradation? An appraisal, Life Sci. 23: 1103 (1978).

55. E.B. Marliss, C.N. Wei, L.L. Dietrich, The short-term effects of protein intake on 3-methylhistidine excretion, Am. J. Clin. Nutr. 32: 1617 (1979).

56. E.G. Afting, W. Bernhard, R. Janzen, J.H. Röthig, Quantitaive importance on non-skeletal muscle N-methylhistidine and creatine in human urine, Biochem. J. 200: 449 (1981).

57. S.G. Massry, J.W. Coburn, D.B.N. Lee, J. Jowsey, C.R. Kleeman, Skeletal resistance to parathyroid hormone in renal failure: Study in 105 human subjects, Ann. Intern. Med. 78: 357 (1973).

58. H.P. Rodemann, A.L. Goldberg, Arachidonic acid, prostaglandin E_2 and $F_{2\alpha}$ influence raies of protein turnover in skeletal and cardiac muscle, J. Biol. Chem. 257: 1632 (1982).

59. S.A. Laidlaw, R. Zipser, T. Tasaki, S.H.W. Wu, J.D. Kopple, Inhibiton of prostaglandin E_2(PGE_2) release by indomethacin (IND) does not decrease muscle protein degradation in acutely uremic ratss, Kidney Int. in press (1986).

60. H. Umezawa, T. Aoyagi, Activites of proteinase inhibitors of microbial origin, in: "Proteinases in Mammalian cells and tissues", A.J. Barred, ed., North Holland, Amsterdam (1977).

61. A. Hershko, A. Ciechanover, Mechanisms of intracellular protein breakdown, Annu. Rev. Biochem. 51: 335 (1982).

WATER, ELECTROLYTE AND ACID-BASE DISTURBANCES IN ACUTE RENAL FAILURE

G. Conte, S. Federico, A. Dal Canton and V.E. Andreucci

Dept. Nephrology, 2nd Faculty of Medicine

University of Naples, Italy

URINE OUTPUT IN ARF

A complete anuria(a few milliliters of urine in 24 hrs) is rare in ARF. It may occur in bilateral complete ureteral obstruction, in renal cortical necrosis, in acute glomerulonephritis and in bilateral renal artery occlusion(Andreucci et al., 1984).

It is customary to call "oliguria" a urine output of less than 500 ml/day or less than 20 ml/hour(it is advisable, in severely ill patients, to record hourly urine output) (Andreucci et al., 1984).

Oliguria may be observed both, in 'prerenal ARF' and in 'Acute Tubular Necrosis'(ATN or 'renal ARF'). In 'prerenal ARF' it is the combined result of the fall in GFR and the increased tubular reabsorption (a physiologic response of intact kidney to hypoperfusion secondary to the decrease in effective blood volume). In ATN oliguria is due to the fall in GFR (Andreucci et al., 1984).

In 'nonoliguric ARF' urine output is greater than 500 ml/day. The cause of a greater urine volume in some patients with ARF is not completely known. The 'nonoliguric' condition has been attributed to (A) reduced tubular reabsorption of sodium, (B) reduced tubular reabsorption of water and (C) nephron heterogeneity (Gordon and Schrier, 1984).

(A) Reduced tubular reabsorption of sodium.

The ischemic and/or toxic insult, by causing severe cellular injury, may greatly diminish sodium transport in the proximal tubule and thick portion of the ascending limb of Henle; the decreased sodium reabsorption may lead to a great sodium delivery to the distal nephron that may overwhelm distal tubular capacity in reclaiming sodium. The result will be a marked natriuresis and, consequently, a marked water excretion. An increase in fractional excretion of filtered sodium(FENa) is observed in both 'oliguric' and 'nonoliguric' ATN. But there is no prove that it is greater in 'nonoliguric' type of ARF (Gordon and Schrier, 1984).

(B) Reduced tubular reabsorption of water.

Laboratory tests reveal abnormalities in water conservation in 'nonoliguric' ARF: low urinary density and osmolality, U/P Osm of 1. A nephrogenic origin of this defect in water conservation has been demonstrated in experimental models of "nonoliguric ARF"(Gordon et al.1982;Anderson et al.1982)probably due to a severe defect in medullary interstizial tonicity,secondary to a decrease in solute reabsorption in the Henle's loop(Gordon and Schrier,1984)

(C)Nephron heterogeneity.

It is possible that in "nonoliguric" ARF there is a subset of nephrons that has not been damaged by the ischemic or toxic insult;these nephrons would continue to mantain filtration and urine flow thereby accounting for the greater urine output in this type of ARF.In favour of this hypotesis is the experimental observation of Fine(1981) who obtained either oliguric or nonoliguric form of ischemic ARF by using different anesthetic agents in rats;in the oliguric form the kidney appeared composed of a homogeneous population of severely damaged nephrons; in the "nonoliguric" form a heterogeneous population of nephrons was observed,with two-thirds of severely damaged nephrons and one-third of completely normal nephrons.

HYPONATREMIA IN ARF

Mild salt depletion does not cause hyponatremia. The osmolality in the extracellular fluid volume (ECV) is maintained normal by the combined actions of three factors:thirst,ADH secretion and concentrating-diluting mechanism of the kidney(Narins et al.1982). Thus,any time a mild deficit of sodium occurs,the resulting hypotonicity in ECV will inhibit both thirst and ADH secretion,leading to an equivalent and immediate renal loss of water. Thus isotonicity is established again at the cost of mild ECV contraction. Under such circumstances should hyponatremia be observed,it will usually be a iatrogenic hyponatremia secondary to i.v. infusion of salt-free solutions. Sometimes the excessive hydration is due to increase in water intake.

Severe salt depletion,on the contrary,causes hyponatremia.In condition of marked ECV contraction, in fact, the priority of maintaining a normal osmolality in the ECV is sacrificed in order to minimize ECV contraction; the three water- retaining forces are stimulated rather than inhibited; the resulting hyponatremia reflects severe hypovolemia (Narins et al, 1982). "Prerenal"ARF is secondary to severe ECV depletion due to loss of sodium-containing fluids through the gastrointestinal tract (because of severe sweating, burns) or the kidneys (because of salt-losing nephritis, loop diuretics, etc.);under such circumstances the hypothalamic-renal factors are stimulated leading to renal retention of ingested water; hyponatremia is therefore observed reflecting the hypovolemia. Hypotonicity and hyponatremia will be worsened if salt-free solutions are given by mouth and/or by i.v. infusion in these patients with 'prerenal' ARF (Andreucci et al, 1984 chapter 7 and 21).

A decrease in 'effective' arterial blood volume may also occur in edematous states, such as congestive heart failure (because of reduced cardiac output), cirrhosis with ascites (because of reduction in peripheral resistance) and nephrotic syndrome or severe burns (because of a reduction in total blood volume due to protein losses). (The 'effective' arterial blood volume is defined as the relative fullness of the arterial tree as determined by cardiac output, peripheral vascular resistance and total blood volume). These are situations of ECV expansion in which the reduced 'effective' blood volume will cause a disproportionate retention of ingested water; the result will be a hypervolemic hyponatremia (Narins et al, 1982; Andreucci et al, 1984 chapter 7). The resulting renal hypoperfusion will cause 'prerenal ARF' (Andreucci,1984 chapters 1 and 2) which is reversed by hemodynamic improvement and re-expansion of 'effective' arterial blood volume (Andreucci, 1984 chapter 21).

HYPERNATREMIA IN ARF

Very frequently ECV depletion is due to losses of hypotonic fluids (sodium concentration lower than that of plasma); this is the case with the fluid loss by vomiting or nasogastric suction(Na in gastric juice = 60 mmol/liter), by diarrhea or intestinal drainage(Na in small bowel juice = 105 mmol/liter, in ileal fluid=129 mmol/liter, in cecal fluid= 80mmol/liter) by excessive sweating(Na in sweat = 45 mmol/liter). If these losses remain unreplaced or partially replaced by relatively hypertonic solution(such as normal saline,which contains 154 mmol/liter of Na), a 'prerenal ARF' with hypernatremia will result(Narins et al, 1982;Andreucci et al, 1984 chapter 7). This hypovolemic hypernatremia will be worsened by associated conditions of water loss, such as increase in insensible water(e.g.because of hyperpnea). The occurence of hypervolemic hypernatremia is usually iatrogenic; thus, it is observed when metabolic acidosis is treated with hypertonic solutions of sodium bicarbonate.

HYPERKALEMIA IN ARF

Hyperkalemia is quite frequent in ARF. Particularly in oliguric ARF it derives from potassium retention. A iatrogenic component is frequently associated due to an excessive potassium administration as oral intake, stored blood transfusion, i.v. infusion of potassium-containing solutions, or K-penicilline administration (Andreucci et al, 1984,chapter 7). A redistribution of potassium between intracellular and extracellular spaces, (because of metabolic acidosis or hypercatabolic states), may further contribute to the hyperkalemia observed in ARF. Thus a severe life-threatening hyperkalemia is usually observed in postsurgical or posttraumatical ARF (Andreucci,1984 chapter 12).

A fatal hyperkalemia may occur in diabetic patients following i.v. infusion of glucose solutions without insulin; the sudden hyperglycemia, in fact, will cause an osmotic movement of cellular water(containing potassium) to the extracellular fluid. This phenomenon does not occur in normal subjects because of rapid secretion of aldosterone and insulin with the consequent cellular re-entry of potassium (Godfarb et al,1976; Narins et al,1982).

HYPOKALEMIA IN ARF

Hypokalemia may occur even in oliguric ARF. It is secondary to potassium losses with potassium-containing fluid,by vomiting or nasogastric suction(K in gastric juice = 9 mmol/liter), intestinal drainage(K in small bowel juice = 5 mmol/liter), diarrhea(in diarrhea states stool may contain from 10 to 100 mmol/liter of K), severe sweating(K in sweat = 4.5 mmol/liter). This hypokalemia is expression of potassium depletion. Sometimes, however, potassium depletion may be associated with normokalemia or even hyperkalemia because of simultaneous severe metabolic acidosis and the consequent redistribution of K from the intracellular space to the extracellular fluid (Andreucci et al, 1984,chapter 7).

ACID-BASE BALANCE IN ARF

The acid-base status may be of some help in evaluating the etiology of ARF: a metabolic acidosis may result from diarrhea or intestinal fistulas ((the'anion-gap' may be normal,the lost bicarbonate being replaced by chloride overreabsorbed by proximal tubules of the hypoperfused kydney); metabolic alkalosis may result from vomiting, nasogastric suction, diuretic therapy. In ATN, however, when the renal damage has occurred, acid retention will always lead to metabolic acidosis that may only be blunted by persisting vomiting or nasogastric suction. Under such circumstances the 'anion-gap' will be invariably increased (Andreucci et al, 1984 chapter 7).

In ATN a severe metabolic acidosis is always seen in conditions of overproduction of organic or inorganic acids. This occurs in lactic acidosis, in diabetic ketoacidosis and in hypercatabolic states. Thus, a particularly severe metabolic acidosis is observed in rhabdomyolysis-induced ARF due to the great amount of hydrogen ions and their associated anions released from tissue destruction (McCarron et al, 1979; Andreucci,1984 chapter 12).

HYPOCALCEMIA IN ARF

Hypocalcemia is frequent in ARF and is responsible for the secondary hyperparathyroidism commonly observed in ARF (Kokot, 1984). The fall in serum calcium is due to phosphate retention (because of the impaired renal function), low blood levels of vitamin D and a skeletal resistance to the calcemic action of PTH (Massry et al, 1974). A marked hypocalcemia is typically observed in the oliguric phase of rhabdomyolysis-induced ARF: the severe hyperphosphatemia, due to phosphate retention (because of the renal shutdown) as well as phosphate release by skeletal muscle (because of their excessive breakdown), will cause calcium salt deposition in traumatized muscles which leads to the fall in serum levels of calcium(Meroney et al, 1956; Akmal et al, 1978; Andreucci, 1984 chapter 12). Hypocalcemia with hyperphosphatemia is also observed in patients with acute lymphoblastic leukemia and ARF (due to acute nephrocalcinosis) following cytolytic therapy (Andreucci, 1984 chapter 2; Andreucci et al, 1984 chapter 7).

HYPERCALCEMIA IN ARF

Hypercalcemia is typically observed in the diuretic phase of rhabdomyolysis-induced ARF. This hypercalcemia has been attributed to resolution of soft-tissue calcification, increased calcium resorption from bone and increase in gut calcium absorption. In these patients plasma levels of PTH have been found low, normal and high (Kokot, 1984) and plasma levels of vitamin D normal or high (Andreucci, 1984 chapter 12).

REFERENCES

Andreucci, V.E., Federico, S., Memoli, B., and Usberti, M., Clinical diagnosis in acute renal failure, in: "Acute Renal Failure. Pathophysiology, Prevention and Treatment", V.E. Andreucci, ed., Martinus Nijhoff Publ., Boston(1984), chapter 7, p.189.

Andreucci, V.E., Pathophysiology of ischemic/toxic acute renal failure, in: "Acute Renal Failure. Pathophysiology, Prevention and Treatment", V.E. Andreucci, ed., Martinus Nijhoff Publ. Boston(1984), chapter 1, p.1.

Andreucci, V.E., Different forms of ischemic/toxic acute renal failure in humans, in: "Acute Renal Failure. Pathophysiology, Prevention and Treatment", V.E. Andreucci, ed., Martinus Nijhoff Publ., Boston(1984), chapter 2, p.51.

Andreucci, V.E., Myoglobinuria and acute renal failure, in: "Acute Renal Failure. Pathophysiology, Prevention and Treatment", V.E. Andreucci, ed., Martinus Nijhoff Publ., Boston(1984), chapter 12, p.251.

Andreucci, V.E., Conservative management and general care of patients with acute renal failure, in: "Acute Renal Failure. Pathophysiology, Prevention and Treatment", V.E. Andreucci, ed., Martinus Nijhoff Publ., Boston(1984), chapter 21, p.403.

Gordon, J.A. and Schrier, R.W., Non-oliguric acute renal failure, in: "Acute Renal Failure. Pathophysiology, Prevention and Treatment", V.E. Andreucci, ed., Martinus Nijhoff Publ., Boston(1984), chapter 10,p.221.

Gordon, J.A., Anderson, R.J., Peterson, L.K., 1982, Water metabolism after cis-platinum in the rat., Am. J. Physiol., 243: F36.

Godfarb, S., Cox, M., Singer, I., Goldberg, M., 1976, Acute hyperkalemia induced by hyperglicemia: Hormonal mechanism., Ann. Intern. Med., 84: 426.

Narins, R.G., Jones, E.R., Stom, M.C., Rudnick, M.R., Bastl, C.P., 1982, Diagnostic strategies in disorders of fluid electrolyte and acid-base homeostasis., Am. J. Med., 72: 496.

Finn, W.F., 1981, Nephron heterogeneity in polyuric acute renal failure., J. Lab. Clin. Med., 98: 21.

Anderson, R.J., Gordon, J.A., Peterson, L.K., Gross, P., Ellis, M., 1982, The renal concentration defect following non-oliguric acute renal failure in the rat., Kidney Int., 21: 583.

McCarron, D.A., Elliott, W.C., Rose, J.S., Bennett, W.M., 1979, Severe mixed metabolic acidosis secondary to rhabdomyolysis., Am. J. Med., 67: 905.

Kokot, F., Endocrine system in acute renal failure, in: "Acute Renal Failure. Pathophysiology, Prevention and Treatment", V.E. Andreucci, ed., Martinus Nijhoff Publ., Boston(1984), chapter 5, p.167.

Massry, S.G., Arieff, A.I., Coburn, J.W., Palmieri, G., Kleeman, C.R., 1974, Divalent ion metabolism in patients with acute renal failure: Studies on the mechanism of hypocalcemia., Kidney Int. 5: 437.

FILTRATION PRESSURE AND GLOMERULAR PERMEABILITY IN $HgCl_2$-ACUTE RENAL FAILURE IN THE DOG

Raymond Vanholder, Pierre Paul Lambert*, and Norbert Lameire

Renal Division, University Hospital
Gent, Belgium
Queen Elisabeth Foundation, Brussels, Belgium

There are essentially four mechanisms that can explain the filtration fall that is observed during experimental acute renal failure : tubular back-leakage, tubular obstruction, a decrease of glomerular permeability and a fall in effective filtration pressure due to hemodynamic changes. The studies that make an attempt to characterize these different mechanisms are rare and focus in most of the cases on the maintenance phase but not on the initiation phase of acute renal failure.

The present series of studies was undertaken in 10 dogs to evaluate polyvinylpyrrolidone (PVP) macrolecular sieving curves, in an attempt to determine whether changes in glomerular hemodynamics play a role in the early filtration fall within the first three hours after the induction of toxic acute renal failure by the injection of $HgCl_2$ in the dog.

For this purpose, 3 mg/kg $HgCl_2$ were administered intravenously as a bolus injection, and clearance studies were obtained one, two and three hours thereafter. Renal blood flow was calculated from PAH clearances that had been corrected for PAH-extraction and hematocrit. I^{125} PVP macromolecular sieving curves were obtained in the control period and 3 hours after the mercury injection. The macromolecular separation, based on the molecular radius, was obtained by chromatography on Sephadex G 2000, and sieving coefficients were calculated as described previously[1].

There was a gradual decline of both glomerular filtration rate (GFR) and renal blood flow (RBF) within the first three hours after the mercury injection, GFR decreasing from 75.5±3.5 to 43.4±2.8 ml/min.100 g KW (Δ%: -43%, $p<0.01$), and RBF from 552.1±32.9 to 343.7±27.0 ml/min.100 g KW (Δ%: -37%, $p< 0.01$). Concomitantly, a diuretic effect was observed with a rise of the fractional sodium excretion and of the osmolar excretion. The evolution of the I^{125}-PVP sieving curves is illustrated in table 1: there was a significant shift upwards and to the right for macromolecules with an Einstein-Stokes radius of more than 2.3 nm.

Table 1. I^{125}-PVP fractional clearances

Einstein-Stokes radius (nm)	Control	3 hrs after $HgCl_2$	Φ_{exp}/Φ_{contr}
2.0	1.01±0.02	1.00±0.02	0.99
2.2	0.98±0.02	0.99±0.02	1.01
2.4	0.91±0.02	0.98±0.02**	1.08
2.6	0.80±0.02	0.90±0.02**	1.13
2.8	0.65±0.02	0.79±0.02**	1.22
3.0	0.50±0.02	0.64±0.02**	1.28
3.2	0.36±0.02	0.49±0.02**	1.36
3.4	0.26±0.01	0.35±0.02**	1.35
3.6	0.18±0.01	0.24±0.02**	1.33
3.8	0.12±0.01	0.15±0.01*	1.25
4.0	0.08±0.01	0.11±0.01	- [a]

[a]Values too small to allow a valid calculation.
*$p<0.05$, **$p<0.01$ vs. control.

A first possible explanation for a similar shift to the right would be the presence of tubular back-leakage of small molecules, such as inulin and creatinine. In the normal kidney, inulin as well as PVP are excreted by the filtration process, and are not reabsorbed nor secreted on the tubular level. If in acute renal failure, passive back-leakage of inulin were present without back-leak of the larger macromolecules, it can be supposed that macromolecular PVP sieving coefficients would be overestimated. Similar results have been presented previously by Myers and co-workers as evidence for the presence of back-leak in the case of ischemic post-surgical acute renal failure in man[2,3]. In these studies, it was observed that the sieving curve was projected more to the right in acute renal failure, compared to the curve obtained in prerenal insufficiency as well as in control conditions. Moreover, the sieving coefficients exceeded unity for the smallest macromolecules, a situation that seems highly improbable under any other condition than back-leak. At the same time, it was observed that the relation between the control and the experimental sieving coefficients tended to rise to a plateau value for the larger macromolecules.

In the present study, the situation was not entirely the same, in spite of a similar shift to the right of the sieving curve. First, the sieving coefficients had no tendency to rise above unity, even for the smallest macromolecules (Table 1). Second, the relation between experimental and control sieving coefficients (Φ_{exp}/Φ_{contr}) showed no plateau values for the largest macromolecules. Consequently, the shape of the sieving curve gave little support in favor of an eventual tubular back leak.

There were other results in the present study that were also in disagreement with the back-leak hypothesis. First, the relation between creatinine and inulin clearance remained always near to unity (Fig. 1).

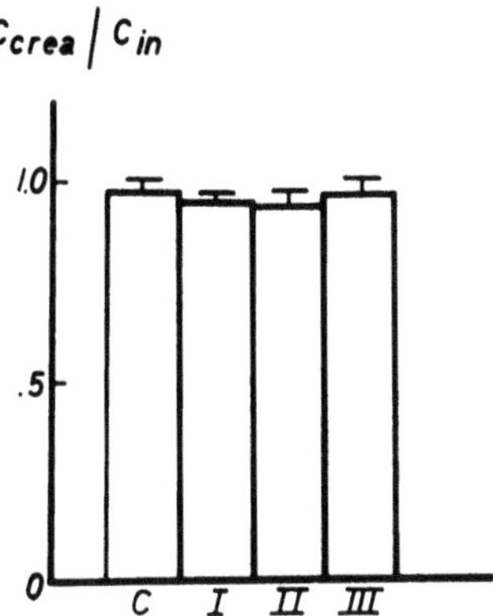

Fig. 1. Evolution of the relation C_{crea}/C_{in} during the first three hours after $HgCl_2$.
C: control; I-III: 1-3 hrs after $HgCl_2$.

Furthermore, the PAH-extraction remained normal as well during the whole experiment (Fig. 2). In the case of tubular back-leak, one should expect a fall of the extraction in parallel with the tubular lesions.

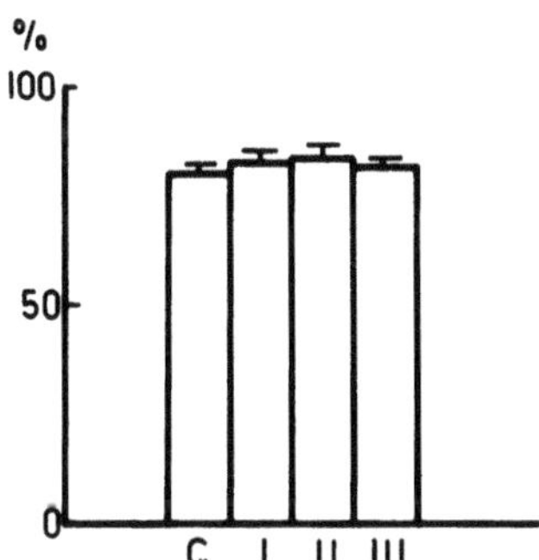

Fig. 2. Evolution of PAH-extraction. C: control; I-III: 1-3 hrs after $HgCl_2$.

All these results are in agreement with several studies in $HgCl_2$ acute renal failure in the rat, where also no arguments in favor of tubular back-leak could be found[4-6].

An eventual shift in the sieving curve could also be attributed to hemodynamic reasons, since its shape is influenced by the relative contribution of diffusion and convection in the filtration process. Several situations could explain a shift upward and to the right[7]: 1) in the case of a fall in blood flow without change in filtration; 2) when the effective filtration pressure decreases; 3) when the protein concentration of the blood, and consequently also the colloid osmotic counterpressure increases; 4) finally, when the glomerular permeability increases.

From our results, it is clear that neither filtration fraction nor colloid osmotic pressure are increased three hours after $HgCl_2$ (Table 2).

Table 2. Evolution of mean glomerular colloid osmotic pressure (Π_G) and filtration fraction (FF).

	Π_G (mm Hg)	FF (%)
Control	21.6±0.4	29±3
3 hrs after $HgCl_2$	22.5±0.5	28±2

It is also highly improbable that glomerular permeability would augment in the case of a filtration fall. Consequently, there remains only one theoretical explanation for the observed changes, namely a fall in filtration pressure.

The evolution of the hemodynamic parameters playing a role in the filtration process can also be calculated by a mathematical model developed by Dubois et al[8]. This makes it possible to calculate the effective filtration pressure (EFP), the glomerular permeability (Kf) and its two constituants, the pore radius of the glomerular membrane (R) and the filtration surface per unit of length ($Ap/\Delta x$).

It has been preferred to express the evolution of these hemodynamic parameters in a relative (i.e. percentual) way rather than in absolute numbers, since the exact values of Kf and EFP remain unknown at present. Up till now, extremely wide ranging values have been found depending on the investigation method, either micropuncture[9], the study of the isolated glomerulus[10,11], or the study of sieving curves[12]. The micropuncture method, which is most currently used, is only representative for the superficial glomeruli. For all these reasons, we have preferred to express our experimental data as a percent of the control data.

Kf and its two constituants R and $Ap/\Delta x$ remained unaltered, but there was a marked fall in effective filtration pressure by 40 %, in parallel with the fall in GFR. This decrease in effective filtration pressure can be attributed to two different mechanisms, either a fall of the filtration pressure due to hemodynamic factors, or a rise in intratubular pressure due to obstruction. The present study does not allow a distinction between these two possibilities. Several previous studies from our group have however demonstrated a strict parallelism between RBF and GFR[13-15], as illustrated in Table 3. This suggests that hemodynamic changes are at least in part responsible for the fall in filtration pressure within the first three hours after mercuric chloride.

Table 3. Percent changes of GFR and RBF, 3 hrs after $HgCl_2$.

	GFR (%)	RBF (%)
$HgCl_2$ alone	-43	-38
Mannitol 5 % (0.75 ml/min.kg)	- 3	- 4
Saline (3 ml/min.kg)	- 3	- 1
Bilateral carotid clamping	- 4	-15
Verapamil (0.005 mg/kg.min-I.R.)	-19	-18
Captopril (300 µg/kg-I.V.)	-21	+ 3
Dazoxiben (0.5 mg/kg-I.V.)	-37	-41
Saline (0.75 ml/min.kg)	-42	-37
Suprarenal aortic clamping	-56	-62

In summary, the initiation phase of toxic acute renal failure due to mercury is characterised by a fall in filtration and renal blood flow, and by a shift of the PVP-macromolecular sieving curve to the right. Tubular backleak is excluded at this stage. On theoretical and mathematical grounds, the change of the sieving curve can only be explained by a fall in effective filtration pressure. This can be attributed, either to tubular obstruction, or to a hemodynamic change. Other results obtained by our group demonstrate a remarkable parallelism between GFR and RBF, and suggest that hemodynamic factors are at least in part responsible for this decrease of the effective filtration pressure.

REFERENCES

1. VANRENTERGHEM Y., VANHOLDER R., LAMMENS-VERSLYPE M. and LAMBERT P.P.: Sieving studies in "urea-induced nephropathy" in the dog. Clin. Science, 58, 65-75, 1980.

2. MYERS B.D., CHUI F., HILBERMAN M. and MICHAELS A.S.: Transtubular leakage of glomerular filtrate in human acute renal failure. Am. J. Physiol., 237, F319-F325, 1979.

3. MYERS B.D., HILBERMAN M., SPENCER R.J. and JAMISON R.L.: Glomerular and tubular function in non-oliguric acute renal failure. Am. J. Med., 72, 642-649, 1982.

4. DI BONA G.F., MAC DONALD F.D., FLAMENBAUM W., DAMMIN G.J. and OKEN D.E.: Maintenance of renal function in salt loaded rats despite severe tubular necrosis induced by $HgCl_2$. Nephron, 8, 205-220, 1971.

5. FLAMENBAUM W., MAC DONALD F.D., DI BONA G.F. and OKEN D.E.: Micropuncture study of renal tubular factors in low dose mercury poisoning. Nephron, 8, 221-234, 1971.

6. OLBRICHT C., MASON J., TAKABATAKE T., HOHLBRUGGER G. and THURAU K.: The early phase of experimental acute renal failure. II. Tubular leakage and the reliability of glomerular markers. Pflügers Arch., 372, 251-258, 1977.

7. BRENNER B.M., BOHRER M.P., BAYLIS C. and DEEN W.M.: Determinants of glomerular permselectivity: insights derived from observations in vivo. Kidney Int., 12, 229-237, 1977.

8. DU BOIS R., DECOODT P., GASSEE J.P., VERNIORY A. and LAMBERT P.P.: Determination of glomerular intracapillary and transcapillary pressure gradients from sieving data. I. Mathematical model. Pflügers Arch., 356, 299-316, 1975.

9. NAVAR L.G., BELL P.D., WHITE R.W., WATTS R.L. and WILLIAMS R.H.: Evaluation of the single nephron glomerular filtration coefficient in the dog. Kidney Int., 12, 137-149, 1977.

10. SAVIN V.J., PATAK R.V., MARR G., HERMRECK A.S., RIDGE S.M. and LAKE K.: Glomerular ultrafiltration coefficient after ischemic renal injury in dogs. Circ. Research, 53, 439-447, 1983.

11. OSGOOD R.W., PATTON M., HANLEY M.J., VENKATACHALAM M., REINECK J. and STEIN J.: In vitro perfusion of the isolated dog glomerulus. Am. J. Physiol., 244, F349-F354, 1983.

12. LAMBERT P.P., AEIKENS G. and BERGMANN P.: Microrheology, water permeability and permselectivity for macromolecules in the renal glomerulus. In: The paracellular pathway. Ed. S.E. Bradley and E.F. Purcell, Josiah Macy Jr. Foundation, 1982, pp. 97-117.

13. VANHOLDER R., LEUSEN I. and LAMEIRE N.: Influence of isotonic mannitol and saline in $HgCl_2$-induced acute renal failure. Nephron, 23, 744-748, 1983.

14. VANHOLDER R., MATTHYS E., LEUSEN I. and LAMEIRE N.: Effect of premercurial resetting of intrarenal vascular resistance on $HgCl_2$-induced acute renal failure. J. Clin. Lab. Med., in press.

15. VANHOLDER R. and LAMEIRE N.: Effect of captopril on $HgCl_2$-induced acute renal failure (ARF). Abstracts of the IXth international congress of nephrology, Los Angeles, 1984, p. 338A.

SUPEROXIDE RADICALS (SR) IN THE PATHOPHYSIOLOGY OF ISCHEMIC ACUTE RENAL FAILURE (ARF)

Rossana Faedda, Andrea Satta, G. Franco Branca, Franco Turrini, Bruno Contu, and Ettore Bartoli

Istituto di Patologia Medica, Università di Sassari
Viale San Pietro 12,07100 Sassari (Italy)

INTRODUCTION

Several factors including hypoxia, lysomal enzymes release, endotoxins and kinins have been involved in the pathogenesis of ARF[1]. Among these, hypoxia represents the initiating event of a series of biochemical reactions which culminate in the production of oxidative radicals[2]. The most important are the superoxide ions (O_2^-) and the free radicals which result from their interactions with other molecules. These substances can injure cells by peroxidating the lipid membranes. The organism however has efficient enzymatic and non enzymatic systems which can oppose and control the production of free radicals and superoxide anion. These systems are represented by superoxide dismutase, catalase and glutathione peroxidase which can detoxicate the SR, the hydrogenperoxide and the lipid peroxides[3,4]. Among the other physiological scavangers glutathion, vitamin E and C, cysteine and probably uric acid have great importance[5]. The biological sequence occurring during ischemia is schematically represented in Fig.1. During hypoxia there is a rapid consumption of ATP with a rise in intracellular AMP concentration, subsequently metabolized to adenosine, inosine and finally hypoxanthine, which accumulates in the ischemic tissue and represents the substrate of xanthine(X) dehydrogenase and X- oxidase Certain authors postulate that the fundamental biochemical phase during hypoxia, is represented by X-dehydrogenase activity, while in the reoxygenation phase the activity of Xoxidase prevails, producing hydrogen peroxide and SR, responsible for the maintenance of the ischemic damage. In accordance with these data, several authors have found a clear reduction of the vascular permeability with a rapid functional recovery of the ischemic organ after its pretreatment with allopurinol, dimethylsulphoxide (DMSO), superoxide dismutase (SOD), catalase or with substances inhibiting the X-oxidase[6,7,8]. The present study is aimed at verifying the speed in recovery of the glomerular function in course of a ARF after pretreatment with DMSO and SOD using a simple experimental protocol on rats, in which one kidney could act as a control of the controlateral organ which was protected from the effect of reoxygenation.

METHODS

The experiments were performed on 57 Wistar rats weighing 250 to 400 g.

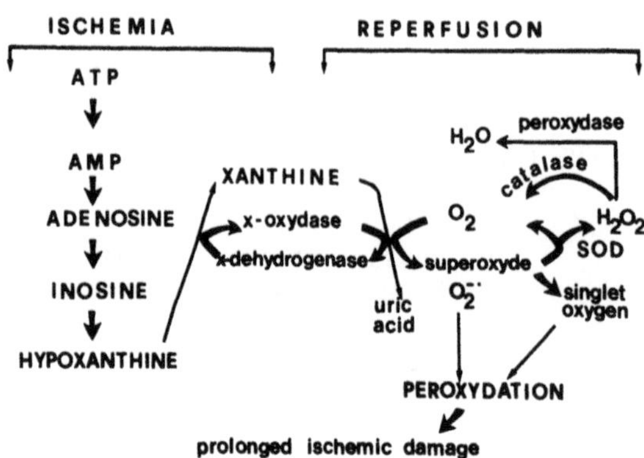

Fig. 1.
The figure schematically shows the biochemical steps activated during ischemia and reoxygenation. Oxygen is generated by X-oxidase induced by the increased substrate formation (cascade on the left side). The oxygen gives rise to SR, which are either protonated (upward sequence on the right) or acted upon by lipids (downward sequence).

After a 12 hour fast, they were anestethized with Thiopenthal-Na (50 mg/Kg). On a surgical table at 37°C, a tracheal tube was inserted and catheters placed in the jugular vein, femoral artery and ureters. The renal arteries were dissected free of the surrounding tissue and exposed. After quantitatively replacing the surgical losses, a maintenance infusion of an artificial isotonic solution containing normal concentrations of Na bicarbonate, NaCl, KCl and glucose was given. It contained ^{131}I-Hypaque in concentrations suitable for clearance measurements. The infusion rate of isotonic fluids was then adjusted to 3 ml/hr to achieve and maintain extracellular volume expansion. At steady state, two clearance periods were performed on both kidneys simultaneously. The two renal arteries were then clamped 5 minutes one from the other, to induce ischemia in 10 rats (group 1). The infusion of fluid and glomerular markers was drastically reduced to a minimum. Thirty minutes after the induction of ischemia, DMSO (200 mg/Kg) was given i.v. 1 min before till 3 min after releasing the clamp of one of the two renal arteries. Five minutes were allowed for the substance to be filtered, then the other renal artery was opened. The recovery period of the glomerular function was timed on both kidneys and clearance periods were performed in the early recovery phase. In a second set of 17 animals (group 2), once the basal clearances were performed, ischemia was induced in a right kidney while the left one was left unclamped. The arterial clamp was released 30 min later and measurements were performed again during the recovery time. Once the baseline urine flow had been reattained, SOD (30 mg/Kg) was given i.v. and 30 min later ischemia was induced in the left kidney. Even in this case the same procedure described above was followed. The maintenance infusion rate was 1 ml/hr. On plasma and urinary samples the electrolyte concentration was measured with flame photometer and the radioactivity with a well-type gamma counter. The urinary flow ($\dot{V}$), glomerular filtration (GFR) and Sodium excretion (UNa.V) were measured. In a final set of 23 rats a similar procedure was followed, but the kidneys were removed immediately after the 30' ischemia or after 2', 5', 15', 30' from the reoxygenation. Both cortex and medulla were removed for tissue glutathion measurements. Seven of the 23 animals were pretreated with BCNU (carmustine, 5 mg/Kg intraperitoneally) and Diamide 75 mg/Kg i.v. These agents prevent the regeneration of GSH through reducing reactions. Therefore they should enhance the damage occurring during reperfusion. The data were processed statistically, means and standard errors of the mean (SEM) calculated. Significance between means was tested by paired "t" test, between regression coefficients by covariance analysis.

RESULTS

The experimental model used enables us to evaluate in each animal the difference between a control kidney, not protected from the substances examined, and an experimental kidney, exposed to these same substances. The results are reported in Table 1. After reperfusion the control kidneys showed a functional recovery of diuresis after 25.0±8.6 minutes in the 1st group and 21.2±5.3 in the 2nd. Four kidneys showed anuria. In the kidneys protected with DMSO and SOD the recovery occurred respectively after only 15.8±6.8 and 12.8±4.7 minutes, $P<0.05$. In the recovery phase the initial GFR measured was not different in left and right kidneys. Subsequently the recovery was definitely more rapid in the treated kidneys. With DMSO the recovery rate was 5.2% per minute of the basal GFR, as opposed to the 3.4% of the control kidney, while with SOD it was 3% as opposed to 1% of control, $P<0.05$ (Fig.2). The covariance analysis showed a significant difference in the slope of the recovery of GFR, $\dot{V}$ and UNa $\dot{V}$ ($P<0.05$) demonstrating that both DMSO and SOD had had a protective effect on the experimental kidney promoting a quick diuresis and a rapid functional recovery. The glutathion concentration was not significantly different between the two kidneys, even though it followed a trend similar and parallel to the modifications in renal emodynamics. The GSH levels, reduced during the ischemical phase, increased progressively in the reoxygenation phase (Fig.3), confirming that the enzyme can be used as a marker of the post-ischemic damage.

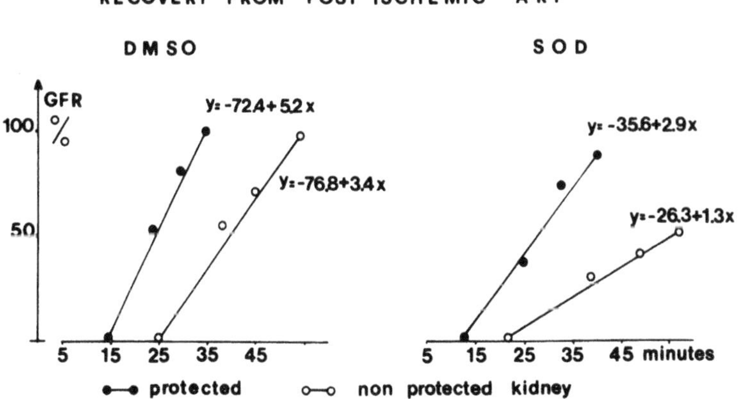

Fig. 2. GFR is in the ordinate expressed as a percentage of the baseline preischemic value. In abscissa the time after reperfusion is reported. The closed circles refer to the protected, the open circles to the control kidney. Regression lines and equations were computed from mean values indicated by symbols.

Table 1. Effects of SR scavengers on recovery from ARF

	V μl/min		GFR μl/min		UNa μEq/ml	
	U	P	U	P	U	P
Effects of DMSO						
Baseline	9.1±1.2	9.5±1.5	240±34	271±44	139±22	157±28
Recovery	9.4±1.8	12.3±3.3	139±22	159±24	138±25	151±12
sequence	12.2±2.9 *	18.5±2.5	177±49 *	229±29	119±31 *	157±15
	18.3±6.6 *	22.1±5.6	236±71 *	274±37	142±43 *	188±22
Effect of SOD						
Baseline	14.6±0.8	16.1±4.6	1134±134	1228±204	177±53	162±70
Recovery	8.0±1.7	9.0±2.1	342±142	401±125	155±21	178±19
sequence	10.7±0.9	13.3±3.8	469±185 *	794±88	161±10	170±22
	14.6±2.6	13.8±3.4	578±248 *	845±35	168±19	179±23

The table reports means and standard deviations of the values for urinary flow rate (V), glomerular filtration rate (GFR) and urinary sodium concentration (UNa). The data were obtained before and after ischemia in the control unprotected kidney (U) and in the paired organ protected (P) with DMSO or SOD. Asterisks show the significance by paired "t" test.

Confirming these data, in the 7 rats treated with Diamide + BCNU the GSH levels remained extremely low for over 30 min after reperfusion (Fig.3).

DISCUSSION

The pathophysiology of experimental ARF is still a matter of controversy[9]. The model based on renal artery clamping corresponds to the more common clinical forms of the disease[10]. Hypoxia represents the initiating event of the biochemical cascade which culminates with the production of SR responsible for the ischemic damage[11, 13].

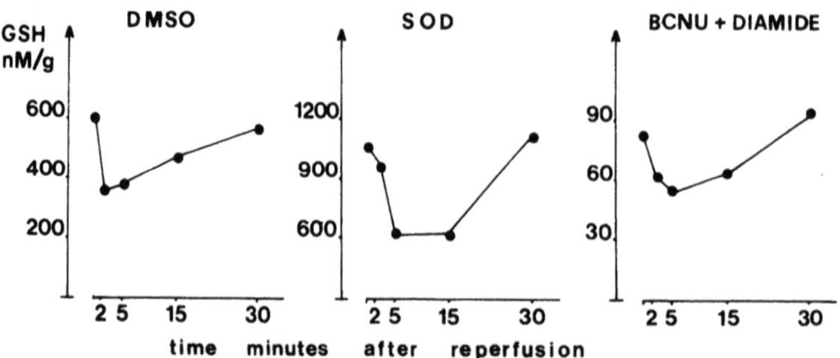

Fig. 3. In the ordinates are concentrations of glutathion (GSH) nM/g of kidney tissue, measured at the times after reperfusion reported in abscissa. Time zero is the 30th minute of ischemia without clamp release. Note that the scales of the ordinates are different for the three substances tested, such that the values of BCNU + Diamide are about one tenth those with SOD.

The most important source of superoxide seems to be the xanthine-oxidase enzyme, activated during ischemia by the conversion of xanthine-dehydrogenase from certain proteases stimulated by the high intracellular calcium concentration. In our study we assessed the glomerular functional recovery after i.v. administration of radical scavangers, using an experimental model of ischemic ARF in rats. The data demonstrate that DMSO and SOD exert a significant protective effect, inducing a faster diuretic response and a definitely higher functional recovery. An indirect proof was given by the trend of the glutathion concentration, which increased progressively in the 20 minutes after reoxygenation, parallel to the physiological and emodynamic recovery. Probably DMSO and SOD blocked the enzymatic steps leading to toxic and cytolytic substances. In conclusion, our data confirms the hypothesis that the ischemic damage occurs even at the moment of reperfusion of the organ and that it results, at least in part, from the release of SR. Substances able to prevent their formation or to accelerate their removal (DMSO, SOD) reduce the entity of the damage in the animal and could prove helpful clinically. The opposite effect of BCNU and Diamide supports this explanation.

AKNOWLEDGEMENT

This study was supported by the "Assessorato all'Igiene e Sanità della Regione Autonoma della Sardegna", Italy.

REFERENCES

1. J.M. McCord, Oxygen-derived free radicals in post-ischemic tissue injury, New Eng.J.Med. 312:159 (1984).
2. F.Z.Meerson, V.E.Kagan, Y.P.Kozlov, L.M.Belkima and Y.V.Arkhipenko, The role of lipid peroxidation in pathogenesis of ischemic damage and the anti-oxidant protection of the heart, Basic Res.Cardiol. 77:465 (1982).
3. W.A.Pryor, The formation of free radicals and the consequences of their reactions in vivo, Photochem.Photobiol. 28:787 (1978).
4. B.E.Leibovitz, B.V.Siegel, Aspects of free radical reactions in biological system: aging, J.Gerontol. 35:45 (1980).
5. B.N.Ames, R.Cathrat, E.Schwiers, P.Hochstein, Uric acid provides an antioxidant defense against oxidant and radical- caused aging and cancer: a hypothesis, Proc.Natl.Acad.Sci. USA 78, 6858 (1981).
6. M.Shlaper, P.F.Kane, V.Y.Wiggins, M.M.Kirsh, Possible role for cytotoxic oxygen metabolites in the pathogenesis of cardiac ischemic injury, Circulation 66:85 suppl.1 (1982).
7. J.R.Stewart, W.H.Blackwell, S.L.Crute, V.Loughlin, M.L.Hess, L.S. Greenfield, Prevention of myocardial ischemia: reperfusion injury with oxygen free radical scavengers, Surg.Forum 33:317 (1982).
8. A.S.Casale, G.B.Bulkley, B.H. Bulkley, J.T. Flaherty, V.L.Gott, T.S. Oxygen free radical scavengers protect the arrested, globally ischemic heart upon reperfusion, Surg.Forum 34:313 (1983).
9. D.E.Oken, Acute renal failure (vasomotor nephropathy): Micropuncture studies on the pathogenesis mechanisms, Ann.Rev.Med. 26:307 (1975).
10. N.Parekh, U.Veith, Renal hemodynamics and oxygen consuption during post-ischemic acute renal failure in the rat, Kidney Intern. 19:306 (1981).

11. J.M.McCord, I.Fridovich, The reduction of cytochrome C by milk xanthine-oxidase, J.Biol.Chem. 243:5753 (1968).
12. C.E.Jones, J.W.Crowell, E.E.Smith, Significance of increased blood uric acid following extensive hemorrhage, Am.J.Physiol. 214:1374 (1968).
13. D.A.Parks, G.B.Bulkley, N.D.Granger, S.R.Hamilton, J.M.McCord, Ischemic injury in the cat small intestine: Role of superoxide radicals, Gastroenterology 82:9 (1982).

SERINE AND METALLO PROTEINASES IN ACUTE RENAL FAILURE

Roland M. Schaefer[1], Christopher Wanner[2], and Walter H. Hörl[2]

Department of Medicine, Division of Nephrology

Universities of [1]Wuerzburg and [2]Freiburg, FRG

INTRODUCTION

Recent studies have demonstrated frank proteolytic activity in plasma fractions of patients with acute renal failure (ARF) following traumatic injuries and/or septicemia [1-3]. Therefore, it was assumed that proteases play a key role in the catabolic state of ARF [4]. Since hemodialysis may even cause a further release of leukocyte proteinases, which has been widely documented for elastase [5-7], one was frightened that the very measure to relieve the burden of ARF might contribute to the catabolism of this state. Therefore, the present study was performed to further characterize this proteolytic activity in the plasma of such patients.

MATERIALS AND METHODS

16 patients (13 males, 3 females) suffering from acute renal failure, aged 56.3 $\pm$ 4.9 years (mean $\pm$ SEM, range 18-84) were studied. Four patients were admitted with multiple traumatic injuries, 10 patients underwent abdominal or thoracic surgery. One patient suffered from hemorrhagic shock and one patient from myocardial infarction. In 12 patients the clinical course was complicated by septicemia. The parenteral nutrition of these patients consisted of 40-70 % glucose in combination with insulin, essential and non-essential amino acids (1 g/kg/day) achieving a minimal daily caloric intake of 3,000 kcal. Antibiotic and/or antimycotic drugs were administered according to culture sensitivities.

Hemodialysis was performed 3-4 hours daily using hollow fiber dialyzers. Ultrafiltrates of patients with ARF were obtained from the dialyzer prior to hemodialysis during a period of 10 minutes.

Phosphorylase kinase was incubated with these ultrafiltrates for 12 and 24 hours at a temperature of 37°C [8]. Samples of 20 µl were subjected to polyacrylamide gel electrophoresis in the presence of $NaDodSO_4$ according to Porzio and Pearson [9]. Plasma protein precipitation by trichloric acid (TCA) was performed as previously described [2]. The protein concentration was measured by the method of Lowry et al. [10]. Leukocyte isolation was achieved by a combination of dextran sedimentation, differential centrifugation, and hypotonic lysis. Disruption of the leukocytes was brought about by a freeze and de-freeze procedure. Extracts of white cells were incubated with phosphorylase kinase for 6 hours.

RESULTS

Non-TCA precipitable protein was measured in the plasma of healthy controls and patients with various forms of renal failure. This low-molecular-weight protein fraction has been reported to be a sensitive marker of catabolism [2,4,7]. It has been assumed that this fraction represents proteins, peptides and/or amino acids generated by proteolytic degradation of plasma proteins normally cleared by the kidney. Fig. 1 shows non-TCA precipitable plasma protein levels under various conditions. Healthy controls reached levels of 0.25 $\pm$ 0.02 mg/ml, whereas patients with chronic renal failure undergoing long-term hemodialysis displayed concentrations of 1.10 $\pm$ 0.10 mg/ml. Patients with non-septic ARF showed values of 1.65 $\pm$ 0.11 mg/ml. The highest levels of non-TCA precipitable protein were found in patients with ARF and sepsis (2.72 $\pm$ 0.23 mg/ml).

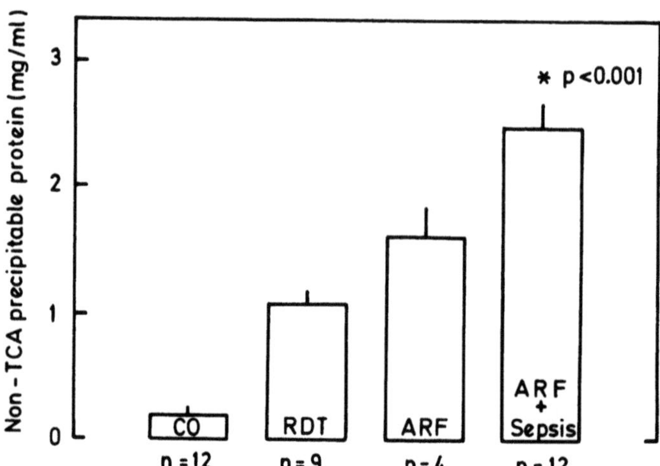

Fig. 1: Non-TCA precipitable protein of healthy controls or patients on regular dialysis treatment (RDT) and of ARF patients with and without sepsis.

Granulocyte extracts obtained from healthy controls were incubated with phosphorylase kinase. After 6 hours there was a predominant degradation of the alpha subunit of this enzyme (Fig. 2A). When an ultrafiltrate obtained from a patient with ARF and sepsis during the first 10 minutes of the extracorporeal treatment, was incubated with phosphorylase kinase a predominant digestion of the gamma subunit occured (Fig. 2B).

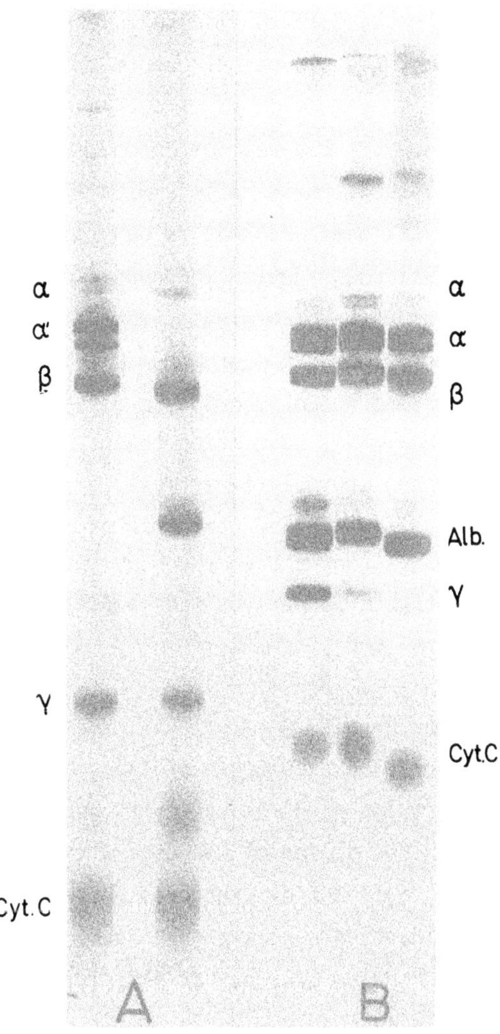

Fig. 2A: Effect of an extract from purified human granulocytes, obtained from healthy subjects, on the degradation of the subunits of phosphorylase kinase.

Fig. 2B: Effect of an ultrafiltrate from a patient suffering from ARF and sepsis on the digestion of the subunits of phosphorylase kinase.

DISCUSSION

During the last several years further insight into the mechanisms of protein catabolism in ARF has been accumulated. Enhanced protein degradation of skeletal muscle could be shown in acutely uremic rats [11-13]. This finding is in agreement to our observation of increased proteolytic activity in the plasma of patients suffering from post-traumatic ARF [1-3]. Additional evidence has been provided by the occurance of peptide/protein split products in the plasma (Fig. 1), decreased trypsin binding capacity of the plasma [2,3] and in-vitro degradation of the test-enzyme phosphorylase kinase by ultrafiltrated plasma fractions concentrated dialysate and urine fractions from catabolic patients suffering from ARF [2]. Furthermore, Hörl et al. described a metallo proteinase in the plasma of patients with acute and chronic renal failure [8].

Fig. 2B shows the proteolytic cleavage of phosphorylase kinase in the presence of an ultrafiltrate from a patient with ARF and sepsis. The prominent splitting of the gamma subunit is completely different from the pattern of proteolytic degradation induced by extracts of purified human granulocytes (Fig. 2A), which predominantly digest the alpha subunit of phosphorylase kinase. A phenomenon that is in good agreement with the fact that purified human granulocyte elastase also preferentially degradates the same subunit [14], suggesting that leukocytes do not contribute to the enhanced proteolytic activity of the plasma in the state of ARF and sepsis. The finding that this activity could be inhibited by EDTA [8] suggests that the enhanced proteolytic activity of the plasma in these patients is derived from a metallo proteinase, whose origin is up to now undefined.

CONCLUSIONS

High levels of non-TCA precipitable proteins and the cleavage of phosphorylase kinase provide good evidence that there is frank proteolytic activity in the plasma of patients with ARF and sepsis. The fact that extracts derived from disrupted white cells display a different pattern of digestion suggests that leukocyte proteinases do not contribute to the enhanced proteolytic activity of plasma fractions in ARF.

ACKNOWLEDGEMENTS

This work was supported by the Deutsche Forschungsgemeinschaft, Ho 781/3-4. The excellent technical assistance of Miss U. Putsche and Mrs. M. Röder is greatly appreciated. The authors also acknowledge the excellent secreterial assistance of Miss C. Maiberger for preparing the manuscript.

REFERENCES

1. W.H. Hörl, A. Heidland, Enhanced proteolytic activity - cause of protein catabolism in acute renal failure, Am. J. Clin. Nutr. 33: 1424-1427 (1980).
2. W.H. Hörl, J. Stepinski, C. Gantert, M. Hörl, A. Heidland, Evidence for the participation of proteases on protein catabolism during hypercatabolic renal failure, Klin. Wochenschr. 59: 751-759 (1981).
3. W.H. Hörl, J. Stepinski, R.M. Schaefer, C. Wanner, A. Heidland, Role of Proteases in hypercatabolic patients with renal failure, Kidney Int. 24 (suppl 16): S-37 - S-42 (1983).
4. A. Heidland, W.H. Hörl, Contribution of proteases to hypercatabolism in acute renal failure, in Nephrology, edited by Robinson RR, New York, Berlin, Heidelberg, Tokyo, Springer Verlag, 1984, Vol. I, pp 763-775.
5. W.H. Hörl, M. Jochum, A. Heidland, H. Fritz, Release of granulocyte proteinases during hemodialysis, Am. J. Nephrol. 3: 213-217 (1983).
6. W.H. Hörl, A. Heidland, Evidence for the participation of granulocyte proteinases on intradialytic catabolism, Clin. Nephrol. 21: 314-322 (1984).
7. W.H. Hörl, H.B. Steinhauer, P. Schollmeyer, Plasma levels of granulocyte elastase during hemodialysis: Effects of different dialyzer membranes, Kidney Int. 28: 791-796 (1985).
8. W.H. Hörl, C. Wanner, F. Thaiss, P. Schollmeyer, Detection of a metalloproteinase in patients with acute and chronic renal failure, Am. J. Nephrol. 6: 6-13 (1986).
9. M.A. Porzio, A.M. Pearson, Improved resolution of myofibrillar proteins with sodium dodecyl sulfate-polyacrylamide gel electrophoresis, Biochim. Biophys. Acta 490: 27-35 (1977).

10. O.H. Lowry, N.J. Rosebrough, A.L. Farr, R.J. Rondall, Protein measurements with the folin reagent, J. Biol. Chem. 193: 265-275 (1951).

11. R.M. Flügel-Link, J.B. Salusky, M.R. Jones, J.D. Kopple, Protein and amino acid metabolism in posterior hemicorpus of acutely uremic rats, Am. J. Physiol. 244: E 615 - E 623 (1983).

12. E.W. Mitch, A.S. Clark, Muscle protein turnover in uremia, Kidney Int. 24 (suppl. 16): S 2 - S 8 (1983).

13. A.J. Garber, Skeletal muscle protein and amino acid metabolism in experimental chronic uremia in the rat: Accelerated alanine and glutamine formation and release, J. Clin. Invest. 62: 623-632 (1978).

14. R.M. Schaefer, A. Heidland, W.H. Hörl, Role of leukocyte proteinases and proteinase inhibitors in the catabolism of acute renal failure, Kidney Int. (suppl.) in press (1986).

EFFECTS OF ENDOTOXIN ON HEMODYNAMICS OF ISOLATED DOG KIDNEY

Nadine Bourgeois, Charles Reuse, Jean-Marie Boeynaems, Michel Staroukine and Jean-Louis Vanherweghem

Université Libre de Bruxelles
(Hôpital Erasme and Hôpital Brugmann)
Brussels, Belgium

INTRODUCTION

Endotoxin have been incriminated in the pathogenesis of acute renal failure in liver disease[1,2]. The altered renal function has been attributed to intense renal vasoconstriction and to a fall in renal perfusion pressure. Many authors[3,4,5,6,7,8,9] postulated that the vasoconstriction was due to both a direct local action of endotoxin on the renal vascular bed and to secondary systemic release of vasocontrictor agents during the systemic hypotension. In an attempt to separate the systemic hemodynamic effects of endotoxin from a direct action of these substances on the kidney, we studied the influence of exogenous endotoxin on isolated dog kidney perfusions.

MATERIAL AND METHOD

The kidney perfusions were conducted as follows: after the intravenous injection of 250 mg heparin, bilateral nephrectomy was performed in eight 14-20 kgs Mongrel dogs, under pentobarbital (30 mg/kg) anesthesia. Both kidneys of each animal were then individually connected to 2 separate Nizet's pump oxygenators [10] and perfused simultaneously. Each pump oxygenator was primed with 450 cc of heparinized blood obtained from a common pentobarbital anesthetized 25-35 kgs Mongrel dog. Arterial pressure into the circuit was kept constant at 120 mmHg as well as blood temperature at 37°C.

The oxygenator receiving the experimental kidney (EK) was primed by 450 ml arterial blood in which 100 mg of endotoxin (LPS E. COLI B4:111 provided by DIFCO), diluted in 20 cc NaCl 9°/°, were added within the minutes following the beginning of the perfusion. Five minutes after this pulse, constant infusion of 200 mg of the same toxin, diluted in 60 cc NaCl 9°/°°, was begun for 2 hours, at the rate of 1.6 mg/min. The control kidney (CK) was primed with 450 cc arterial blood in which 20 cc NaCl 9°/°° were added within the 5 minutes of the beginning of the perfusion and a infusion of 60 cc NaCl 9°/° was started 5 minutes later.

Care was taken to alternate right and left organs in successive experiments.

One hundred mg of creatinine were added to each aliquot of priming blood at the beginning of the perfusion.

Renal blood flow was directly measured at the renal vein. Blood samples and urine collections were regularly obtained during the 3 hours of perfusion.

Creatinine determination was made by colorimetric determination according to the Jaffe reaction. Plasma renin activity was determined by the angiotensin I generation rate after 15 minutes incubation of plasma at 37° in presence of 4.64 mg Na2 EDTA, 0.5 mg phenantroline and 0.2 mg neomycine sulfate per ml. Angiotensin I was measured by radioimmunoassay. Plasma renin substrate was measured according to the method of Tree[11] except that angiotensin I determination was performed by radioimmunoassay. Plasma angiotensin II was measured by a modification of the radioimmunoassay method of Düsterdick and Mc Elwee[12]. Six Keto Prostaglandin $F_1\alpha$ (6 Keto $PGF_1\alpha$) and Thromboxane B_2 (TX B_2) were measured by radioimmunoassay directly in the plasma (20 microl), 3H-labeled tracers of 6 Keto $PGF_1\alpha$ or TX B_2 (11.000 dpm), antiserum (final dilution :$10^{-4}$for 6 Keto $PGF_1\alpha$, 6 x 10^{-5} for TX B_2) and bovine gammaglobulins (0.25 mg/dl) in Tris-HCl buffer (pH 7.4, 50 mM) were incubated in a total volume of 0.4 ml for 60 minutes at room temperature. Then 0.4 ml of a cold 25M solution of polyethylene-glycol was added to separate bound and free antigen. The pellet was dissolved in 0.1 ml 0.1 M NaOH and counted in liquid scintillation. Standards of 6 Keto $PGF_1\alpha$ and TX B_2 were obtained from Upjohn Diagnostics. Three H 6 Keto $PGF_1\alpha$ and TX B_2 were purchased from Amersham.

Statistical calculations were conducted according to Wilcoxon's rank sum tests for paired data[13], each measurement being compared to the paired measurements simultaneously obtained in the control kidney.

RESULTS

As shown in figure 1, vasodilatation occurred in the control kidney immediately after the start of the artificial perfusion.

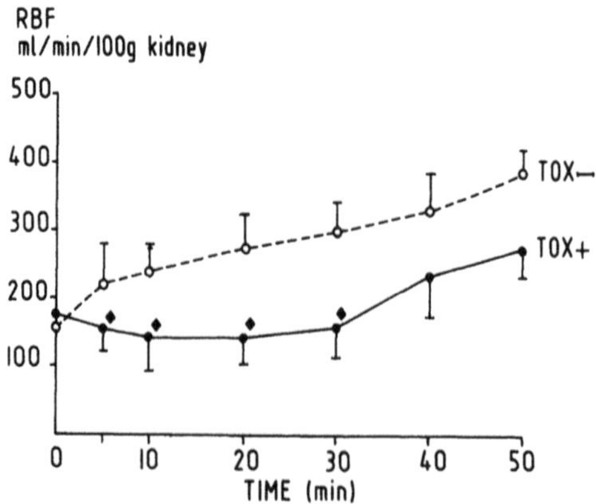

Fig. 1. Renal blood flow (RBF) of isolated dog kidney following the admnistration of 100 mg endotoxin at the start of the artificial kidney perfusion. Results are given by the means ± SEM (n=8). Dotted line represents the control kidneys (♦ $p \leq 0.01$).

The renal blood flow in the kidney receiving endotoxin slightly decreased in the course of the first half hour and was significantly ($p \leq 0.01$) lower than in the control kidney (EK: 252 ± 73 vs CK: 329 ± 67 ml/min/100 g kidney).

After 1 hour, and despite the continuous infusion of endotoxin, vasodilatation occurred in EK in a similar way as in CK. After 2 hours of artificial perfusion, there was no more significant difference for renal blood flow between EK and CK (EK: 366 ± 62 vs 393 ± 76 ml/min/100 g kidney; $p > 0.05$) (fig.2).

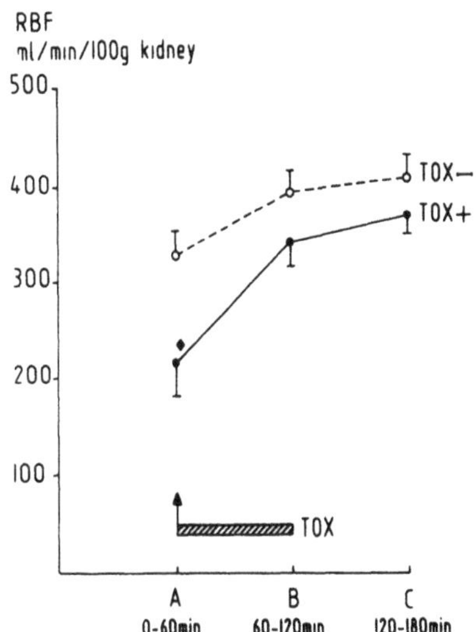

Fig. 2. Effects of endotoxin on renal blood flow (RBF) of isolated dog kidney. Results are given by the means ± SEM (n=8). The dotted line represents the control kidneys. The arrow indicates the continuous infusion of endotoxin (1.6 mg/min) (◆ $p \leq 0.01$).

During the first half hour EK was anuric while CK already exhibited a small diuresis (0.7 ± 0.3 ml/min/100g kidney) with a glomerular filtration rate of16 ± 4 ml/min/100g kidney. After one hour, diuresis appeared also in EK and there was no significant difference for glomerular filtration rate between EK and CK.

No significant difference was observed in renin activity, neither in substrate levels, angiotensin levels, nor in 6 Keto $PGF_{1}\alpha$ or TX B_2 between EK and CK (Table I). Six Keto $PGF_{1}\alpha$ progressively increased during the course of the artificial perfusion in both kidneys while TX B_2 remained stable.

Table 1. Effects of endotoxin on isolated dog kidney. Renin angiotensin system and 6 Keto $PGF_{1}\alpha$ and $TX\ B_2$ synthesis. Results are expressed by the means ± SEM (n=8).

		EK	CK
RENIN ACTIVITY ng A_1/ml/h	Period A	24.8 ± 6.8	20.2 ± 8.1
	Period B	39.5 ± 16.5	24.5 ± 9
	Period C	1.1 ± 0.5	12.8 ± 5.5
RENIN SUBSTRATE ng A_1/ml	Period A	129 ± 39	139 ± 57
	Period B	76 ± 28	47 ± 22
	Period C	7 ± 5	1 ± 1
ANGIOTENSIN II pg/ml	Period A	1549 ± 340	1798 ± 583
	Period B	1945 ± 336	3207 ± 568
	Period C	1056 ± 317	1186 ± 214
6 KETO $PGF_{1}\alpha$ ng/ml	Period A	3.9 ± 2.3	1.9 ± 0.6
	Period B	12.5 ± 0.7	9.5 ± 2.4
	Period C	26.4 ± 8.5	23.5 ± 7.5
$TX\ B_2$ ng/ml	Period A	5.0 ± 0.8	10.6 ± 2.3
	Period B	6.4 ± 1.6	7.6 ± 2.4
	Period C	11.0 ± 2.5	11.0 ± 5.4

DISCUSSION

Our data show that high doses of exogenous endotoxin induced a transient decrease in renal blood flow with anuria in isolated dog kidney in which the blood pressure was artificially kept at a constant level of 120 mmHg. These data support the suggestion that endotoxin could actually have a direct effect on renal hemodynamics[1,3]. In our experiments, this renal vasoconstrictive effect of endotoxin is not mediated neither by the renin angiotensin system nor by cyclooxygenase products of arachidonic acid. A direct effect of endotoxin on kidney vasculature may thus be postulated.

Despite the high doses of endotoxin we used and despite of its continous infusion we were unable to demonstrate a sustained toxic effect of endotoxin on the kidney. Indeed the characteristic vasodilatation of isolated dog kidney[9] appeared after one hour in the kidney receiving endotoxin as well as in the control kidney. We have nevertheless to underline some particularities of our experimental model: vasodilatation classically occurs in the course of the isolated dog kidney perfusion, due to a progressive accumulation of prostaglandins in the perfusing blood [14,15]. This could explain the escape of the isolated dog kidney from the influence of potent vasoconstrictive agents such as angiotensin or endotoxin.

ACKNOWLEDGEMENTS

This work was supported by "Fonds de la Recherche Scientifique Médicale" (contract n° 3.4555.82); during this work, Nadine Bourgeois was a fellow of the "Fondation Erasme".

REFERENCES

1. H. LIEHR AND A. JACOBS, Endotoxin and renal failure in liver disease, in: "The kidney in liver disease", M. Epstein, ed., Elsevier Biomedical, New York, Amsterdam, Oxford (1983).

2. P. CORATELLI, G. PASSAVANTI, I. MUNNO, D. FUMAROLA and A. Amerio, New Trends in Hepatorenal Syndrome, Kidney Int. 28 (suppl 17):s-143 (1985).

3. L. HINSHAW, G. BRADLEY AND C. CARLSON, Effect of endotoxin on renal function in the dog, Am. J. Physiol. 196 (5): 1127 (1959).

4. L. HINSHAW, W. SPINK, J. VICK, E. MALLET and J. FINSTAD, Effect of endotoxin on kidney function and renal hemodynamics in the dog, Am. J. Physiol. 201 (1): 144 (1961).

5. J. GILLENWATER, E. DOOLEY and E. FROHLICH, Effect of endotoxin on renal function and hemodynamics, Am. J. Physiol. 205 (2): 293 (1963).

6. S. WILKINSON, V. ARROYO, B. GAZZARD, H. MOODIE, R. WILLIAMS, Relation of renal impairment and haemorrhagic diathesis to endotoxemia in fulminant hepatic failure, Lancet: 521 (1974).

7. S. WILKINSON, B. PORTMANN, D. HURST and R. WILLIAMS, Pathogenesis of renal failure in cirrhosis and fulminant hepatic failure, Postgrad. Med. J. 54: 503 (1975).

8. C. CLEMENTE, J. BOSCH, J. RODES, V. ARROYO, A. MAS, S. MARGALL, Functional renal failure and haemorrhagic gastritis associated with endotoxinemia in cirrhosis, Gut 18: 556 (1977).

9. M. LEVY, A. LISZAUER, M. WEXLER, Renal blood flow in normal dogs and in dogs with experimental liver cirrhosis following the acute continuous infusion of endotoxin, Can. J. Physiol. Pharmacol. 61: 1396 (1983)

10. A. NIZET, The isolated perfused kidney:possibilities, limitations and results, Kidney Int. 7: 1 (1975).

11. R. TREE, Measurement of plasma renin substrate in man, J. Endocr. 56: 159A (1973).

12. G. DÜSTERDIECK and G. Mc ELWEE, Estimation of angiotensin II in human plasma by radioimmunoassay. Some applications to physiological and clinical states, Eur. J. Clin. Invest. 2: 32 (1971).

13. T.SWINSON, Statistics at square one, XVII - Some non parametric tests, Br. Med. J. 2: 632 (1976).

14. H. ITSKOWITZ, N. TERRAGNO and J. Mc GIFF, Effects of renal prostaglandin on distribution of blood flow in the isolated canine kidney. Circulation Res. 34: 770 (1974).

15. J.L. VANHERWEGHEM, J. DUCOBU and A. d'HOLLANDER, Effects of indomethacin on renal hemodynamics and on water and sodium excretion by the isolated dog kidney, Pflügers Archv. 357: 243 (1975).

INTRACELLULAR ACID-BASE AND ENERGY METABOLISM IN OLIGURIC ACUTE RENAL FAILURE (OARF)

A. Guariglia, C. Antonucci, U. Arduini, S. Del Canale, E. Coffrini, P. Vitali and E. Fiaccadori

Istituto di Clinica Medica e Nefrologia - Parma

Direttore: Prof. Alberico Borghetti

INTRODUCTION

Acute renal failure is often associated with a condition of metabolic acidosis. However, extracellular acid-base parameters do not seem to be fully representative of the entity of retained acids, since it is the intracellular compartment which is mainly involved in buffering of the acid load (1-2).
Bone and soft tissues (e.g. skeletal muscle)have been reported as major sites of intracellular buffering.
Significant participation of cell metabolic buffers in this process has been demonstrated: it is likely due to the effect of increased cell H^+ activity on several important cell metabolic pathways (3-4).
Moreover, intracellular acidosis may disrupt the equilibrium between production and utilization of high-energy phosphate compounds (5).
The aim of the present study was thus to evaluate, by means of direct tissue analyses, the main indices of skeletal muscle acid-base and energy metabolism in five patients presenting acute oliguric renal failure (OARF).
Metabolic parameters were evaluated at the onset of the syndrome, in the acidemic state, and after alkali treatment, either by standard and/or haemodialytic procedures.

PATIENTS AND METHODS

Five patients affected by OARF (urine volume < 500 ml/24 h) were admitted to the present study. In all patients clinically evident signs of malnutrition, extrarenal disease,sepsis, hypovolemia and hypoxia were excluded.
Data of all patients, relative to age, sex, OARF aetiology, duration of oliguria before the study, as well as renal function

Table 1. Clinical data of OARF patients.

PATIENTS	AGE years	SEX	OARF AETIOLOGY	OLIGURIA days	BUN g‰	Creat. mg%
1) R.E.	28	M	Rhabdomyolysis	4	1.35	19.5
2) F.E.	70	F	Myeloma kidney + FANS	3	0.55	9.0
3) T.D.	74	F	Obstr.uropathy	2	0.70	7.0
4) S.R.	48	F	Acute interst. nephritis	5	1.38	17.2
5) R.I.	71	M	Obstr.uropathy	5	1.50	17.6

indices (BUN and Creatinine) at the time of admission are reported in Table 1. In all patients blood was drawn from femoral vessels for acid-base and routine analyses. Thereafter repeated muscle needle biopsies from quadriceps femoris, according to Bergström (6), were performed (phase A). Muscle samples were then analyzed for the following parameters:

- acid-labile CO_2 (TCO_2), hence intracellular bicarbonate(HCO_{3i}) and pH (pH_i) (7).
- adenylate compounds (ATP-ADP-AMP)(8) from which energy charge potential (ECP=ATP+0.5ADP/ATP+ADP+AMP) (9).
- phosphocreatine (PCr) and creatine (Cr), and thus total creatine (TCr) as a reference index of muscle mass (8).

The same experimental procedures were carried out after a full correction of extracellular acid-base parameters was achieved (after 6-8 days) (phase B). Adequate protein and caloric intake (35 KCal/Kg b.w./24 h; 300 KCal/gN) both orally or i.v. infusion, was maintained for the entire period of study.
In patients 1-2 (persistent OARF) the normalization of acid-base parameters was obtained by means of daily haemodialysis (HD). In patients 3-4-5 HD was performed only in the acute phase, thereafter only standard alkali therapy was administered. In all patients a parallel improvement of BUN and creatinine was achieved.

STATISTICS

Values are expressed as mean $\pm$ SD. In each patient the significance of the differences between A and B phases was assessed by means of the Student's "t" test for paired data.

RESULTS

Acid-base and electrolyte values referring both to the acute (A) and recovery (B) phase are reported in Table 2.

Table 2. Blood acid-base and electrolyte indices before (A) and after (B) therapy.

PATIENTS		pH_a	$PaCO_2$ mmHg	HCO_3 mmol/l	Na mmol/l	K mmol/l	Cl mmol/l
1	A	7.35	31	16.6	127	4.4	98
	B	7.42	37	24.0	136	4.6	100
2	A	7.35	33	18.5	141	4.6	106
	B	7.36	36	20.8	142	3.9	98
3	A	7.33	28	14.5	136	4.6	102
	B	7.45	39	27.3	140	4.1	100
4	A	7.29	37	18.0	120	7.6	94
	B	7.44	35	24.0	138	4.1	103
5	A	7.28	35	16.0	139	6.9	105
	B	7.38	40	24.0	142	4.7	93

The main indices of intracellular acid-base equilibrium in OARF patients, as compared to age-matched control subjects are listed in Table 3. OARF patients are characterized by a decrease of both HCO_{3i} and pH_i which, however, was not related to the extracellular acid-base changes (see H_i/H_e gradient). Main parameters of cell energy metabolism are reported in Table 4 and compared to age-matched control subjects.

Table 3. Intracellular acid-base indices in phase A.

PATIENTS	HCO_{3i} mmol/l H_2O_i	pH_i	H_i nmol/l H_2O_i	H_i/H_e
1	5.9	6.67	214	4.75
2	3.8	6.56	275	6.11
3	5.0	6.80	158	3.36
4	8.7	6.92	120	2.35
5	8.8	6.88	132	2.53
MEAN	6.4	6.76	179	3.82
± SD	2.0	0.13	57	1.40
CONTROLS(n=11)				
MEAN	11.7	7.05	89	2.22
± SD	1.1	0.05	4	0.31

Table 4. Muscle energy metabolism parameters.

PATIENTS	ATP*	PCr* *mmol/Kg DW	TCr*	ATP/TCr	PCr/TCr	ECP
1	24.9	71	113	0.22	0.63	0.938
2	20.8	76	143	0.14	0.53	0.912
3	21.8	60	115	0.19	0.52	0.931
4	18.6	48	95	0.19	0.52	0.924
5	18.7	51	100	0.19	0.51	0.928
MEAN	20.9	61	113	0.19	0.54	0.927
± SD	2.3	10	16	0.02	0.04	0.008
CONTROLS(n=10)						
MEAN	24	74	120	0.21	0.62	0.938
± SD	1	6	16	0.02	0.04	0.007

Patient 1 presented normal levels of all indices considered. The other patients were characterized by a constant decrease of PCr/TCr ratio; ATP/TCr and ECP levels fell within lower values of normal range or were reduced.

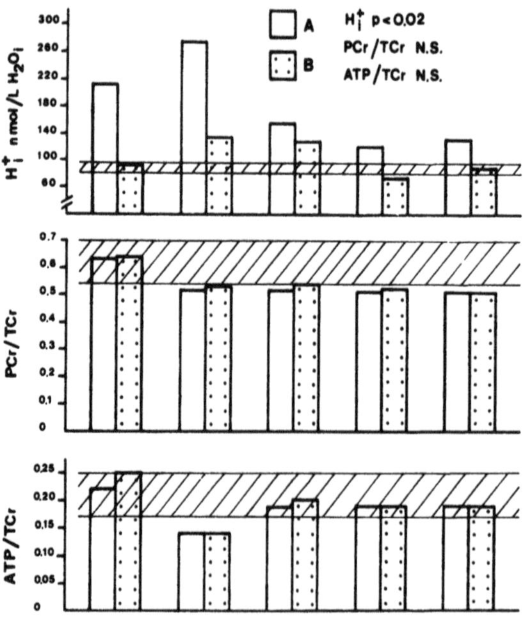

Fig. 1. Intracellular H^+ and energy metabolism indices in phase A and B are illustrated. Despite a significant improvement of intracellular acidity, ATP/TCr and PCr/TCr were unchanged. Normal range is expressed by shaded areas.

The recovery of extracellular acid-base equilibrium was followed by a parallel improvement of intracellular indices; on the contrary no changes of high energy phosphate compound levels were detected (Figure 1).

DISCUSSION

The present data would suggest that acidosis-associated OARF is characterized by important derangements of cell acid-base and energy metabolism.
Skeletal muscle cells appear to be actively involved in the buffering of the acute acid load as demonstrated by the pH_i shift towards acidosis. Moreover the cell compartment seems to be more seriously affected than the extracellular fluid as demonstrated by the constant finding of an increased H_i/H_e ratio. Proton accumulation may also be responsible for the parallel impairment of energy metabolism indices.
In fact, the finding of reduced PCr levels can be ascribed both to the physiological PCr breakdown, in order to prevent ATP depletion (see below) and to a direct action of PCr as a metabolic buffer (5), according to the well established reaction ($PCr+H^++ADP \longrightarrow Cr+ATP$).
Acidosis has been experimentally reported to interfere with normal glycolytic rhythm, by inhibiting rate-limiting enzymes such as phosphorilase-b-kinase and phosphofructokinase (5): this may ultimately lead to impaired ATP production as demonstrated by our data.
However, apart from the limiting effects of acidosis, the action of other factors must be taken into account to explain the present results.
In fact, a lack of correlation between H_i^+ increase and reduced ATP and PCr levels was observed, together with the finding that alkali therapy corrected only the acid-base indices and not high-energy phosphate compound content.
Recovery mechanisms of impaired energy metabolism thus appear somewhat blunted. This may suggest that:

- other perturbing factors related to the condition of acute uremia are involved;
- they cannot be corrected solely by routine treatment;
- their action can also continue when there is apparent functional recovery.

Among these factors, special mention should be given to the catabolic state characteristic of this syndrome (10).
In fact, similar metabolic patterns have been reported in previous studies of severely ill patients, where reduced substrate availability and/or utilization were attributed to a catabolic state (11).
Similarly, decreased energy charge potential, as seen in the present study, would suggest that biochemical signs of catabolism, together with a condition of intracellular acidosis, can be considered among the main determinants of the deranged metabolism found in OARF patients.

REFERENCES

1. Schwartz W.B.,Orning K.J., Porter R.: The internal distribution of hydrogen ions with varying degrees of metabolic acidosis. J. Clin. Invest. 36: 373 (1957).
2. Swan R.C., Pitts R.F.: Neutralization of infused acid by nephrectomized dogs. J. Clin. Invest. 34: 205 (1955).
3. Cohen R.D., Iles R.A.: Intracellular pH. CRC Crit. Rev. Clin. Lab. Sci. 101 (1975).
4. Relman A.S.: Metabolic consequences of acid-base disorders. Kidney Int. 1: 347 (1972).
5. Hultman E., Sahlin K.: Acid-base balance during exercise. In "Exercise and sport sciences reviews". Hutton R.S. - Miller D.I. eds. Franklin Institute Press. Philadelphia pg. 41-128 (1980).
6. Bergström J.: Muscle electrolytes in man. Scand J. Clin. Lab. Invest. 14: (suppl. 68) 1 (1962).
7. Fiaccadori E., Guariglia A., Arduini U., Del Canale S., Mori G., Reni F., Vitali P., Borghetti A.: Intracellular bicarbonate and pH determination in rat skeletal muscle from acid-labile CO_2 measurement by dead-stop end-point potentiometric titrations. Eur. Rev. Med. Pharm. Sci. 1: 1 (1986).
8. Harris R.C., Hultman E., Nordesjö L.O.: Glycogen,glycolytic intermediates and high energy phosphates determined in biopsy samples of musculus femoris of man at rest. Scand J. Clin. Lab. Invest. 33: 109 (1974).
9. Atkinson D.E.: The energy charge of the adenylate pool as a regulatory parameter. Interaction with feed-back modifiers. Biochemistry 7: 4030 (1968).
10. Kopple J.D., Cianciaruso B.: The role of nutrition in acute renal failure. In: "Acute renal failure: pathophysiology, prevention and treatment". Andreucci V. ed.,Martinus Nijhoff Publishing, Boston. p. 423-446 (1984).
11. Bergström J., Boström H., Fürst P., Hultman E., Vinnars E. Preliminary studies of energy-rich phosphagens in muscle from severely ill patients. Crit. Care Med. 4 (4): 197, (1976).

PLASMA AND SKELETAL MUSCLE FREE AMINOACIDS IN ACUTE RENAL FAILURE

Almerico Novarini, Isabella Simoni, Rossana Colla, Antonio Trifirò*, Achille Guariglia°, Emilio Sani, and Alberto Montanari

Istituto di Semeiotica Medica; * Stazione Sperimentale per le Conserve Alimentari; ° Istituto di Clinica Medica e Nefrologia
Parma, Italy

Abnormalities in protein metabolism are well known in acute renal failure (ARF) (1, 2). When renal function is acutely reduced or completely abolished, two phenomena contribute to derange protein metabolism: first, acute protein catabolism occurs inducing negative nitrogen balance, overproduction of urea and other nitrogen catabolites; second, these latter substances accumulate in the body, due to defective renal excretion, possibly contributing through their toxic effect to enhance proteolysis. In addition, if ARF is accompanied or is caused by catabolizing events (severe bleeding, surgery, sepsis, rhabdomiolysis), a further stimulus to protein breakdown contributes to a tremendous, acute malnutrition (1, 2). It is generally thought that the severity of protein catabolism may influence the clinical course of ARF (1). Acute malnutrition in ARF may be easily demonstrated by net loss of muscle mass (1, 2) and from a biochemical point of view by severely negative balance, fall of serum proteins and finally by changes in plasma amino acids (AA) levels, with reduction of essential AA (1). However, plasma free AA concentrations are not fully representative of the whole body pool of free AA, the concentrations of which are by far higher in intracellular water (ICW) than in plasma (3). Muscle tissue is the largest homogeneous cellular tissue in the body, thus containing the largest amount of free AA. Every catabolic condition is characterized primarily by increased net muscle protein degradation, which in turn causes increased flow of free AA to other organs, mainly to the liver. Accelerated muscle proteolysis is reflected also by changes in muscle free AA concentrations, as it has been demonstrated under several conditions, such as surgical trauma, sepsis, diabetes mellitus (4, 5, 6, 7). On the other hand it has been shown that sufficient and equilibrated concentrations of cellular free AA are needed to fully regulate equilibrium between muscle protein synthesis and breakdown (8).

There is no available information on muscle free AA in human ARF. In this paper, we report preliminary results on free AA levels in plasma and skeletal muscle, obtained by needle biopsy, of patients with ARF.

MATERIALS AND METHODS

We studied five patients (4 males), aging 34-82, body weight 70±13 kg with ARF (2 tubulonecrosis, 1 stone obstructive uropathy, 1 myeloma, 1 acute glomerulonephritis) and 9 healthy control subjects. Table I reports main laboratory data of ARF patients. None of them had clinical or biochemical signs of sepsis, shock, tissue destruction, hemorrhage, significant external fluid losses nor other acute, superimposed or preexisting, catabolizing events. Their protein or I.V. AA intake was 35-45 gr per day with 1600-2100 kCal. 3 out of 5 received a daily infusion of 15 gr AA and 800-1200 kCal. as dextrose; AA or dextrose infusion had been stopped at least 12 hours before the study. None of the patients had been submitted to dialysis; the study was performed 3-6 days after the onset of ARF. Diabetes mellitus or liver cirrhosis were excluded in every patient. Each subject was submitted to the study under postabsorptive conditions.

Table 1. Main hematological and biochemical data in 5 patiens with ARF (m±SD)

UREA mg/dl	141 ± 30
CREATININE mg/dl	8.4 ± 2.8
CREATININE CLEARANCE ml/m'	8 ± 7
URIC ACID mg/dl	8.5 ± 0.3
Na^+ mmol/l	138 ± 6
K^+ mmol/l	4.6 ± 0.6
Cl^- mmol/l	98 ± 11
Ca mg/dl	8.7 ± 0.8
Pi mg/dl	6 ± 2.6
ARTERIAL pH	7.35 ± 0.06
HCO_3^- mmol/l	18.1 ± 2.7
pCO_2 mmHg	33 ± 4
pO_2 mmHg	79 ± 16
Hb g/dl	12 ± 2.3
WHITE CELLS/cmm	9500 ± 3200
TOTAL PROTEIN g/dl	6.2 ± 1
ALBUMIN g/dl	3.6 ± 0.8

Muscle biopsy and analysis technique. Muscle biopsy of the

quadriceps was carried out using needle described by Bergström (9, 10). Each muscle sample, weighing 30-60 mg, was rapidly divided into two fragments. The first was immediately weighed and homogenized with 6% cold sulfosalicylic acid; plasma was precipitated with 3% cold sulfosalicylic acid. AA were measured using the Carlo Erba 3A29 Automatic Aminoanalyzer. The AA concentrations were expressed as umol/kg of muscle wet weight (AA_m) or per kg of plasma water (AA_{ECW}). GLN and GLU and muscle ASP were found to be unstable during storage; ASN and CYS peaks in muscle were well separated only in some subjects. Therefore, GLN and GLU acid are not included in the results, while ASP, ASN and CYS are reported only in plasma. In the second muscle fragment, total muscle water (TW) and muscle fat free dry solids (FFS) weight were measured. The fragment was then treated with alkali for measurement of the muscle Cl (Cl_m, mmol/kg FFS). The partition into extra (ECW) and intracellular (ICW) water was estimated by the chloride method (3, 7, 9, 10). Details of AA analysis and calculations have been published elsewhere (7). The statistical significance was calculated using Student's t-test for unpaired data when the population variances were the same (F-test at 5% of significance). When the variances were different, the analysis was made according to the Wilcoxon test.

RESULTS

TW, ECW, ICW and muscle Cl in ARF and control subjects are reported in table 2 . The rise in TW is solely due to the increased ECW, according to an expansion of whole body extracellular volume in ARF.

Table 2. Muscle Cl and Total Extracellular and Intracellular water (m±SD)

	Clm mmol/kgFFS	TW kg/kgFFS	ECW_{Cl} kg/kgFFS	ICW_{Cl} kg/kgFFS
CONTROLS (n=9)	98±21	3.49±0.21	0.73±0.20	2.77±0.21
ARF (n=5)	167±26	4.20±0.68	1.58±0.45	2.62±0.72
p	0.001	0.02	0.001	

Table 3 summarizes free AA concentrations in plasma ECW and muscle ICW. In ECW, only GLY, MET, PHE and total aromatic AA (AAA) are normal, while all other AA are significantly reduced. In muscle ICW the concentrations of several AA (THR, SER, GLY, VAL, ILE, LEU, total BCAA, PHE, ORN, total AAA) are elevated. The resulting intra/extracellular gradients (table 4) are significantly increased in ARF. The PHE/TYR ratio is elevated in both ICW and ECW.

Table 3. Amino acid levels in plasma (ECW) and muscle intracellular water (ICW) in controls (C n=9) and ARF patients (n=5) (m±SD) (umol/kg ECW or ICW)

	ECW			ICW		
	C	ARF	p	C	ARF	p
THR	119±32	64±7	0.005	623±244	1101±420	0.02
SER	123±32	78±20	0.02	1063±496	2123±506	0.005
GLY	199±56	163±92		1731±589	2941±1257	0.05
ALA	295±31	178±52	0.001	3247±1098	5009±2342	
VAL	215±42	155±14	0.02	368±82	559±110	0.005
CYS	48±15	130±59	0.05			
MET	22±6	22±8		53±12	145±120	
ILE	76±13	44±17	0.005	103±30	313±162	0.005
LEU	132±31	95±10	0.05	226±36	525±224	0.02
TYR	63±21	33±10	0.02	154±36	239±149	
PHE	49±14	48±13		120±39	275±93	0.005
PHE/TYR	0.77±0.17	1.51±0.24	0.001	0.77±0.17	1.27±0.28	0.005
ORN	78±19	41±10	0.005	566±173	965±374	0.02
LYS	180±33	115±16	0.005	1017±292	1488±1297	
HIS	92±11	62±10	0.001	553±191	1370±993	
ARG	91±23	65±14	0.05	686±259	801±591	
BCAA	423±82	294±31	0.01	681±88	1398±390	0.001
AAA	113±33	81±24		252±93	514±240	0.02

Table 4. Intra/extracellular gradients for some amino acids in ARF

	C (n=9)	ARF (n=5)	p
VAL	1.72±0.26	3.67±0.73	0.001
ILE	1.41±0.37	8.36±4.13	0.001
LEU	1.85±0.27	5.77±2.52	0.001
TYR	2.65±0.99	7.12±3.88	0.005
BCAA	1.69±0.13	4.95±1.32	0.001
AAA	2.36±1.02	6.45±3.27	0.005

DISCUSSION

Only a small number of patients suffering from ARF were admitted to the study because of the exclusion of the patients in whom ARF was caused or accompanied by severe acute catabolic events, such as surgery, sepsis or bleeding. Therefore, we assume that the present results reflect reliably the influence of acute uremia "per se" on free AA pools in man. Our findings are at variance to those reported by Flügel-Link et al. (1983) in rats with ARF (11). Their animals showed low levels of several AA in

both plasma and ICW; however, these Authors studied rats submitted to surgery (nephrectomy or sham operation), then fasted for 30 hours. Surgery and 30 hours fasting may have largely affected free AA pools in both ARF and sham operated rats. Thus, the relative contribution of ARF and of these catabolic stimuli is not distinguishable. Acute catabolic conditions have been demostrated to be associated with changes of intracellular free AA closely resembling those we show in ARF (4, 5, 6). In both acute catabolic conditions (4, 5, 6) and ARF, elevated muscle concentrations of most AA mainly BCAA, AAA and MET with striking increases in their muscle: plasma ratios are found. The mechanisms involved in this AA "pattern of catabolism" (5) are unclear. It is conceivable that increased flow of AA from catabolic muscle and the functional properties of membrane systems for AA efflux from muscle cells, mainly the leucine preferring system or system L (4, 7, 12), play an important role. Whatever the involved mechanisms, the present data suggest that muscle AA changes and their increased muscle: plasma ratio in ARF result mainly from acute muscle protein catabolism. However this point of view cannot reliably explain our data on plasma AA. In fact, under acute catabolic conditions, several AA are high in plasma too, although at a lesser extent than in muscle (4, 5, 6), rather than reduced, as we observe in ARF. This suggests that AA pools in ARF are affected also by mechanisms other than acute protein catabolism. Normal or reduced circulating levels of some AA despite high muscle concentrations may be explained by impaired renal production. Such a phenomenon may account for plasma depletion of SER, which is mainly produced by the Kidney (13), as well as that of ALA, ARG and ORN (13). However changes of ARG and ORN may also derive from accelerated ureagenesis (11) these AA being involved in urea cycle. In fact the activity of hepatic arginase and ORN aminotransferase is enhanced in experimental ARF (1). Thus, low plasma ARG and ORN could result from both accelerated ureagenesis and impaired renal production. In addition, a prominent role upon low plasma ALA should be played by the liver, where ALA is a major AA substrate for gluconeogenesis (15). Physiologically renal tissue produces large amounts of TYR from PHE (13). Thus, low plasma TYR with normal PHE and elevated PHE/TYR ratio may derive from reduced renal function. However, PHE/TYR ratio is elevated also in trauma (4, 5, 6) and diabetes mellitus (7); furthermore in ARF hepatic degradation of TYR is increased (14). To explain low plasma BCAA in ARF, these AA could be utilized at an increased rate in extramuscular organs, such as liver and brain; also the adipose tissue, where BCAA desamination is irreversible may participate. Furthermore, under acute catabolic conditions the oxidative use of BCAA in muscle is enhanced, despite their increased net flow from muscle (16). How these mechanisms, thought to act upon free BCAA levels, may contribute to the pattern of free BCAA we show in ARF is far from being clarified.
In summary, human ARF is characterized by low concentrations of most AA in plasma, despite high levels in muscle water. This pattern may be related mainly to three mechanisms: first, accelera-

ted net protein degradation with increased oxidation of BCAA in muscle; second, reduction or abolition of metabolic function of the Kidneys; third, enhanced uptake or degradation of AA by extramuscular organs, mainly by the liver.

REFERENCES

1) Kopple J.D., Cianciaruso B., 1984, The role for nutrition in acute renal failure, in: "Acute Renal Failure", V.E. Andreucci ed., Martinus Nijhoff, Boston.
2) Knochel J.P.: Complications of total parenteral nutrition. Kidney International, 27:489 (1985).
3) Bergström J., Fürst P. et al.: Intracellular free aminoacid concentration in human muscle tissue. J. Appl. Physiol. 36: 693 (1974).
4) Elwin D.M., Fürst P. et al.,1981, Effect of fasting on the muscle concentration of BCAA. In: "Metabolism and Clinical Implications of BCAA and BCKA", Elsevier, North Holland.
5) Askanazi J., Fürst P. et al.: Muscle and plasma amino acids after injury. Hypocaloric glucose Vs. Amino acid infusion. Ann. Surg. 191: 465 (1980).
6) Askanazi J., Carpentier J.A. et al.: Muscle and plasma Amino acids following injury. Influence of recurrent infection. Ann. Surg. 192: 78 (1980).
7) Borghi L.,Lugari R. et al.: Plasma and skeletal muscle free amino acids in type I insulin treated diabetic subjects. Diabetes 34, 812 (1985).
8) Fulks R.M., Li J.B. et al: Effects of insulin, glucose and amino acids on protein turnover in rat diaphragm. J. Biol. Chem. 250: 290 (1975).
9) Bergström J.: Muscle electrolytes in man. Scand. J. Clin. Lab. Invest. 14 (suppl. 68): 1 (1962).
10) Montanari A., Borghi L. et al: Skeletal muscle cell abnormalities in acute hypophosphatemia during total parenteral nutrition. Mineral Electrolyte Metabolism 10: 52 (1984).
11) Flügel-Link R.M., Salusky I.B. et al: Enhanced muscle protein degradation and urea nitrogen appearance (UNA) in rats with acute renal failure. Am. J. Physiol. 244: 615 (1983).
12) Christensen H.N.: Organic ion transport during seven decades.The amino acids, Bioch. Biophys. Acta 779: 255 (1984).
13) Tizianello A., Deferrari G.et al: Renal metabolism of amino acids and ammonia in subjects with normal renal function and in patients with CRI. J.Clin. Invest. 65: 1162 (1980).
14) Frohlich J., Hoppe-Seyler G. et al: Possible sites of interaction of acute renal failure with amino acid utilization for gluconeogenesis in isolated perfused rat liver. Eur. J. Clin. Invest. 7: 261 (1977).
15) Felig P.: Amino acid metabolism in man. Ann. Rev. Biochem. 9: 44: 933 (1975).
16) Tischler M.E., Fagan J.M.: Response to trauma of protein, amino acid, and carbohydrate metabolism in injured and uninjured rat skeletal muscles. Metabolism Clin. Exp., 32, 853 (1983).

INFLUENCE OF SOME UREMIC TOXINS ON OXYGEN CONSUMPTION OF RATS IN VIVO AND IN VITRO

M.Hohenegger, H.Echsel, M.Vermes, and H. Raneburger
Institute of General and Experimental Pathology
University of Vienna, Austria

INTRODUCTION

Hypothermia has been reported as a symptom of uremic patients.[1,9,11] Body temperatures between 33 and 34 °C are regularly observed in rats, 24 hours after bilateral nephrectomy.[10] This phenomenon was studied by our group during the last years and the following results were obtained:

1. Hypothermia is secondary to a severe reduction of the metabolic rate because nephrectomized rats, maintained at a normal body temperature by housing them in a thermostat, did not improve oxygen consumption.[10]
2. Hypothermia and hypometabolism occur at a normal pO_2 of arterial blood, a rather elevated blood pressure[10] and a normal cardiac output (unpublished results).
3. Correction of extracellular pH in uremia by bicarbonate treatment does not ameliorate the metabolic situation.[1o]
4. Pretreatment with triiodothyronine (T_3) over a period of 3 days does not prevent the reduction of oxygen consumption following nephrectomy.[6] As such a pretreatment prevents the reduction of the metabolic rate in cyanide, fluoride and digitoxin intoxication, the lacking effect of T_3 in uremia may be considered to some degree as a specific phenomenon.[4]

In a further series of experiments we investigated whether some of the so-called uremic toxins were able to induce a similar reduction of oxygen consumption in normal rats.

MATERIAL AND METHODS

Male Sprague-Dawley rats, weighing between 15o and 3oo g were employed. After a fasting period of 24 hours the toxins were applied intraperitoneally, dissolved in Krebs-phosphate buffer, pH 7.4, volume o.5 to 1.o ml/1oo g body wt. Toxins were given as single doses, alone or in different combinations (see below). Controls received the solvent only. In most cases rats with and without T_3 pretreatment[6] were investigated. Oxygen consumption was measured over a period of at least 6 hours following toxin injections by employing a diaferometer[1o] or a digital respirometer according to Gutmann.[2] In several experiments arterial systolic blood pressure was recorded on the tail by using Doppler's ultrasound technique.

In vitro respiration of rat diaphragma and liver slices was measured by employing the conventional Warburg technique. Air was the gas phase. Substrate free Krebs-phosphate buffer, pH 7.4, was used as incubation medium as described previously.[5] In some experiments plasma from rats, nephrectomized 48 hours before, was employed as incubation medium.

RESULTS

The general metabolic data from rats, 24 and 48 hours after nephrectomy are summarized in table 1.

Table 1

Metabolic data of bilaterally nephrectomized rats

24 hours after nephrectomy	48 hours after nephrectomy
Oxygen consumption:	
minus 4o - 5o %	minus 6o %
Body temperature:	
33 - 34 oC	32 oC
BUN:	
12o - 14o mg/dl	26o - 3oo mg/dl
Blood pH (cardiac puncture)	
7.2	7.o

Reduction of oxygen consumption was maximal 2 - 3 hours after application of the toxins and generally disappeared few hours later. Lowered blood pressure was never observed during these periods.

In vitro none of these substances alone or in different combinations (3o mg/dl each) reduced oxygen consumption of diaphragma or liver slices. Plasma of uremic rats (pH 7.5 by contact with air) was also without any effect on tissue respiration, irrespective of the fact whether the tissues were taken from normal or uremic rats. A brief summary of the in vitro experiments is given in table 4.

Table 4

Uremic toxins having no influence on respiration of rat diaphragma and liver slices

Concentration in the incubation medium (Krebs-phosphate buffer,pH 7.4, 37°C): 3o mg/dl each

Single substances:	Acetoine, m-Cresol, p-Cresol, Indole, Methylguanidine, Putrescine
Combinations:	Acetoine + p-Cresol + Methylguanidine + Putrescine ; p-Cresol + Methylguanidine

DISCUSSION

In bilaterally nephrectomized rats reduced oxygen consumption and hypothermia are constant findings. In human uremia these symptoms are well known but are obviously lacking in many cases. It has been supposed[11] that hypothermia might be masked by infection which can also induce fever in uremic subjects. Systematic measurements of oxygen consumption in human uremia have unfortunately not performed yet.

The underlaying mechanism for uremic hypometabolism is not known. According to our investigations it is not the consequence of hypothermia, cardiovascular failure or hypoxemia of the arterial blood. Consequently the reduced metabolic rate in uremia may be induced either:

1) by a primary defect of cellular metabolism due to uremic

toxins,

or

2) by a disturbance of microcirculation, so that even in the presence of normal arterial oxygen saturation tissue pO_2 (tpO_2) might be low.

The latter possibility would be compatible with the observation of reduced deformability of red blood cells in uremia.[8] A definite decision, however needs direct measurement of tpO_2. In our laboratory tpO_2 of muscle (measured according to Kessler et al.[7]) had been found without essential alterations in nephrectomized rats.

Uremic toxins are generally present in body fluids in low concentrations being in the range of µmol/l (for review see Giordano[1]). Among these substances indole only was able to reduce oxygen consumption of normal rats at a low dose of 5 mg/kg body wt. However, combinations of other toxins without effect when given alone at high concentrations were effective when applied in combination at a low dose each. As the number of so-called uremic toxins is important a lot of combinations has to be tested for obtaining complete information which substances were really dangerous for the uremic patient. The mechanism for enhanced toxicity by combination and interaction of substances is complex and best known for several interactions between drugs.[3] For the case of uremic toxins such interactions are poorly understood at the moment. An obvious result of this study was the discrepancy between in vivo and in vitro results. In vitro, substances acting in vivo, may probably be absent or lacking in adequate concentrations (H^+ ions, hormones, etc.). Disturbances of microcirculation would not be detectable by in vitro experiments where tissues are optimally supplied with oxygen by diffusion.

From all toxins tested indole only induced a significant reduction of the metabolic rate when given at a low dose of 5 mg/kg body wt.(table 2).

Table 2

Effect on oxygen consumption of a single dose of uremic toxins i.p. in rats

	Oxygen consumption 1/kg/24 hours, $\bar{x} \pm$ SD	
	Without T3 pretreatment	With T3 pretreatment
Controls	47.5 ± 5.5 (n=9)	62.2 ± 4.1 (n=1o)
Indole, 5 mg/kg	34.1 ± 7.o (n=9)	38.4 ± 8.9 (n=1o)
p	< o.o1	< o.o1

Ineffective: Acetoine, m-Cresol, p-Cresol,Putrescine,
Methylguanidine: 5o - 1oo mg/kg body wt.

Other substances (see table 2) had no effect, even when given at a ten- to twentyfold higher dose.

Several but not all combinations of these substances, given at a dose of 1o mg/kg body wt. each, actually reduced oxygen consumption. Some examples are presented in table 3.

Table 3

Effect on oxygen consumption of uremic toxins given in combination, 1o mg/kg each i.p., in T_3 pretreated rats

	Oxygen consumption 1/kg/24 hours, $\bar{x} \pm$ SD
Controls (n=6)	75.4 ± 1o.5
p-Cresol + Methyl-guanidine + Putrescine (n=8)	59.7 ± 7.7
p	< o.o1
Controls (n=8)	64.o ± 5.5
m-Cresol + Methyl-guanidine (n=8)	46.2 ± 2.4
	< o.o1

Ineffective: Methylguanidine + Putrescine;
m-Cresol + Putrescine

SUMMARY

According to our present knowledge hypometabolism and hypothermia in uremia are most probably due to direct actions of toxic substances at the cellular level. A cardiovascular etiology seems less possible. A similar reduction of oxygen consumption as observed in uremia can be produced by 5 mg/kg body wt. indole i.p. Acetoine, m- and p-cresol, methylguanidine and putrescine do not reduce oxygen consumption even at tenfold higher doses. Some combinations of these substances, however, are effective when given only 1o mg/kg body wt. each. The effects in vivo cannot be reproduced by employing in vitro systems.

REFERENCES

1. C.Giordano, The biochemical basis of uremic toxicity, Int.J.Ped. Nephrol. 3:239-25o (1982)
2. K.Gutmann, Measuring oxygen consumption with an all-electronic multirange digital respirometer, Oecologia 56:14o (1983)
3. P.D.Hanstein, Arzneimittel-Interaktionen, Hippokrates Verlag, 2nd Ed., Stuttgart (1981)
4. M. Hohenegger, Wirkungen der akuten Urämie, Azidose und Alkalose auf Energiehaushalt und Fettstoffwechsel, Funkt.Biol.Med. 1:148-156 (1982)
5. M.Hohenegger,and M.Brezina, Some aspects of renal energy and lipid metabolism in newborn rats, Biol.Neonate 46:177-185 (1984)
6. M.Hohenegger, R.Kramar, P.Om, M.Weissel,and R.Watschinger, Influence of triiodothyronine, amphetamine, and dinitrophenol(DNP) on the reduced metabolic rate in uremic and acidotic rats, Exp.Pathol. 22: 37-42 (1982)
7. M.Kessler, D.W. Lübbers, B.A.Krumme, K.Schönleben,and H.Bünte, Oxygen tension in different tissues, Bibl.Anat. 16:146-149 (1977)
8. Y.Kikuchi, T.Koyama, Y.Koyama, S.Tozawa, T.Arai, M.Horimoto,and Y. Kakiuchi, Red blood cell deformability in renal failure, Nephron 3o:8-14 (1982)
9. J.P.Knochel,and D.W.Seldin , The pathophysiology of uremia, in: The Kidney, B.M.Brenner, and F.C. Rector jr. ed., Saunders Company, Philadelphia (1976)
1o. P.Om,and M.Hohenegger, Energy metabolism of acute uremic rats, Nephron 25:249-253 (198o)
11. G.Schreiner,and J.F.Maher, Uremia:Biochemistry,Pathogenesis and Treatment, Ch.C.Thomas Editors, Springfield (1961)

ACKNOWLEDGMENTS

These investigations were supported by Fonds des Burgmeisters der stadt Wien fur die medizinisch-wissenschaftliche forschung und Österreichisher fonds zur Förderung der wissenchaftlichen Forschung, Projekt 3346.

GLUCOSE METABOLISM IN ACUTE RENAL FAILURE

C. Giordano, P. Castellino, M. Pluvio, and N.G. De Santo

Istituto di Medicina Interna e Nefrologia 1st Medical Faculty

University of Napoli, Italy

INTRODUCTION

Fasting hyperglycemia as well as a prolonged elevation of plasma glucose after both oral (OGTT) and intravenous glucose tolerance test (IVGTT) has been observed in acute uremic patients and in experimentally induced acute uremia in animals (1,2,3).

This is associated with elevated fasting insulin levels and an enhanced insulin response to the administered glucose (2,4,5). Recent studies have suggested that glucose intolerance in ARF is primarily caused by insulin resistance in peripheral tissues (5). In particular, muscle tissues have been shown to play a major role in glucose disposal and in the pathogenesis of insulin resistance. However little information is currently available on insulin sensitivity in acute uremic patients. Moreover little is known on the metabolic utilization of glucose during hyperinsulinemia in ARF. More specifically, it is not clear if both glucose oxidation and glucose storage (an index of glycogen synthesis) are impaired in acute uremic patients as suggested by in vitro studies on muscle preparation from acute uremic rats (3).

PATIENT POPULATION

Six control subjects and six patients with acute renal failure participated in the study; (53+4 and 48+3 years of age respectively). All uremics (mean 107+5%) and control (mean 104+5%) were within 20% of the ideal body weight, based on the medium frame of the Metropolitan Life Insurance Table (1959). The mean serum urea nitrogen and creatinine concentration averaged 128+12 mg/dl and 8+1 mg/dl, respectively; plasma potassium was 4.9 meq/L in uremic subjects. There was no family history of diabetes mellitus or other endocrine disease. Four of the six uremic patients were restudied after resolution of acute renal failure (serum urea and creatinine levels 20+2 and 1.2 mg/dl, plasma potassium 4.2+0.3, urine volume 1.2+0.4 Liter/day). Tests were performed at 0800 hour after an overnight fast. The purpose and potential risk of the study were explained to all subjects and a voluntary consent was obtained prior to their participation.

PATIENT POPULATION

Six control subjects and six patients with acute renal failure participated in the study; (53+4 and 48+3 years of age respectively). All uremics (mean 107+5%) and control (mean 104+5%) were within 20% of the ideal body weight, based on the medium frame of the Metropolitan Life Insurance Table (1959). The mean serum urea nitrogen and creatinine concentration averaged 128+12 mg/dl and 8+1 mg/dl, respectively; plasma potassium was 4.9 meq/L in uremic subjects. There was no family history of diabetes mellitus or other endocryne disease. Four of the six uremic patients were restudies after resolution of acute renal failure (serum urea and creatinine levels 20+2 and 1.2 mg/dl, plasma potassium 4.2+0.3, urine volume 1.2+0.4 Liter/day). Tests were performed at 0800 hour after an overnight fast. The purpose and potential risk of the study were explained to all subjects and a voluntary consent was obtained prior to their participation.

METHODS

Euglycemic Insulin Clamp Studies

Polyethilene catheters were inserted in a forehand vein and in an antecubital vein. The hand was heated at 70°C to ensure arterialization of the venous blood. Following the collection of at least three basal samples a primed continuous infusion of insulin was administered to acutely rise and maintain plasma insulin concentration at 100 U/ml above basal levels. Plasma glucose levels were measured every 5 minutes and a 20% glucose infusion was periodically adjusted to maintain euglycemia (6). Plasma glucose was measured by a Beckman glucose analyzer 2. Plasma insulin and glucagon levels were measured by radioimmunoassay.

Continuous Indirect Calorimetry

A plastic ventilated hood was placed over the head of the subjects and made air tight around the neck. A slight negative pressure was maintained in the hood by continuous aspiration. The Oxygen and Carbon dioxide content of the air flowing out of the hood was continuously measured by a Beckman Metabolic Cart (7).

RESULTS

Basal insulin concentration was slightly higher in uremic in comparison to control subjects (14+3 vs 11+4 uU/ml) and returned to normal after recovery of renal function (9+3 uU/ml). During the euglycemic insulin clamp studies the steady state insulin concentration was slightly higher in acute uremics in comparison to controls (115+7 vs 92+ uU/ml) and declined to 96+ uU/ml in the clamp studies performed during the recovery phase. This was reflected by a lower insulin clearance in uremics in comparison to controls (415+48 vs 505+ ml/m^2 min; P<0.05) and was restored to normal with the recovery of renal function (480+55 ml/m^2 min). Also glucagon levels were increased in uremics in comparison to controls (235+33 vs 456+33 pg/ml; P<0.01). Fasting plasma glucose concentration averaged 84+mg/dl in controls and 89+4 mg/dl in uremics. The mean glucose concentration during the 40 to 100 min of the insulin clamp was 86+3 in controls and 88+2 mg/dl in uremics, the coefficients of variation were 4.3% and 4.8%, respectively. The average rate of glucose utilization from 40 to 120 min was markedly reduced in uremics in comparison to controls (2.6+0.3 vs 4.7+0.4 mg/kg min; P<0.01) (Fig 1).

Four of the six patients were restudied after resolution of renal insufficiency; in these patients the rate of glucose utilization averaged 2.8±0.4 mg/Kg min in the anuric phase and rose to 3.9±0.5 mg/Kg min in the recovery (Fig 2).

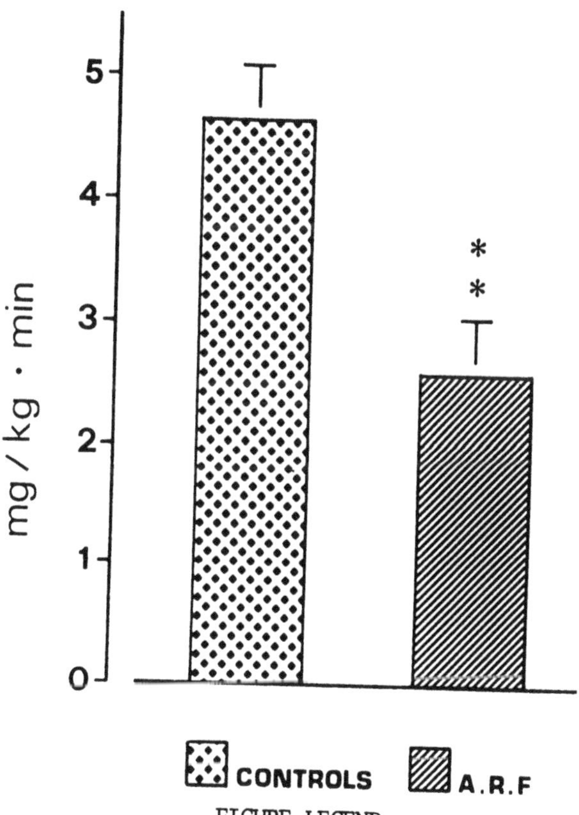

FIGURE LEGEND

FIG 1: Insulin mediated glucose metabolism in acute uremics and controls Values are in mg/Kg min ± SEM. ** P <0.01.

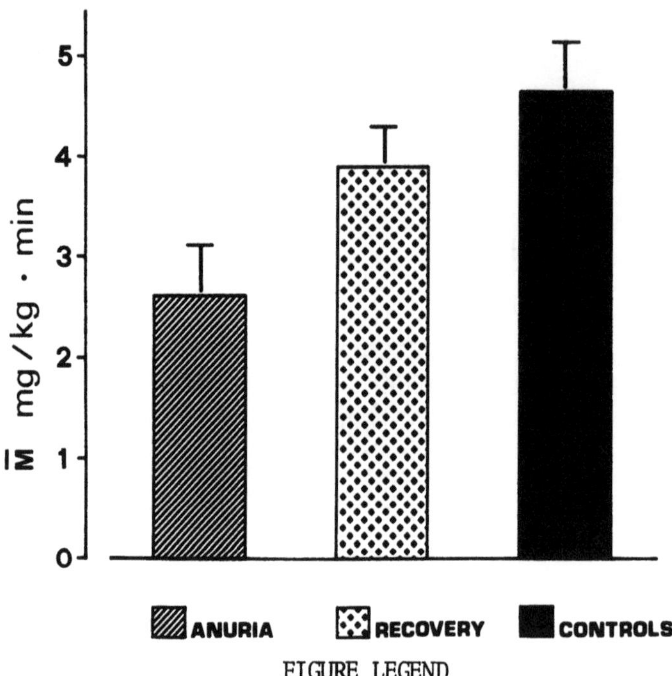

FIGURE LEGEND

FIG 2: Insulin mediated glucose metabolism in acute uremic patients during anuric and recovery period and controls. All values are in mg/Kg min $\pm$ SEM.

The indirect calorimetry data from 6 control subjects and 3 uremics are summarized in Table 1.

TABLE 1. Summary of Indirect Calorimetry Data in 6 controls and 2 patients with ARF. Glucose and oxidation are expressed in mg/Kg.min. RQ= Respiratory Quotient. *P< 0.01 vs basal.

	N	BASAL			INSULIN CLAMP		
		Gluc. Ox	Lipid Ox	RQ	Gluc. Ox	Lipid Ox	RQ
CONTROLS	6	0.82±0.04	0.79±0.07	.81	1.80±0.10	0.38±0.03	.92
A.R.F. anuria	3	0.76±0.03	0.83=0.04	79	1.20±0.06	0.58±0.06	.84
recovery	3	0.80±0.06	0.81±0.08	.81	1.55±0.02	0.48±0.09	.88

In controls, hyperinsulinemia was associated with a significant rise in glucose oxidation that went from 0.82±0.04 to 1.80±0.10 mg/Kg min (P<0.01). A concomitant inhibition of lipid oxidation was also observed: 0.79±0.07 vs 0.38±0.03 mg/Kg min. This was reflected by a rise in the respiratory quotient that went from 0.81 to 0.92.

In acute uremia the basel values of glucose and lipid oxidation were not significantly different from controls. However in the insulin stimulated state both the rise in glucose oxidation and the inhibition in lipid oxidation were markedly impaired. These abnormalities were almost completely reversed with the recovery of renal function.

DISCUSSION

Hyperglycemia during fasting as well a prolonged glucose elevation after an OGTT an/or IVGTT has been observed in acute uremic patients and in experimentally induced acute uremic animals (1,2,3). This is associated with elevated fasting insulin concentrations and sustained hyperinsulinemia after glucose administration (2,4,5). Moden et al (5) performed intravenous glucose tolerance test in anesthetized nephrectomized and sham operated rats.

Fasting plasma glucose concentration was higher in uremic rats in comparison to controls and this was associated with a slower decline in plasma glucose levels following the administration of the intravenous load. However the concomitant insulin response was greater in uremic animals than in controls. Therefore the primary event in glucose intolerance in acute uremia, as well as in chronically uremic patients, does not seem to be an impairment in insulin secretion but an ineffective response of target tissues to insulin. This impairment in insulin action may reside in any of the following abnormalities: 1) incomplete suppression of hepatic glucose production 2) reduced uptake of glucose by the liver and the splanchnic area 3) impaired peripheral utilization of glucose. To our knowledge, the first two possibilities have not been investigated in acute uremic patients and therefore no definite conclusion can be made. However, some insight can be gained from experiments in vitro (5) in which a normal suppression of hepatic glucose production was observed in isolated perfused liver preparations from acute uremic rats during hyperinsulinemia. Similar conclusion were obtained by De Fronzo et al (8) who investigated the suppression of hepatic glucose production during hyperinsulinemia in chronic uremic patients.

With regard to glucose uptake by the splanchnic bed, Katz et al (9) have recently demonstrated that the splanchnic area does not play a major role in the disposal of both an intravenous and an oral glucose load and that most of the administered glucose escapes the splanchnic bed and is metabolized by peripheral tissues. Similar results were also obtained during an intravenous glucose administration in chronic uremic patients by De Fronzo et al (10). Thus it seem unlikely that either incomplete suppression of hepatic glucose production or a reduced splanchnic glucose uptake may be the major determinants of the abnormalities in glucose tolerance observed in acute uremia. Therefore, the interest has focused on the role of peripheral tissues in the disposal of glucose in ARF. To address this question, we have investigated the insulin mediated glucose metabolism in patients with acute renal failure employing the euglicemic insulin clamp technique as described by De Fronzo et al (6).

This technique provides a reliable index of tissues sensitivity to insulin within a physiologic range of hyperinsulinemia. In the present study insulin mediated glucose uptake was markedly impaired in acute uremic patients in comparison to controls. Peripheral tissues have been shown to play a major role in the disposal of glucose administered during hyperinsulinemia, and particularly muscle tissues are likely to be the primary site of insulin resistance in acute uremia.

Similar results were obtained by Clark and Mondon (11,5) who showed that insulin stimulated glucose uptake by perfused hind quarters of acute uremic rat is reduced. May et al (12) have investigated the insulin mediated glucose metabolism in epitrochlearis muscle preparation from sham operated and acutely uremic rats. They observed that the insulin mediated glucose uptake measured with D 2-^{3}H glucose was markedly impaired in uremics. The maximal rate of glucose uptake was decreased by 24% but the insulin concentration that elicited the half maximal stimulation of glucose uptake was similar in control and ARF rats. This indicates depressed insulin responsiveness with no alteration in insulin sensitivity (13), and is consistent with a post-receptor defect in insulin action. Interestingly, a similar post receptor impairment in insulin action was observed by DeFronzo et al (14) in patients with chronic renal failure. With regard to the possible mechanism responsible for insulin resistance, this can reside in an impairment in glucose oxidation, glycolysis or glucose storage as glycogen. In the present study both glucose oxidation, measured by indirect calorimetry, and glucose storage, measured as the difference between total glucose uptake and glucose oxidation, were markedly impaired in acute uremia. The mechanism responsible for this decline in insulin stimulated glucose oxidation cannot be described to an inhibition of pyruvate kinase and pyruvate dehydrogenase activity and are at present poorly understood (12, 15).

May et al (12) have also observed an alteration in glycogen synthesis measured as the amount of D-^{14}C glucose incorporated into glycogen during hyperinsulinemia in epitrochlearis muscle preparation of acute uremic rats. This is consistent with an alteration in glycogen synthetase activity who was observed by May (12) and Horl (16). Heidland et al (16,17) also showed that glycogen metabolism in ARF is not dependent on the adrenergic regulation and is stimulated by serine. In contrast a normal activity of the glycolitic pathway has been shown in muscle and liver preparation from acute uremic rats (12,15). Finally, lactate release has been shown to be normal in ARF (11,12) and this consistent with a normal glycolytic activity and a decrease in glucose oxidation. This suggest that in acute renal failure the primary defect is not in the transport mechanism of glucose since this would be expected to reduce glycolysis, glucose oxidation and glycogen synthesis in a comparable degree.

REFERENCES

1. Reaven, G.M., Wwisinger, J.R., Swenson, R.S.: Insulin and glucose metabolism in renal insufficiency. Kidney Int. 1974 (S1); 6:S63-S69.
2. Briggs, J.D., Buchanam, K.D., Luke, R.G., McKiddie, M.T.: Role of insulin in glucose intolerance in uremia. Lancet 1967; 1:462-464.
3. DeFronzo, R.A., Andres, R., Edgar, P., Walker, W.G.: Carbohydrate metabolism in uremia: a review. Medicine 1973; 52:469-481.
4. Nitzen, M., Metzer, B.E., Wilber, J.F.: The effect of acute uremia on plasma glucose, insulin and growth hormone in the rat. Life Sci. 1971; 10:671-676.
5. Mondon, C.E., Dolkas, C.B., Reaven, G.M.: The site of insulin resistance in acute uremia. Diabetes 1978; 27:571-576.
6. DeFronzo, R.A., Tobin, A.J., Andres, R.: The glucose clamp technique. A method for the quantification of beta cell sensitivity to glucose and of tissues sensitivity to insulin. Am. J. Physiol. 1979; 237:E214-E223.
7. Thiebaud, D., Jacot, E., DeFronzo, R.A., Maeder, E., Jaquier, E., Felber, J.P.: Effect of graded doses of insulin on total glucose oxidation, and glucose storage in man. Diabetes 1982; 31:957-963.
8. DeFronzo, R.A., Smith, D., Alverstrand, A.: Insulin action in uremia. Kidney Int. 1983; 24(S16):S102-S114.
9. Katz, L.D., Glickman, M.G., Rapaport, S., Ferranini, E., DeFronzo, R.A: Splanchnic and peripheral disposal of oral glucose in man. Diabetes 1983; 32:675-679.
10. DeFronzo, R.A., Alverstrand, A., Smith, D., Hendler, R., Hendler, E., Wahren, J.: Insulin resistance in uremia. J. Clin. Invest. 1981; 67:563-568.
11. Clark, A.S., Mitch, W.E.: Muscle protein turnover and glucose uptake in acute uremic rats. J. Clin. Invest. 1983; 72:836-845.
12. May, R.C., Clar, A.S., Goheer, M.A., Mitch, W.E.: Specific defect in insulin mediated muscle glucose and protein metabolism in acute uremia. Kidney Int. 1985; 28:490-497.
13. Kahan, C.R.: Insulin resistance, insulin insensitivity and insulin unresponsivness: A necessary distinction. Metabolism 1978; 27(S2):1893-1902.
14. Smith, D., DeFronzo, R.A.: Insulin resistance in uremia mediated by post binding defects. Kidney Int. 1982; 22:54-62.
15. Mayer, K.P., Hoppe-Seyler, G., Talke, H., Frolich, J., Schollmeyer, P., Gerok, W.: Enzimatic and metabolic studies on carbohydrate metabolism in rat liver during acute uremia. Europ. J. Clin. Invest. 1973; 3:201-207.
16. Horl, W.H., Stepinski, J., Heidland, A.: Carbohydrate metabolism and uremia. Mechamism for glycogenolysis and gluconeogenesis. Klon. Wschr. 1908; 58:1051-1064.

DRUG-INDUCED ACUTE RENAL FAILURE

A CLINICAL INSIGHT INTO THE PATHOPHYSIOLOGY OF DRUG-INDUCED ACUTE RENAL FAILURE

Luigi Minetti, Raffaele Galato, Loredana Radaelli, Carlo Rovati and Massimo Seveso

Division of Nephrology
Ca'Granda Hospital
Milano, Italy

INTRODUCTION

A major subset of drug-induced acute renal failure (DI-ARF) is the drug-induced acute tubular necrosis (DI-ATN). Drug-induced acute interstitial nephritis, acute glomerulonephritis, and acute renal vasculitis are other subsets of DI-ARF, that unlike DI-ATN are immunologically mediated. They present morphologic and functional changes quite similar to those of corresponding idiopathic forms. Likewise, the drug-induced acute tubular necrosis (DI-ATN) is currently believed to show clinical, histological and functional features not distinguishable from those of post-ischemic ATN (IS-ATN). Whereas it appears that prolonged renal ischemia is the most common pathogenetic factor of the latter, direct nephrotoxin exposure is the etiologic factor commonly encountered in patients developing DI-ATN.

Experimental murine and canine models of ATN can be categorized in three general groups: 1) in the toxic type, including mercury-, uranyl nitrate-, glycerol-induced forms, at the micropuncture studies the majority of surface tubules result devoided of fluid and usually exhibit a normal or low luminal hydrostatic pressure; 2) in the ischemic type, in which ARF follows total arterial clamping or norepinephrine infusion, the proximal tubules are distended with fluid and have a remarkably high luminal pressure that would be expected to stop the filtration process; 3) in the third group, produced by methemoglobin or globin injections, an admixture of the abnormalities of the two above-mentioned types of ATN can be observed, some nephrons displaying overt obstruction while others are collapsed and have distinctly low tubular pressures[1].

The features of tubular damage in human ATN were made clear by the microdissection studies of J. Oliver[2]. In the ischemic type of ATN tubular cell necrosis is patchy and affects short lengths of tubules, the straight segments of the proximal tubule being the most vulnerable. Disruption of necrotic tubule segments may occur (tubulorrhexis). In nephrotoxic ATN the lesion consists of extensive necrosis along proximal tubule, and tubulorrhexis does not occur , unless the injury is severe. In both ischemic and nephrotoxic types the lumina of distal tubules are occupied by casts.

Transtubular backleak, tubular obstruction and glomerular hypofiltration are at once principal consequences of these histopathologic changes and pathogenetic factors of impairment or suppression of renal function and oliguria. The transtubular backleak (i.e., the backleak of tubular fluid across necrotic epithelium into the interstitium) is depending on the severity of the damage[3]. The more severe is the lesion, the earlier and more marked is the obstruction of the terminal straight segment of the proximal tubule by occluding casts (with an ensuing transtubular backleak from more proximal convolutions). The less severe, or later in the course of ATN, is the lesion, the more prominent appear the occluding casts in the distal segments of nephrons (transtubular backleak from the lumen of the thick ascending limb of Henle)[4]. The glomerular hypofiltration, besides being caused by preglomerular vasoconstriction and decrease of hydraulic permeability and surface area available for filtration[5,6], can also ensue from the rise of upstream proximal tubular pressure caused by occluding casts[3].

There are however some questions to be solved. Different degrees of injury do correspond in the setting of ARF to discernible clinical differences? Are there distinct pathophysiologic patterns corresponding to the two types of ATN, post-ischemic and nephrotoxic?

A clinical insight into the pathophysiology of human ATN could be provided from the so-called urinary indexes, that are used in the differential diagnosis of ARF[7]. In the setting of ARF a urinary sodium concentration (UNa^+) less than 20 mEq/L strongly suggests a prerenal cause of renal failure, whereas a value greater than 40 mEq/L indicates intrinsic renal disease; UNa^+ values between 20 and 40 mEq/L may be encountered in all forms of renal failure. As far as the meaning of the urinary sodium concentration (UNa^+) is concerned we can reasonably assume that in the setting of oliguria and/or rapidly increasing creatininemia a high UNa^+ means that sodium tubular reabsorption is very reduced in still functioning nephrons, in distal tubule at least.

Urine-to-plasma creatinine ratios (U/P creat) less than 20 are most commonly observed in ATN, whereas U/P creatinine greater than 40 are usually seen in prerenal azotemia. Significant overlap between groups is encountered with U/P creat of 20 to 40. The U/P creat can also be considered an index of tubular integrity, as it indicates the ability to concentrate urine[8]. The lower the U/P creat., the lesser the ability to concentrate urine.

The fractional excretion of filtered sodium (U/P Na^+ divided by U/P creat x 100 = FE Na^+) may provide early differentiation between prerenal azotemia and ATN; it is less than 1 in most of former cases, and more than 1 in most of latter ones. $FeNa^+$ also reflects the sodium tubular reabsorption, but unlike UNa^+ along the whole tubule. Very high levels of $FENa^+$ mean indeed that sodium reabsorption is reduced in proximal tubule as well.

The use of a ratio obtained by dividing UNa^+ by U/P creat (Renal Failure Index: RFI) as means of differentiating the cause of ARF was suggested by Handa and Marrin[9]. RFI magnifies the inverse relationship between these two indices, since it is higher as higher is UNa^+ and lower as lower is the U/P creat; it is usually less than 1 in prerenal azotemia, and more than 1 in ATN.

In the context of ATN these urinary indexes could reflect not only the severity of the tubular damage, but also its site and extension along the nephron. Different admixtures of tubular obstruction, transtubular backleak and glomerular hypofiltration could bring about different patterns of urinary indexes. The two experimental models, ischemic and toxic, of ATN have different histopathological patterns; they could have also different pathophysiologic patterns. If the two types of human ATN, IS-ATN and DI-ATN, should reproduce the experimental models, they could display different patterns of urinary indexes as well.

To verify this assumption we compared the urinary indexes of drug-induced ATN patients with those of post-ischemic ATN patients.

MATERIALS AND METHODS

In a retrospective analysis of 864 ARF cases, who had been admitted to the Division of Nephrology, Ca'Granda Hospital of Milano from 1969 to 1981, two groups of patients were selected on the basis of the following criteria:

First group (IS-ATN):
- clinical circumstances suggesting a renal ischemic insult;
- diagnosis of ATN on the basis of physical examination, laboratory findings and clinical course.

Second group (DI-ATN):
- clinical circumstances suggesting drug-induced ARF;
- renal biopsy performed in the first ten days of ARF;
- a histological pattern consistent with ATN.

Both groups:
- availability of urinary indexes within the first three days of ARF.

The following urinary indexes were taken into account:
- the urinary sodium concentration: (mEq/L) UNa^+
- the urine-to-plasma creatinine ratio: U/P creat
- the fractional excretion of filtered sodium: $\frac{U/P\ Na^+}{U/P\ creat}\% = FE\ Na^+$
- the "Renal Failure Index": $\frac{U\ Na^+}{U/P\ creat} = RFI$

From each case only the earliest available pattern of urinary indexes was evaluated. The retrospective analysis was limited to the period 1969-1981, as afterwards nearly all the ARF cases, who were admitted, had been treated very early by hypertonic mannitol, high doses of furosemide, and vasodilator hormones.

The patients were divided in oliguric (daily urine volume less than 400 ml) and non-oliguric.

First group (IS-ATN): 109 cases.
A) Oliguric IS-ATN cases (54).
B) Nonoliguric IS-ATN cases (55).

Second group (DI-ATN): 35 cases.
A) Oliguric DI-ATN cases (20).
B) Nonoliguric DI-ATN cases (15).

Drug-induced ATN
Non-oliguric (15 cases): - gentamicin: 7; - contrast media: 5; - cefaloridin: 1; - sulindac: 1; - grafenin: 1
Oliguric (20 cases): - rifampicin: 10; - gentamicin: 6; - cefaloridin: 1; - fenoprofen: 2; - naproxen: 1

RESULTS

Among nonoliguric cases only two DI-ATN patients and one IS-ATN patient showed FE Na^+ less than 1 (DI-ATN: U Na^+ 36, U/P creat 19.3, FE Na^+ 0.59; U Na^+ 20, U/P creat 54.7, FE Na^+ 0.28; IS-ATN: U Na^+ 33, U/P creat 32, FE Na^+ 0.75). Among oliguric cases only one IS-ATN patient showed FE Na^+ less than 1 (U Na^+ 37, U/P creat 32.4, FE Na^+ 0.8). As a result all urinary indexes but one could be considered consistent with diagnosis of intrinsic ARF. The above-mentioned DI-ATN patient, with urinary indexes out of the typical range (U Na^+ 20, U/P creat 54.7 and FE Na^+ 0.28), displayed at renal biopsy a histopathological pattern of acute tubular necrosis, as the other cases of DI-ATN group did.

1) Nonoliguric IS-ATN (55 cases) vs oliguric IS-ATN (54 cases). (Table 1) The difference were statistically significant for all the urinary indexes: U Na^+, $p < 0.001$; U/P creat, $p < 0.005$; FE Na^+, $p < 0.001$; RFI, $p < 0.001$.

2) Nonoliguric DI-ATN (15 cases) vs oliguric DI-ATN (20 cases). (Table 1) The differences were significant only for U Na^+ ($p < 0.025$) and U/P creat ($p < 0.05$).

Table 1. U r i n a r y i n d e x e s (means, SD, range).

	U Na^+	U/P creat	RFI	FE Na^+
POST-ISCHEMIC ATN (IS-ATN: 109 cases)	71.13±26.99 (24÷143)	9.60±6.26 (1.6÷32.4)	10.92± 8.69 (1.03÷40)	7.94± 6.37 (0.75÷30)
OLIGURIC IS-ATN (54 cases)	79.89±27.27 (31÷140)	7.88±6.29 (1.6÷32.4)	14.61± 9.46 (1.14÷40)	10.54± 6.97 (0.8 ÷30)
NONOLIGURIC IS-ATN (55 cases)	62.53±23.99 (24÷143)	11.29±5.80 (2.75÷32)	7.29± 6.01 (1.03÷33.5)	5.40± 4.5 (0.75÷25)
DRUG-INDUCED ATN (DI-ATN: 35 cases)	78.26±27.72 (20÷121)	10.24±9.95 (1.8÷54.7)	15.24±14.40 (0.37÷66.8)	11.01±10.41 (0.28÷47)
OLIGURIC DI-ATN (20 cases)	87.55±21.65 (37÷110)	7.28±5.19 (2.26÷22)	18.47±11.72 (2.5÷44.12)	13.57± 8.73 (1.7÷31.97)
NONOLIGURIC DI-ATN (15 cases)	65.87±30.68 (20÷121)	14.19±13.21 (1.8÷54.7)	10.93±16.79 (0.37÷66.8)	7.6 ±11.73 (0.28÷47)

3) Oliguric DI-ATN (20 cases) vs oliguric IS-ATN (54 cases). (Table 1) No significant differences were observed.

4) Nonoliguric DI-ATN (15 cases) vs nonoliguric IS-ATN (55 cases). (Table 1). No significant differences were observed.

5) All DI-ATN (35 cases) vs all IS-ATN (109 cases). (Table 1) The differences of urinary indexes are statistically significant only for FE Na^+ and RFI ($p < 0.05$).

6) Distribution of oliguric and nonoliguric IS-ATN cases according to U Na^+. 26/54 oliguric (48.1 %) and 13/55 (23.6 %) nonoliguric patients presented U Na^+ higher than 80 mEq/L.

7) Distribution of oliguric and nonoliguric DI-ATN cases according to UNa^+. 15/20 oliguric (75 %) and 5/15 (33 %) nonoliguric patients had U Na^+ higher than 80 mEq/L.

8) Distribution of oliguric and nonoliguric IS-ATN cases according to U/P creat.
42/54 (77.7 %) oliguric and 23/55 (41.8 %) nonoliguric patients showed U/P creat less than 10.

9) Distribution of oliguric and nonoliguric DI-ATN cases according to U/P creat.
16/20 (80 %) oliguric and 7/15 (46.5 %) nonoliguric patients showed U/P creat less than 10.

10) Distribution of IS-ATN vs DI-ATN oliguric cases according to U Na^+ (Fig. 1). 75 % of DI-ATN cases, but only 48 % of IS-ATN cases, displayed U Na^+ higher than 80 mEq/L.

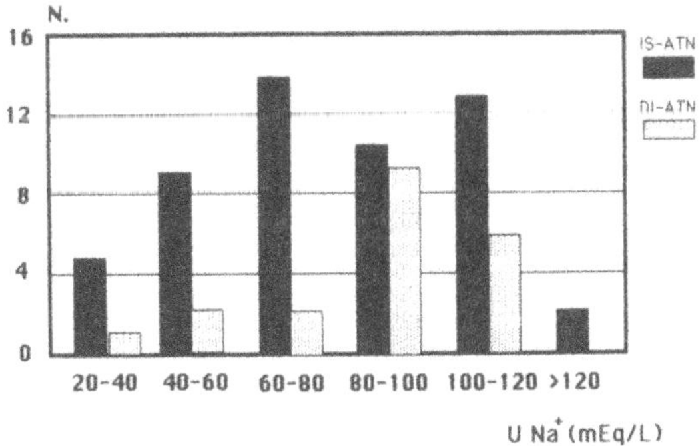

Fig. 1. Oliguric post-ischemic ATN (IS-ATN) patients vs. oliguric drug-induced ATN (DI-ATN) patients.

DISCUSSION

The pathophysiology of human acute tubular necrosis, and its relationship with the histopathological pattern, has been recently investigated by evaluating the kinetics of inulin excretion and the dextran clearance. The time at which inulin excretion peaks after a bonus injection varies from almost normal to greatly prolonged in ATN patients[10]. The delay in the residence time of inulin in the "urinary dead space" (inulin transit time) should be related with the reduction in the velocity of tubular fluid flow in obstructed tubules[11]. Another cause could be a very low rate of formation of glomerular ultrafiltrate, possibly due, at least in part, to an increase in tubular pressure produced by obstructing casts[3].

The presence of a transtubular backleak of filtrate in human postischemic ATN has been inferred from observation of changes of the fractional urinary clearance of dextran molecules of graded size. In surgical patients with overt ATN the ratio Cdextran/Cinulin resulted elevated above control values, therby indicating a dextran clearance higher than the inulin clearance for every size of dextran molecule, conceivably for a disproportionally larger blackleak of smaller inulin molecules as compared with larger dextran molecules[3]. The finding was interpreted as providing compelling evidence of transtubule backleak in human severe postischemic ATN, and it was calculated that approximately 50% of filtered inulin was lost by transtubular backleak[3].

As to the drug-induced ATN we do not now whether it is sharing the same mechanism, and which kind of experimental model it has to be referred to. According to the experimental data there should be different histopathologic and pathophysiological patterns of nephrotoxic ATN. Whereas in the mercuric chloride model backleak of filtrate and tubular obstruction are evident, in the aminoglycoside model backleak and obstruction do not appear to play important roles[12].

Our cases, that were in a range of values consistent with the diagnosis of ATN, displayed some variations of urinary indexes according to the presence of oliguria or non-oliguria. In the setting of ATN, as far as the meaning of the difference between oliguria and nonoliguria is concerned various explanations have been proposed. Oliguria, that is variously defined as urine output of less than 0.5 ml/Kg/h or 240 ml/m2/24 hours or, as in the present study, less than 400 ml/24 hours, at some stage is usual in ATN, but the patient with ARF does not need oliguria to have renal failure[13]. In non-oliguric ARF there is increasing azotemia and creatininemia while the daily urine volume may be "normal". Nephrotoxic ATN has been told to be more often non-oliguric in comparison with post-ischemic ATN.

Non-oliguric ATN is probably synonymous with mild ATN, the GFR remaining above about 5 ml/min throughout[14]. The concept that non-oliguric ATN could be an attenuated form of ATN is supported from many considerations. Formerly, many patients with nephrotoxic ATN and virtually all patients with post-ischemic ATN were oliguric[15], but during the last decade non-oliguric forms have become increasingly prevalent, the non-oliguric patients now constituting a majority among ATN cases[16]. This should be true for both post-ischemic and nephrotoxic forms. The reason could be that, more recently, "protective" agents as mannitol, furosemide and vasodilator hormones have been extensively used in patients at risk of ischemic or nephrotoxic insult. Such agents could attenuate the ensuing ARF with the result of urine flow remaining high and the GFR less depressed It is conceivable that the protective mechanism of furosemide and dopamine is due to a common effect that lowers preglomerular vascular resistance, elevates the transcapillary hydraulic-pressure gradient, and increases the rate of tubule fluid so that necrotic cell debris in the tubule lumen may be dispersed with the result that tubular obstruction is prevented or relieved[3].

A higher incidence of non-oliguric forms in DI-ATN in comparison with post-ischemic ATN cases has not been confirmed by our data, but the material we reported was formed by selected cases. Some experimental models of nephrotoxicity seem to suggest that the severity of the insult is important in this connection. Two models of gentamicin nephrotoxic ATN have been indeed obtained: with low doses of gentamicin a non-oliguric form, with high doses an oliguric one[12]. Also the type of renal injury could be related with the occurrence of oliguria/non-oliguria. For instance, cysplatinum nephrotoxic ATN is caracterized by non-oliguria.

The problem is to understand the meaning of non-oliguria in both IS-ATN and DI-ATN patients: a mild form due to a lesser insult, or an attenuated and abbreviated course because of early medical intervention, or a peculiar kind of structural and pathophysiologic change. As to U/P creat, the differences between oliguric and nonoliguric patients were quite similar in both IS-ATN and DI-ATN groups (they were unlike for U Na^+ instead). In other words, the tubular ability to concentrate urine appeared more reduced in oliguria than in nonoliguria, independently on the type of ATN. The finding seems to agree with the assumption that in oliguric patients there are fewer still functioning nephrons than in nonoliguric ones, and not with the hypothesis of a more severe and extensive damage of individual nephrons. The fact that we did not observe significant differences in urinary indexes between DI-ATN and IS-ATN cases, either in the setting of oliguria or nonoliguria, suggests that in human ATN the histopathological and pathophysiologic features could be similar in both drug-induced and ischemic type. By the way, our DI-ATN group was quite heterogeneous as regards to the etiologic factors. It is doubtful whether the rifampicin-induced ATN (out of our 35 DI-ATN cases 10 were rifampicin-induced) shares a nephrotoxic or ischemic mechanism. The urinary indexes meaning impairment of sodium tubular reabsorption as U Na^+, FE Na^+ and RFI seemed to be more conspicuous in DI-ATN patients. All (both oliguric and nonoliguric) DI-ATN patients displayed significantly higher values of FE Na^+ and RFI in comparison with all IS-ATN patients. Furthermore, oliguric DI-ATN patients showed a greater prevalence of very high U Na^+ levels than oliguric IS-ATN patients (Fig. 1).

CONCLUSIONS

In the setting of either oliguria or nonoliguria there were not significant differences in urinary indexes between post-ischemic ATN and drug-induced ATN.

Since the U/P creat mean values were significantly higher in nonoliguric than in oliguric patients, of both post ischemic ATN and drug induced ATN groups, it is conceivable that nonoliguria could reflect a greater number of still functioning nephrons rather than different sites and lesser severity of the damage in the still functioning nephrons.

The greater prevalence of very high U Na^+ levels in oliguric drug-induced ATN than in oliguric post-ischemic ATN patients, and the significantly higher mean values of FE Na^+ and RFI in all (both oliguric and nonoliguric) drug-induced ATN than in all post-ischemic-ATN patients, seem to suggest that in drug-induced ATN the impairment of tubular sodium reabsorption is more diffuse (proximal and distal tubule) than in post-ischemic ATN.

REFERENCES

1. D.E.Oken, Theoretical analysis of pathogenetic mechanisms in experimental acute renal failure, Kidney Int. 24:16 (1983).
2. J.Oliver, M.MacDowell, A.Tracy, Pathogenesis of acute renal failure associated with traumatic and toxic injury: renal ischemia, nephrotoxic damage and the ischemuric episode, J.Clin.Invest. 30:1305 (1951).
3. B.D.Myers, and S.M.Moran, Hemodynamically mediated acute renal failure New Engl.J.Med. 314:97 (1986)
4. M.Brezis, S.Rosen, P.Silva, F.H.Epstein, Renal ischemia: a new perspective, Kidney Int. 26:375 (1984).
5. J.H.Stein, and L.D.Barnes, Current concepts on the pathophysiology of acute renal failure, Am.J.Physiol. 234:F171 (1978).
6. R.H.Williams, C.E.Thomas, L.G.Navar, A.P.Evan, Hemodynamic and single nephron function during the maintenance phase of ischemic acute renal failure in the dog, Kidney Int. 19:503 (1981).
7. T.R.Miller, R.J.Anderson, S.L.Linas, W.L.Henrich, A.S.Berns, P.A.Gabow, R.W. Schrier, Urinary diagnostic indices in acute renal failure. A prospective study, Annals, Annals Intern.Med. 89:47 (1978).
8. B.D.Myers, D.C.Miller, J.T.Mehigan, Nature of the renal injury following total renal ischemia in man, J. Clin. Invest. 73:329 (1984).
9. S.P.Handa, and P.A.F.Marrin, Diagnostic indices in acute renal failure, Can.Med.Assoc.J. 96:78 (1967).57).
10. B.D.Myers, B.J.Carrie, R.R.Yee, M.Hilberman, A.S.Michaels, Pathophysiology of hemodynamically mediated acute renal failure in man, Kidney Int. 18:495 (1980).
11. S.M.Moran, B.D.Myers, Pathophysiology of protracted acute renal failure in man, J. Clin. Invest. 76:1440 (1985).
12. T.H.Hostetter, B.M.Wilkes, and B.M.Brenner, Renal circulatory and nephron function in experimental acute renal failure, p. 99, in: "Acute renal failure", B.M. Brenner and A.L. Lazarus, eds., W.B. Saunders Co., Philadelphia (1983).
13. M.R.Rudnick, C.P.Bastl, I.B.Elfinbein and R.G.Naris, The differential diagnosis of acute renal failure, p. 176, in: "Acute renal failure", B.M.Brenner and A.L.Lazarus, eds., W.B.Saunders Co., Philadelphia (1983).

14. R.M.Vertel, and J.P.Knochel, Nonoliguric acute renal failure, JAMA 200:119 (1967).
15. N.G.Levinsky, Pathophysiology of acute renal failure, New Engl.J. Med. 296:1453 (1977).
16. R.J.Anderson, S.L.Linas, A.S.Berns, W.L.Henrich, T.R.Miller, P.A.Gabow, R.W.Schrier, Nonoliguric acute renal failure, New Engl.J.Med. 296:1135 (1977).

DRUG-ASSOCIATED ACUTE RENAL FAILURE. A PROSPECTIVE COLLABORATIVE STUDY OF 81 BIOPSIED PATIENTS

D. Kleinknecht: Coordinator, Société de Néphrologie,
P. Landais, and B. Goldfarb, Methodologists

Centre Hospitalier, 93105 Montreuil & Hôpital Necker
75730 PARIS 15, France

INTRODUCTION

We recently reported the results of a national prospective collaborative study on drug-associated acute renal failure (ARF)[1,2]. Three hundred and ninety-eight patients with drug-associated ARF were registered in 58 french nephrology units, i.e. 18.3 % of total patients with ARF hospitalized during the same period[1]. We wish to describe here the main features and clinical outcome of the biopsied patients in this series.

PATIENTS AND METHODS

During a one-year period, 81 patients underwent a renal biopsy, i.e. 20.4 % of total patients with drug-associated ARF. Fifty-two were male, 29 female, with a mean age of 57.3 years (range 15-81).

Inclusion criteria were : 1) patients with a rapid increase in serum creatinine from a normal level to more than 200 µmol/l, or of 50 % or more above baseline values for patients with preexisting chronic renal insufficiency, and 2) patients with likely or possible side-effects to drugs, according to the algorithm of Dangoumau et al[3]. Patients with advanced chronic renal failure (serum creatinine level above 300 µmol/l) and doubtful cases were excluded.

RESULTS

The drugs mainly involved were non-steroidal anti-inflammatory drugs (NSAID) and antibiotics (Table 1). Among NSAID, clometacin was the most common offending drug, but many other NSAID were associated with ARF, and one-third of the patients received 2 to 5 different NSAID. Antibiotics ranked just behind NSAID and aminoglycosides, mainly gentamicin, accounted for two-thirds of these cases. Only a few patients developed ARF while receiving beta-lactamines or other antibiotics. Glafenin, contrast media, diuretics (mainly triamterene and thiazides), cisplatin and paracetamol were implicated in most of the remaining cases (Table 1).

Table 1. Drugs involved

Drugs	N	Drugs	N
NSAID	25 (30.9 %)	Beta-lactamines	5
Clometacin	6	Others	3
Pirprofen	3	Glafenin	7 (8.6 %)
Indometacin	2	Contrast media	7 (8.6 %)
Fenoprofen	2	Diuretics	4 (4.9 %)
Ibuprofen	2	Chemotherapy	3 (3.7 %)
Niflumic acid	2	Paracetamol	2 (2.5 %)
Others	8	Others	11 (13.6 %)
Antibiotics	22 (27.2 %)		
Aminoglycosides	14		

Renal pathological findings are detailed in Table 2. The most frequent pathological diagnosis was acute tubular necrosis (ATN), even in the NSAID group. Acute interstitial nephritis (AIN) was found in 20 patients, 9 of them in the NSAID group. Nine patients had interstitial epithelioid granulomas after receiving clometacin, ibuprofen, triamterene and cyclothiazide, tienilic acid and phenindione, fenofibrate, netilmicin, and chlorpropamide with furosemide in combination. Eosinophils were detected within the renal interstitium in three instances. Fourteen patients had an underlying chronic nephropathy without acute lesions. Minimal changes, microangiopathy (due to mitomycin) and tubular obstruction (related to an overdose of piridoxilate) were found in the remaining patients.

Forty-nine patients (60.5 %) had non-oliguric ARF. Nine patients had macroscopic hematuria, including 5 in the antibiotic group and 2 in the NSAID group ; ATN was present in 6/9 cases. Heavy proteinuria within the nephrotic range was observed in 7 patients, 6 of them after taking NSAID ; in the latter, renal pathological diagnoses were either ATN, AIN or minimal changes (two cases each). A hypersensitivity reaction, assessed on clinical, biological and/or pathological criteria, were present in 28 patients, including 20 with AIN and 6 with ATN. Thirty-three patients (40.7 %) required dialysis.

Only 10 patients died (12.3 %). Forty-eight patients either recovered fully or regained previous renal function. In 19 patients, permanent renal damage remained (23.5 %), including one who required chronic hemodialysis.

We compared the main differential features between patients with ATN and AIN. Sex, an older age, and the nature of the primarily involved drug were not significant features. Patients with AIN had more frequently non-oliguric ARF, clinical and biological signs suggesting a hypersensitivity reaction, a prolonged ARF period, and permanent renal damage (Table 3).

The predictive value of hypersensitivity signs was also assessed (Table 4). Blood hypereosinophilia was the best predictive sign for recognizing AIN. The progressive addition of clinical signs to blood hypereosinophilia increased the sensitivity and the negative predictive value of these features, but lowered consequently their specificity and their positive predictive value.

Table 2. Renal pathological findings (N = 81)

Diagnoses	NSAID	Glafe-nin	Anti-biotics	Others	Total
Acute tubular necrosis	13	5	13	11	42[a]
Acute interstitial nephritis	8	1	5	6	20[b]
Underlying chronic nephropathy (CN) without acute lesions	2	-	4	8	14
Minimal changes	2	1	-	-	3
Microangiopathy	-	-	-	1	1
Tubular obstruction	-	-	-	1	1

[a] with vasculitis in 1 patient and previous CN in 5 patients
[b] with previous CN in 1 patient

Table 3. Main differential features between pts with ATN and AIN

	ATN	AIN	P
Non-oliguric ARF	45.2 %	73.7 %	< 0.02
Fever, skin rash and/or arthralgias	19.0 %	55.0 %	< 0.01
Blood hypereosinophilia	11.9 %	55.0 %	< 0.001
ARF period, days	10.9 ± 9.6	22.2 ± 17.8	< 0.01
Death	16.7 %	0.0 %	0.05
Permanent renal damage	21.4 %	60.0 %	< 0.01

Table 4. Predictive value of hypersensitivity signs

	AIN (n = 20)	ATN (n = 42)	X_2	SE	SP	PPV	NPV
Blood hypereosinophilia (E)	55 %	11.9 %	13.14	0.55	0.88	0.69	0.80
E and/or fever	70 %	21.4 %	13.70	0.70	0.79	0.61	0.85
E and/or fever and/or arthralgias and/or hepatocellular damage	75 %	23.8 %	14.75	0.75	0.76	0.60	0.86

SE = sensibility. SP = specificity. PPV = positive predictive value.
NPV = negative predictive value

DISCUSSION

The present report is restricted to the study of the biopsied cases with drug-associated ARF. These results confirm the findings observed in the overall series[1,2], except for the incidence of AIN which increased in biopsied cases (24.7 % vs 4.6 % of total patients with drug-associated ARF). It is likely that, in reports including non-biopsied patients, some cases of AIN may have been unrecognized and classified as ATN without the help of a renal biopsy specimen. On the other hand, it is sometimes hard to decide in biopsied patients whether tubular or interstitial involvement is prominent[4]. The relative high incidence of ATN in drug-induced ARF, even in NSAID cases, is also emphasized in a recent survey[5].

The incidence of renal sequelae in this study is comparable to that found in non-biopsied cases with drug-associated ARF[1,2], but is higher than that reported in previous documented series of nephrotoxic ARF[6,7]. The risk for a residual renal damage was maximal in cases with AIN. Half of these patients had epithelioid cell granulomas within the renal interstitium, which may be poor prognostic indicators[8].

A dramatic improvement in renal function has been observed in individual cases of drug-induced AIN after giving high doses of prednisone or methylprednisolone[4], but no controlled studies are available. Prednisone therapy was prescribed in four of our patients with AIN ; only two of them recovered normal renal function.

CONCLUSIONS

1. Drug-associated ARF is an underestimated cause of permanent renal damage
2. Permanent renal damage is more frequent in patients with AIN than in those with ATN
3. AIN should be recognized by an early renal biopsy, especially in patients with hypersensitivity signs
4. The indication of steroid therapy being controversial, controlled studies would be helpful to evaluate the effect of this treatment.

REFERENCES

1. Société de Néphrologie. D. Kleinknecht, P. Landais and B. Goldfarb. Drug-associated acute renal failure. A prospective multicentre report. Proc. Europ. Dial. Transpl. Ass. 21 : 1002 (1985)
2. Société de Néphrologie. D. Kleinknecht, P. Landais and B. Goldfarb. Les insuffisances rénales aiguës associées à des médicaments ou à des produits de contraste iodés. Néphrologie (1986) (in press)
3. J. Dangoumau, J.C. Evreux and J. Jouglard. Méthode d'imputabilité des effets indésirables des médicaments. Thérapie 33 : 373 (1978)
4. J.P. Grünfeld, D. Kleinknecht and D. Droz. Acute interstitial nephritis, in : "Strauss and Welt's diseases of the kidney", R.W. Schrier, C.W. Gottschalk, eds., Little Brown, Boston (in press)
5. J. Carmichael and S.W. Shankel. Effects of nonsteroidal anti-inflammatory drugs on prostaglandins and renal function. Am. J. Med. 78 : 992 (1985)
6. A. Chapman. Etiologie et pronostic actuel de l'insuffisance rénale aiguë en France. Résultats d'une enquête, in "L'insuffisance rénale aiguë", Expansion Scientifique, Paris (1978)
7. C. Pru, J. Ebben and C. Kjellstrand. Chronic renal failure after tubular necrosis. Kidney Int. 21 : 176 (1982)
8. F. Mignon, J.Ph. Méry, L. Morel-Maroger, B. Mougenot, P. Ronco and J. Roland. Granulomes epithélioïdes de l'interstitium du rein, in "Actualités Néphrologiques de l'hôpital Necker", J. Crosnier, J.L. Funck-Brentano, J.F. Bach, J.P. Grünfeld, eds., Flammarion, Paris (1983).

NEPHROGENIC DIABETES INSIPIDUS AND DISTAL TUBULAR ACIDOSIS IN METHICILLIN-INDUCED INTERSTITIAL NEPHRITIS

Ph. Vigeral, A. Kanfer, S. Kenouch, F. Blanchet, B. Mougenot and J.Ph. Méry

Service de Néphrologie and Laboratoire d'Explorations Fonctionnelles, Hôpital Bichat, and Laboratoire d'Anatomie et de Cytologie Pathologiques, Hôpital Tenon, Paris, France

Acute interstitial nephritis associated with methicillin therapy has been reported in over 100 patients (1) and new cases are usually no more reported. Although its clinical picture has been extensively described (2-5), little attention has been paid to the possible occurrence of functional impairment of the distal tubule. This report deals with two patients with methicillin-induced interstitial nephritis and renal failure in whom distal tubular abnormalities were prominent.

CASE REPORTS

Patient 1. A 52-year-old man was admitted because of acute respiratory failure due to bilateral pneumonia. Gentamicin, 180 mg/day, and ampicillin, 8 g/day, were given. The latter drug was withdrawn on the third day when transtracheal aspiration yielded Staphylococcus aureus. Methicillin, 6 g/day, was then begun and led to disappearance of pulmonary symptoms. Serum creatinine was 101 µmol/l when methicillin was started. Eight days later, it was 280 µmol/l. Daily urinary output was 2 liters. There was no rash and temperature was normal. Proteinuria was 0.30 g/24 h, without hematuria or leucocyturia. Peak and trough levels of plasma gentamicin were 5 µg/ml and 1.1 µg/ml, respectively. All drugs were discontinued and the patient was discharged. He was readmitted six weeks later because of persistent renal impairment. Physical examination was normal : temperature was 37°2 C, there was no edema and blood pressure was 140/80 mm Hg. Daily urinary output was 3 liters. Serum creatinine was 175 µmol/l and creatinine clearance was 45 ml/mn. Plasma sodium was 139 mmol, potassium 4.5 mmol, chloride 106 mmol and bicarbonate 18 mmol per liter with arterial pH of 7.37. Urinary pH was 6. There were no proteinuria, hematuria, leucocyturia or glycosuria and amino-acid excretion was normal. A percutaneous renal biopsy was performed. Light microscopy examination showed tubulo-interstitial nephritis with interstitial inflammatory infiltrate and edema associated with tubular alterations (Figure 1a). Glomeruli and vessels were normal. Immunofluorescent study showed linear IgG and IgM along most tubules, indicating the presence of anti-tubular basement membrane (TBM) antibodies (Figure 1b). Circulating anti-TBM IgG antibodies were detected in the patient's serum . Because of polyuria and metabolic acidosis, the patient was further explored, 10 weeks after onset of nephropathy. Results of concentration test are shown on Table 1 : low urine osmolality, together with high values of urine output and free-water clearance after

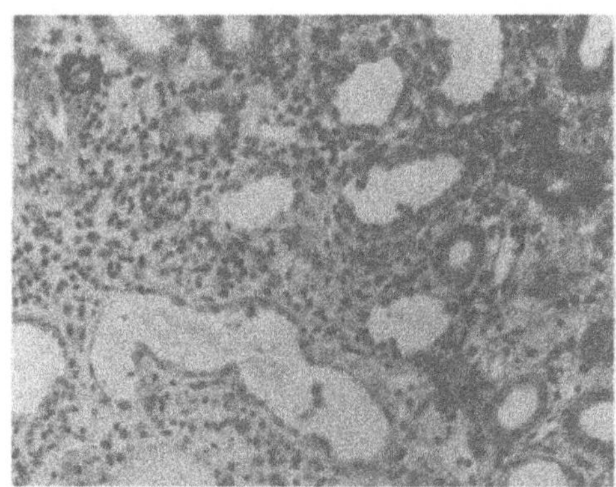
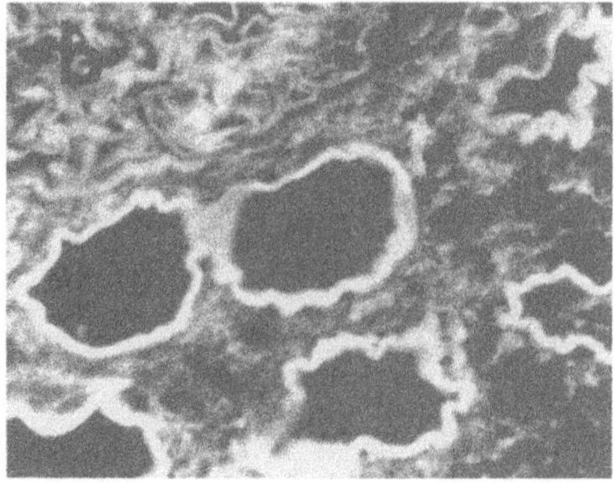

Figure 1. Patient 1 - Renal biopsy

a. Light microscopy : interstitial edema and cellular infiltration surrounding altered tubules with epithelial atrophy (Masson's trichrome, original magnification x 120)
b. Immunofluorescence : linear IgG deposits along cortical tubules (Fluorescein-isothiocyanate conjugated anti-IgG, original magnification x 300)

12 hours of fluid deprivation, demonstrated diabetes insipidus. The high plasma antidiuretic hormone (ADH) level (Normal : 3.6 $\pm$ 0.8 pg/ml) and the persistence of the aforementioned abnormalities after intravenous DDAVP demonstrated its nephrogenic nature. Results of urine acidification (ammonium chloride 5 g orally per day for 3 days) and alcalinization (sodium bicarbonate 400 mmol intravenously for 4 hours) tests are shown on Table 2. An abnormally low urine-blood pCO2 gradient of 16.7 mm Hg (Normal > 30 mm Hg) was observed, suggesting the presence of distal tubular acidosis. Fractional excretion of bicarbonate was 2 %, excluding a proximal tubular acidosis.

Patient 2. A 43-year-old man was admitted because of fever and lumbar pain with psoitis. A diagnosis of Staphylococcus aureus septicemia with left psoas abscess was made. Abscess was percutaneously drained under ultrasonography and antibiotherapy was begun. Netilmicin, 180 mg/day,

Table 1. Patient 1 - Concentration test

	BASELINE VALUES	AFTER FLUID RESTRICTION	AFTER DDAVP
Osmolality (mOsm/kg)			
. Plasma	302	302	300
. Urine	447	528 (>800)	562
Urinary output (ml/mn)	-	1.22 (<0.60)	0.95
Osmolar clearance (ml/mn)	-	2.15	1.78
Free-water clearance (ml/mn)	-	- 0.93 (<-2.0)	- 0.83
Plasma ADH (pg/ml)	-	16.9	> 30

Numbers in parentheses indicate normal values after fluid restriction

Table 2. Patient 2 - Acidification and alcalinization tests

		BASELINE VALUES	AFTER ACIDIFICATION	AFTER ALCALINIZATION
ARTERIAL BLOOD	pH	7.37	7.31	7.46
	pCO_2 (mm Hg)	31.5	26.7	38.9
	HCO_3^- (mmol/l)	18	13.1	27.2
URINE	pH	6	4.95	7.6
	pCO_2 (mm Hg)	-	34.6	55.6

was associated first with oxacillin, 6 g/day for five days, thereafter with methicillin 12 g/day. Serum creatinine was 107 µmol/l on the 11th day of meticillin administration. On the 12th day, high fever associated with chills and a pruriginous rash occurred, and the patient became oliguric. Blood eosinophils were 1040/mm3. Proteinuria, 0.50 g/24 h, and microscopic hematuria were present. There was no eosinophiluria. methicillin and netilmicin were then withdrawn and pertloxacin, 800 mg/day, was introduced. Oliguria lasted 25 days during which the patient received hemodialysis. Thereafter, diuresis increased and renal function progressively improved. A renal biopsy was performed 24 days after onset of renal failure. Light microscopy examination showed the presence of interstitial inflammatory infiltrate with perivascular granulomas, interstitial edema and tubular necrosis. Glomeruli were normal. Immunofluorescent study showed linear IgG and IgM along tubules. Prednisolone, 1 mg/kg/day, was begun. Seven months after onset of nephropathy, the patient was polyuric with a daily urinary output of 4 to 6 liters. Serum creatinine was 213 µmol/l and creatinine clearance was 32 ml/mn. Plasma sodium was 142 mmol, potassium 4.2 mmol, chloride 107 mmol and bicarbonate 21 mmol per liter. A concentration test demonstrated nephrogenic diabetes insipidus with hyposthenuria (Table 3).

Table 3. Patient 2 - Concentration test

	BASELINE VALUES	AFTER FLUID RESTRICTION	AFTER DDAVP
Osmolality (mOsm/kg)			
. Plasma	299	301	304
. Urine	259	263 (>800)	306
Urinary output (ml/mn)	-	1.71 (<0.60)	2.03
Osmolar clearance (ml/mn)	-	1.48	2.04
Free-water clearance (ml/mn)	-	+ 0.23 (<-2.0)	0
Plasma ADH (pg/ml)	7.2	8.2	> 30

Numbers in parentheses indicate normal values after fluid restriction

DISCUSSION

Although clinical picture of meticillin-induced interstitial nephritis has been extensively described, only a few reports have briefly mentioned the possibility of functional tubular impairment (2,6-9). Woodroffe et al. (6) and Border et al. (7) mentioned one patient each with tubular abnormalities that persisted several months after the acute episode. Cogan and Arieff (10) provided evidence of selective distal tubular dysfunction (sodium wasting, acidosis and hyperkalemia) in a single patient with persistent renal insufficiency. The data obtained in our patients clearly demonstrate that important fonctional tubular abnormalities may be the consequence of meticillin-induced interstitial nephritis. Both patients had nephrogenic diabetes insipidus, moderate in patient 1 and severe in patient 2 ; in addition, patient 1 had hyperchloremic metabolic acidosis. Persistent mild renal insufficiency was present in both cases. Since metabolic acidosis and defective urinary concentration ability are features of chronic renal insufficiency (11-13), responsibility of renal failure per se in the tubular abnormalities observed in our patients might be questioned. In this respect, it should be emphazised that vasopressin-resistant hyposthenuria was present in patient 2. Indeed, although hyposthenuria may be present in patients with advanced chronic renal disease and creatinine clearance below 15 ml/mn (13,14), it is not a feature of mild renal insufficiency (15). Likewise, none of the patients with moderate chronic renal failure reported by Conte et al. (16) to have impaired urine concentration ability had hyposthenuria. Experiments in dogs have also demonstrated that renal insufficiency per se does not reduce maximum urine osmolality as long as glomerular filtration rate remains higher that a third of normal (17). Moreover, in both patients, plasma ADH levels were comparable to those observed in two patients with nephrogenic diabetes insipidus reported by Zerbe and Robertson (18) and were much higher than those observed in patients with either acute or chronic renal failure (19). Therefore, it can be assumed that impaired urine concentration ability observed in our patients was due to tubular dysfunction secondary to meticillin-induced chronic tubulo-interstitial lesions rather than to renal insufficiency.

In addition to impaired urine concentration ability, patient 1 had an hyperchloremic metabolic acidosis which seems too severe to be ascribed to the mild decrease in glomerular filtration rate (15). Moreover, bicarbonate loading was followed by an abnormally low increase in urinary pCO_2. Although Fillastre et al. (20) have shown that urinary pCO_2 did not rise enough above arterial pCO_2 in nine patients with chronic renal insufficiency, all their patients had a severe reduction of glomerular filtration rate with creatinine clearance between 5 and 19 ml/mn. Therefore, we do not think that the mild renal insufficiency present in our patient could account for the abnormal response to bicarbonate loading ; indeed, such an abnormal response is considered to be the most sensitive index of decreased distal tubular acidification (21), and several authors considered that it allows a diagnosis of distal renal tubular acidosis even in some patients retaining an intact capacity to lower their urinary pH (22,23).

In conclusion, our observations show that meticillin-induced interstitial nephritis may follow a chronic course and be responsible for protracted distal tubular dysfunctions such as impairment of urine concentration ability and distal tubular acidosis.

REFERENCES

1. G.B. Appel, A decade of penicillin related acute interstitial nephritis - more questions than answers, Clin. Nephrol. 13:151 (1980).

2. D.S. Baldwin, B.B. Levine, R.T. McCluskey and G.R. Gallo, Renal failure and interstitial nephritis due to penicillin and methicillin, New Engl. J. Med. 279:1245 (1968).
3. C. Mayaud, A. Kanfer, O. Kourilsky and J.D. Sraër, Interstitial nephritis after methicillin (letter to the Editor), New Engl. J. Med. 292:1132 (1975).
4. J. Ditlove, P. Weidmann, M. Bernstein and S.G. Massry, Methicillin nephritis, Medicine 56:483 (1977).
5. D. Kleinknecht, A. Kanfer, L. Morel-Maroger and J.Ph. Méry, Immunologically mediated drug-induced acute renal failure, Contr. Nephrol. 10:42 (1978).
6. A.J. Woodroffe, N.M. Thomson, R. Meadows and J.R. Lawrence, Nephropathy associated with methicillin administration. Austr. N. Z. J. Med. 4:256 (1974).
7. W.A. Border, D.H. Lehman, J.D. Egan, H.J. Sass, J.E. Glode and C.B. Wilson, Anti-tubular basement membrane antibodies in methicillin-associated interstitial nephritis. New Engl. J. Med. 291:381 (1974).
8. C.M. Nolan and R.S. Abernathy, Nephropathy associated with methicillin therapy, Arch. Intern. Med. 137:997 (1977).
9. D. Ellis, W.A. Fried, E.J. Yunis and E.B. Blau, Acute interstitial nephritis in children : a report of 13 cases and review of the literature, Pediatrics 67:862 (1981).
10. M.C. Cogan and A.I. Arieff, Sodium wasting, acidosis and hyperkalemia induced by methicillin interstitial nephritis, Amer. J. Med. 64:500 (1978).
11. W.B. Schwartz, P.W. Hall, R.M. Hays and A.S. Relman, On the mechanism of acidosis in chronic renal failure, J. Clin. Invest. 38:39 (1958).
12. H.C. Gonick, C.R. Kleeman, M.E. Rubini and M.H. Maxwell, Functional impairment in chronic renal disease II. Studies of acid excretion, Nephron 6:28 (1969).
13. R.L. Tannen, E.M. Regal, M.J. Dunn and R.W. Schrier, Vasopressin-resistant hyposthenuria in advanced renal disease, New Engl. J. Med. 280:1135 (1969).
14. M.A. Holliday, T.J. Egan, C.R. Morris, A.S. Jarrah and J.L. Harrah, Pitressin-resistant hyposthenuria in chronic renal disease. Amer. J. Med. 42:378 (1967).
15. N.S. Bricker and L. Fine, The renal response to progressive nephron loss, in "The Kidney", B.M. Brenner and F.C. Rector, ed., Saunders, Philadelphia (1981).
16. G. Conte, A. Dal Canton, G. Fuiano, M. Terribile, M. Sabbatini, M. Balletta, P. Stanziale and V.E. Andreucci, Mechanism of impaired urinary concentration in chronic primary glomerulonephritis, Kidney Int. 27:792 (1985).
17. N.S. Bricker, R.R. Dewey, H. Lubowitz, J. Stokes and T. Kirkensgaard, Observations on the concentrating and diluting mechanisms of the diseased kidney, J. Clin. Invest. 38:516 (1959).
18. R.L. Zerbe and G.L. Robertson, A comparison of plasma vasopressin measurements with a standard indirect test in the differential diagnosis of polyuria, New Engl. J. Med. 305:1539 (1981).
19. W. Pruszczynski, H. Caillens, L. Drieu, L. Moulonguet-Doleris and R. Ardaillou, Renal excretion of antidiuretic hormone in healthy subjects and patients with renal failure, Clin. Sci. 67:307 (1984).
20. J.P. Fillastre, R. Ardaillou and G. Richet, pH et pCO2 urinaires en réponse à une surcharge alcaline au cours de l'insuffisance rénale chronique, Nephron 6:91 (1969).
21. M.L. Halperin, M.B. Goldstein, A. Haid, M.D. Johnson and B.J. Stinebaugh, Studies on the pathogenesis of type 1 (distal) renal tubular acidosis as revealed by the urinary pCO2 tensions, J. Clin. Invest. 49:596 (1974).
22. D. Battle, M. Grupp, M. Gaviria and N.A. Kurtzman, Distal renal tubular acidosis with intact capacity to lower urinary pH, Amer. J. Med. 72:751 (1982).

23. M.L. Halperin, M.B. Goldstein, R.M.A. Richardson and B.J. Stinebaugh, Distal renal tubular acidosis syndromes : a physiopathological approach, Amer. J. Nephrol. 5:1 (1985).

CONTRAST-INDUCED ACUTE RENAL FAILURE

Vito M. Campese and Kunitoshe Iseki

Division of Nephrology, Department of Medicine
University of Southern California
Los Angeles, California 90033

INTRODUCTION AND INCIDENCE

Acute renal failure (ARF) can occur after radiologic procedures involving administration of contrast agents for angiography, intravenous urography (IVU), oral cholecystography, cholangiography and computerized tomography (CAT). However, the true incidence of this untoward effect is unknown. Large retrospective reviews, indicate that the incidence of contrast induced acute renal failure in the general population is low, being probably, greater for angiography (0.53%) than for IVU or CAT (0.15%) (1). In some series, the incidence of ARF after angiographic studies was as high as 13% (2-3). The greater incidence of renal complications following angiography may be the result of higher intrarenal concentration of contrast agent or of cholesterol embolization. These retrospective analysis, however, tend to underestimate the true incidence of this complication, since they include only the more serious cases requiring further medical attention but not the majority of cases with only mild and transitory rise in serum creatinine.

There are, unfortunately, only few prospective studies addressing this issue. In these studies the criteria usually used to determine renal failure is a rise in serum creatinine greater than 1 mg/dl or doubling of serum creatinine. These studies indicate that the prevalence of contrast induced renal failure may vary in relation to type of procedure (i.e., angiography vs IVU and/or presence of risk factors. In these prospective studies and in the absence of well identified risk factors, the incidence of contrast induced ARF is approximately 0.6% after IVU and 2% after angiography (1).

The incidence of this complication appears to be increasing. This is partially due to increased physician awareness of this complication and partially to the ever increasing use of radiological procedures with contrast agents even in patients with definite risk factors for contrast induced ARF.

RISK FACTORS

The prevalence of contrast induced ARF varies in relationship with the presence of risk factors (See Table I). Some of these factors are presently well recognized as definite predisposing conditions for ARF. Among those are, prexisting renal insufficiency, volume depletion, diabetes mellitus, multiple myeloma, hypoxia and previous radiocontrast induced ARF.

There is, however, a multitude of other factors which have been occasionally found to be present in concomitance with the onset of contrast induced acute renal failure and that are, therefore, considered as possible risk factors.

TABLE 1

RADIOCONTRAST-INDUCED ACUTE ENAL FAILURE
RISK FACTORS

Definite Risk Factors

1. Pre-existing Renal Failure
2. Volume Depletion
3. Diabetes Mellitus
4. Multiple Myeloma
5. Hypoxia
6. Previous Radiocontrast Induced ARF

Possible Risk Factors

1. Arteriosclerotic Vascular Disease
2. Congestive Heart Failure
3. Concomitant Administration of Other Nephrotoxic Agents
4. NSAID
5. Advanced AGe
6. Contrast Load
7. Ionic Composition and Osmolality of Contrast Agent
8. Cardiovascular Instability
9. Impaired Liver Function
10. Hypercalcemia
11. Vasculitis
12. Proteinuria
13. Uricosuria

Pre-existing Renal Failure

Pre-existing renal failure is undoubtedly the major risk factor for contrast induced ARF. Most of the retrospective surveys of this complication support this notion. More than 90% of the cases reported in the literature involve patients with previously impaired renal function. In the last few years a few prospective studies have addressed this problem and they have clearly demonstrated that there is a significant correlation between the incidence of contrast induced ARF and the degree of pre-existing renal failure. This incidence is of 1-2% in patients with mild renal insufficiency (serum creatinine < 1.5 mg/dl) (4-10); it is approximately 20% in patients with moderate renal failure (serum creatinine between 1.5 and 4.5) (4,11) and it increases to 63% in patients with serum creatinine than 4.5 mg/dl, (Fig 1) (4,11-2).

In the majority of these cases renal function returns to baseline levels. However, a substantial number of patients may experience acute oliguric renal failure and some of them may require permanent hemodialysis.

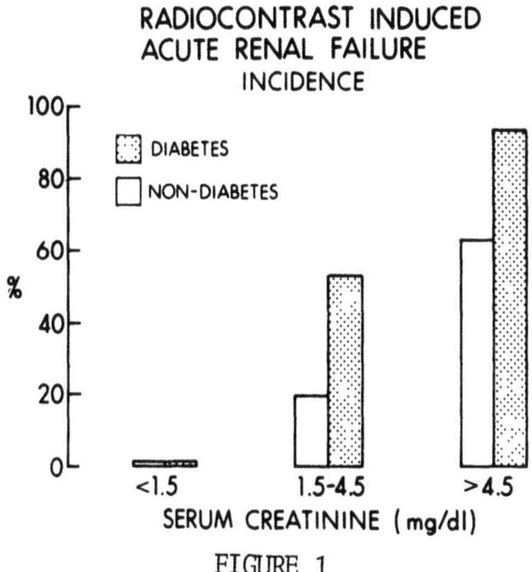

FIGURE 1

Prevalence of Radiocontrast Induced Acute Renal Failure in Diabetic and Non-Diabetic patients with various degrees of renal insufficiency

Volume Depletion

Both clinical and experimental evidence support the notion that volume depletion may be a risk factor for the development of contrast induced acute renal failure (7,13).

Intarenal injection of diatrizoate in sodium depleted dogs decreased renal blood flow by 42% as compared to a fall of 12% in volume repleted dogs (14). These data indicate that sodium depletion accentuates the magnitude and duration of the vasoconstrictive phase of the renal blood flow response to injection of contrast medium and this may be an added risk factor in already predisposed patients.

This is not to say, however, that contrast induced ARF cannot occur in the absence of volume depletion. Indeed, renal failure following IVU or angiography can occur in well hydrated patients (1,4-5, 11, 15-16), however, adequate hydration prior to radiocontrast studies should be always performed since it can reduce the incidence and the severity of this complication.

Diabetes Mellitus

Diabetes mellitus is well recognized risk for developing contrast induced ARF. The large majority of cases of contrast induced ARF reported in the literature involves diabetic patients. Recent prospective studies have clearly indicated that diabetic patients in the absence of renal failure do not appear to be at increased risk (4,16) (Fig 1). However, in the presence of renal insufficiency, diabetic patients appear to be at greater risk than non-diabetic patients with similar degrees of renal insufficiency. Our review of several published prospective studies has shown that the incidence of ARF is of 53% (26 out of 49 cases) in patients with serum creatinine between 1.5 and 4.5 mg/dl and of 94% (30 out of 32 cases) in patients with serum creatinine greater than 4.5 mg/dl (4,9-10,16-18).

Patients of less than 40 years of age with type I diabetes mellitus appear to be even at greater risk of developing contrast induced ARF and more than 50% of them may have irreversible renal damage (16).

Multiple Myeloma

Multiple myeloma is a well recognized risk factor for the development of contrast induced ARF (19). The incidence of this complication in myeloma patients has decreased substantially since the recognition that volume depletion is a concurrent extremely important factor and since the introduction of newer contrast materials such as diatrizoate and its isomers which have less protein binding capacity than the older contrast agents (20). Myers and Whitten (21) described only 2 cases of ARF out of 201 patients with multiple myeloma who underwent IVU, and both of these cases had preexisting renal insufficiency. Thus, even though multiple myeloma has still to be considered a risk factor, it is clear that if appropriate precautions are taken to avoid studies in volume deplete patients or in subject with already impaired renal function, the incidence of this complication will remain very low.

Hypoxia

Hunt et al (22) have shown that diatrizoate has significant direct toxic effect on rabbit proximal tubule cells and it potentiates the degree of tubule cell injury induced by hypoxia. These experimental findings strongly suggest the possibility that the combination of these two factors in clinical situations might be particularly detrimental to the kidneys and warrant the need for caution in using these agents in all clinical situations that may lead to renal tissue hypoxia.

Other Possible Risk Factors

In table I we have listed a multitude of other factors which have been shown to be present in some cases of contrast induced ARF. A cause - effect relationship for most of these factors has not been clearly established.

PATHOGENESIS

The pathogenesis of contrast induced acute renal failure is not clear. However, several mechanisms have been implicated.

Tubular Injury

Several lines of evidence indicate that radiocontrast agents may be directly toxic to proximal renal tubule epithelial cells. First, urinary excretion of several brush border enzymes such as LDH, SGOT, CPK, catalase and alkaline phosphatase increase after administration of radiocontrast agents (23-24). PAH extraction is also impaired (23,25). Second, Humes et al (26) have shown that diatrizoate produced significant declines in K^+, ATP, total adenine nucleotides, tubular basal and uncoupled respiratory rates and an increase in Ca^{++} content in rabbit proximal tubule segments, demonstrating a direct toxic effect of this compound on renal tubular cells; these toxic effects are more prominent during hypoxia. Meglumine, a cation frequently added to diatrizoate containing radiocontrast media, also manifested a moderate renal effect on renal epithelial cells and aggravated the tubular injury produced by diatrizoate (26). Third, renal cortical mithochondrial oxygen consumption supported by succinate and pyruvate-malate was inhibited in a dose-dependent manner by diatrizoate (22). Finally, hypertonic contrast agents induce vacuolization in the cytoplamsa of the renal proximal tubular cells, similar to the "Osmotic Nephrosis" described after administration of mannitol (27-28). Similar changes have been found after administration of low osmolality agents, such as metrizamide, hexabrix and iopamidol (26). These changes appear to be non specific and not directly related to the development of renal toxicity.

Tubular Precipitation of Proteins

It has been suggested that intratubular precipitation of radiocontrast agents with proteins may result in intratubular obstruction and be partly responsible for the radiocontrast induced ARF.

This mechanism is thought to be the major factor responsible for radiocontrast induced acute renal failure in patients with multiple myeloma (20), but its importance in causing renal failure in other clinical conditions is unclear. No correlation has been found between urinary protein excretion and degree of renal impairment in these patients (11,16). Ionic contrast agents can cause a 1,000 fold increase in urinary albumin excretion during the first hour after nephroangiography (29). The nonionic metrizamide caused the same degree of albuminuria than the ionic agents (30). Iohexol, however, has been shown to produce less albuminuria and probably cause less incidence of renal failure (29). More recently, White et al (31) have shown in vitro that diatrizoate interacts with renal tubule and membrane components, to produce a denser and more precipitable tubule protein pellet which may ultimately result in intrarenal obstruction. Other studies have also shown that radiocontrast media precipitate with Tamm-Horsfall proteins (32). These studies support the notion that intratubular precipitation of radiocontrast protein aggregates may contribute to the pathogenesis of radiocontrast induced acute renal failure.

Changes in Renal Hemodynamics

Radiocontrast agents cause immediate and pronounced changes in renal hemodynamics that may play an important pathophysiologic role in the genesis of radiocontrast induced acute renal failure. These agents cause an initial transient vasodilation followed by more prolonged vasoconstriction and decrease in renal blood flow. The decrease in renal blood flow correlates with the osmolality of the contrast media and can be induced by administration of hyperosmolar saline (33). Newer low osmolality contrast media, such as sodium meglumide (1102 mOsm/1) (34) or metrizamide (593 mOsm/1) (35) caused less decrease in renal blood flow than diatrizoate (1455 mOsm/1). The vasconstrictive response is unique for the renal circulation; all other vascular beds respond with vasodilatation. Blockage of the renin-angiotensin system with the renal artery infusion of saralasin, did not alter the magnitude but it decreased the duration of the vasoconstrictive response (13). Recent studies have shown that calcium is important in the vasoconstrictive phase associated with radiocontrast administration. In fact, verapamil, diltiazem or EGTA, significantly reduced the magnitude and duration of renal vasconstriction (36). Sodium depletion accentuates both the magnitude and duration of the vasoconstrictive phase of the renal blood flow response to radiocontrast media (14).

Contrast agents have also been shown to cause rigidification and clumping of red blood cells leading to increased blood viscosity (37). This factor, combined with the decrease in renal blood flow, may cause renal ischemia and decreased glomerular filtration rate. Newer contrast agents with lower osmolality are less likely to cause rigidification of red blood cells and to impair renal microcirculation.

Katzberg et al (38), have demonstrated that administration of contrast media in normal euvolemic dogs, caused a reduction in both glomerular filtration rate and filtration fraction, which coincided with the decrease in renal perfusion. These hemodynamic effects were attenuated by the use of low osmolality and non-ionic contrast agents. These investigators interpreted these hemodynamic changes to indicate an increase in intratubular pressure caused by the hypertonicity of contrast media, rather than renal vasoconstriction.

Uricosuria

Since contrast media increase uricosuria, it has been postulated that this mechanism may be important in the pathophysiology of contrast induced ARF (16). The evidence supporting this concept is, however, not very strong.

Oxaluria

Contrast media increase the urinary excretion of oxalate and it has been suggested that this may play a role in the genesis of radiocontrast-induced ARF (6). Like for the uricosuria, the evidence supporting this notion is weak.

Immunological

Occasionally, acute renal failure may ensue as a consequence of hypersensitivity reaction to radiocontrast agents (39-40). In these cases, ARF is associated with skin rash, eosinophilia, bronchospasm etc. However, this is an infrequent occurrence; therefore, immunologic mechanisms do not appear to play an important pathophysiologic role in most patients with radiocontrast induced ARF.

It has been suggested that radiocontrast agents can precipitate allograft rejection. In one study, 20 of 22 patients with this complication improved after intravenous administration of methylprednisolone (41,42). Serum complement was abnormal in the majority of these patients suggesting a mechanism involving activation of the complement system (43).

CLINICAL COURSE

In the great majority of cases, radiocontrast-induced ARF is characterized by a transitory non oliguric renal failure. Serum creatinine usually rises within 24 hours following the procedures, peaks on the fourth or fifth day and returns to baseline values by the 10-14th day.

Oliguric occurs in approximately 10% of cases and is more frequent in patients with pre-existing moderate to severe renal insufficiency and in diabetics. In patients with advanced renal failure, particularly in dia-

TABLE 2

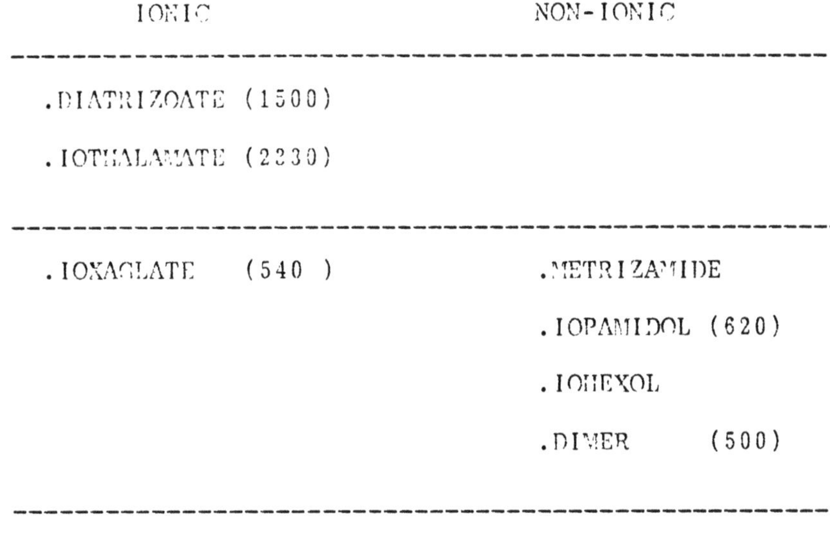

IONIC	NON-IONIC
.DIATRIZOATE (1500)	
.IOTHALAMATE (2230)	
.IOXAGLATE (540)	.METRIZAMIDE
	.IOPAMIDOL (620)
	.IOHEXOL
	.DIMER (500)

In Brackets are the Osmolalities (mmol/kg H_2O)

betics, permanent renal failure may ensue in approximately 50% of cases. The diagnosis of radiocontrast induced renal failure is usually assessed by a rise in serum creatinine within 24-48 hours after the procedures. Hartmann et al (24) have suggested that measurement of urinary excretion of alkaline phosphate on the day of the contrast medium injection and on the following day, can be useful for the early detection of tubular lesions caused by radiocontrast agents. This brush-border enzyme is considered to be a much more sensitive index of renal tubular damage. A positive nephrogram at 24 hours is also considered an indicator of nephrotoxicity.

Urinary indices may be of some help in the diagnosis. Fang et al (45) have observed consistently low urinary sodium and fractional excretion of sodium (FE_{Na}) during the oliguric phase of ARF in 12 patients. Shafi et al (11), however, did not find consistently low FE_{Na} in patients with contrast induced ARF.

In patients with complex clinical disorders, the diagnosis may occasionally be not straight forward and other possibilities have to be considered. Cholesterol embolization may occur as a result of angiographic studies in patients with severe arteriosclerotic vascular disease. In these cases the diagnosis of contrast induced ARF can be mistakenly made (46-47).

Low-Osmolality and Non-Ionic Contrast Media

Most radiological contrast media used for the last 30 years are sodium or meglumine salts of substituted triiodinate benzoic acid. These salts in solution dissociate into one anion (the benzoic acid derivative) and one cation (sodium or meglumine). Since the solutions used for radiocontrast studies are highly concentrated, it derives that the osmolality of these solutions is extremely high (Table 2). Since most of the side effects of radiocontrast agents are due to the very high osmolality, attempts have been made to develop non-ionic low-osmolality agents.

The first of these agents to be introduced was metrizamide. This agent, however, is prepared in lyophilized powder, which needs to be dissolved at the time of each study, and is approximately 25 times more expensive than the conventional contrast agents. More recently, two non-ionic low osmolality contrast agents (iopamidol and Iohexol) and one ionic low-osmolality (ioxaglate) (47) and one non-ionic dimer (48) have been developed. These newer agents have certain definite advantages. They are painless, and they cause less vasodilation, cardiac depression and blood cell aggregates than the conventional hyperosmolar agents.

It has been speculated that these newer contrast agents may have less renal toxicity; however, the data supporting this concept are still scanty. Multicenter randomized studies are needed to ascertain whether the incidence of ARF in high risk patients is substantially reduced by these newer more expensive (3-5 times) agents.

REFERENCES

1. Byrd, L., Sherman, R.L.: Radiocontrast-induced acute renal failure: A clinical and pathophysiologic review. Medicine 58:270-279, 1979.
2. Older, R.A., Miller, J.P., Jackson, D.C., Johnsrude, I.S., Thompson, W.M.: Angiographically induced renal failure and its radiographic detection. Am. M. Roentgenol. 126:1039-1045, 1976.
3. Swartz, R.D., Rubin, J.E., Leeming, B.W., Silva, P.: Renal failure following major angiography. Am. J. Med. 65:31-37, 1978.
4. Van Zee, B.E., Hoy, W.E., Talley, T.E., Jaenike, J.R.: Renal injury associated with intravenous pyelography in nondiabetic and diabetic patients. Ann. Intern. Med. 89:51-54, 1978.
5. Diaz-Buxo, J.A., Wagoner, R.D., Hattery, R.R., Palumbo, P.J.: Acute renal failure after excretory urography in diabetic patients. Ann. Intern. Med. 83:155-158, 1975.
6. Gelman, L.M., Rowe, J.W., Coggins, C.H.: Effects of an angiographic contrast agent on renal function. Cardiovasc. Med. 4:313-320, 1979.
7. Eisenberger, R.L., Bank, W.D., Hedglock, M.W.: Renal failure after major angiography. Am. J. Med. 68:43-46, 1979.
8. D'elia, J., Alday, M., Gleason, R., Malarick, C., Clouse, M., Kaldany, A., Weinrauch, L.: Acute renal failure following angiography. Prospective study of 150 patients, preliminary results. Proc. Clin. Dial. Transplant Forum 8:123-124, 1978.
9. Cramer, R.C., Parfrey, P.S., Hutchinson, T.A., Baran, D., Melanson, D.M., Ethier, R.E., Seely, J.F.: Renal function following infusion of radiologic contrast material. A prospective controlled study. Arch. Intern. Med. 145:87-89, 1985.
10. Kumar, S., Hull, J.D., Lathi, S., Cohen, A.J., Pletka, P.G.: Low incidence of renal failure after angiography. Arch. Int. Med. 141: 1268-1270, 1981.
11. Shafi, T., Chou, S., Porush, J.G., Shapiro, W.B.: Infusion intravenous pyelography and renal function. Arch. Intern. Med. 138:1218-1221, 1978.
12. Milman, N., Gottlieb, P.: Renal function after high-dose Urography in patients with chronic renal insufficiency. Clin. Nephrol. 7:250-254, 1977.
13. Dudzinski, P.J., Petrone, A.F., Persoff, V., Callaghan, E.E.: Acute renal failure following high dose excretory urography in dehydrated patients. J. Urol. 106:619-621, 1971.
14. Larson, T.S., Hudson, K., Mertz, J.I., Romero, J.C., Knox, F.G.: Renal vasoconstrictive response to contrast medium. The role of sodium balance and the renin-angiotension system. J. Lab. Clin. Med. 101:385-391, 1983.
15. Barshay, M.D., Kaye, J.H., Goldman, R., Coburn, J.W.: Acute renal

failure in diabetic patients after infusion pyelography. Clin. Nephrol. 1:35-39, 1973.
16. Harkonen, S., Kjellstrand, C.: Contrast nephropathy. Am. J. Nephrol. 1:69-77, 1981.
17. Teruel, J.L., Marcen, R., Onaindia, J.M., Serrano, A., Quereda, C., Ortuno, J.: Renal function impairment caused by intravenous urography. A prospective study. Arch. Int. Med. 141:1271-1274, 1981.
18. Weinrauch, L.A., Healy, R.W., Leland, O.S., Goldstein, H.H., Kassissieh, S.D., Libertino, J.A., Takacs, F.J., D'Elia, J.A.: Coronary angiography and acute renal failure in diabetic azotemic nephropathy. Ann. Intern. Med. 86:56-59, 1977.
19. Ansari, Z., Baldwin, D.S.: Acute renal failure due to radiocontrast agents. Nephron 17:28-40, 1976.
20. De Fronzo, R.A., Humphrey, R.L., Wright, J.R., Cook, C.R.: Acute renal failure in multiple myeloma. Medicine 54:209-223, 1975.
21. Myers, G.H., Witten, D.M.: Acute renal failure after excretory urography in multiple myeloma. Am. J. Roentgenol. 113:583-588, 1971.
22. Hunt, D.A., Molden, M.C., Humes, H.D.: The effect of radiocontrast agent diatrizoate, on the function of critical renal membranes. 18th Ann. Meet. Am. Soc. Nephrol., Dec. 15-18, 1985, 153A.
23. Talner, L.B., Rushman, H.N., Coel, M.N.: The effect of renal artery injection of contrast material on urinary enzyme excretion. Invest. Radiol. 7:311-322, 1972.
24. Hartmann, H.G., Braedel, H.E., Jutzler, G.A.: Detection of renal tubular lesions after abdominal aortography and selective renal arteriography by quantitative measurements of brush-border enzymes in the urine. Nephron 39:95-101, 1985.
25. Norby, L.H., DiBona, G.F.: The renal vascular effects of meglumine diatrizoate. J. Pharmacol. Exp. Ther. 193:932-940, 1975.
26. Humes, H.D., Hunt, D.A., Tekkanat, K., Holden, M.C.: Toxic effects of n-methylglucosamine on rabbit proximal tubule segments. Am. Soc. Clin. Invest., 1985.
27. Moreau, J.F., Droz, D., Noel, L.H., et al: Tubular nephrotoxicity of water-soluble iodinated contrast media. Invest. Radiol. 15 (Suppl) S54-S60, 1980.
28. Katzberg, R.W., Schulman, G., Meggs, L.G., Caldicott, W.J.H., Damiand, M.M., Hollenberg, N.K.: Mechanism of the renal response to contrast medium in dogs: Decrease in renal function due to hypertonicity. Invest. Radiol. 18:74-80, 1983.
29. Golman, K., Almen, T.: Contrast media-induced nephrotoxicity. Survey and present state. Invest. Radiol. 20:S92-S97, 1985.
30. Holtas, S., Golman, K., Tornquist, C.: Proteinuria following nephroangiography VIII. Comparison between diatrizoate and tohexol in rats. Acta. Radiol. (Suppl) 362:53-56, 1980.
31. White, M.D., Hunt, D.A., Humes, H.D.: Ability of the radiocontrast agent, diatrizoate, to precipitate renal tubules and membranes. 18th Ann. Metting of American Soc. Nephrol. Dec. 15-18, 1985, 163A.
32. Schwartz, R.H., Berdon, W.E., Wagner, H.E., Becker, J., Baker, O.H.: Tamm-horsfall urinary mucoprotcin precipitation by urographic contrast agents. Am. J. Roentgenol 108:698-701, 1970.
33. Katzberg, R.W., Morris, T.W., Burgener, F.A.: Renal renin and hemodynamic responses to selective renal artery catheterization and angiography. Invest. Radiol. 12:381-388, 1977.
34. Russell, S.B., Sherwood, T.: Monomer/dimer contrast media in the renal circulation: Experimental angiography. Br. J. Radiol. 47:268-271, 1974.
35. Morris, T.W., Katzberg, R.W., Fischer, H.W.: A comparison of the hemodynamic response to metrizamide and meglumine/sodium diatrizoate in canine renal angiography. Invest. Radiol. 13:74-78, 1978.
36. Bakris, G.L., Burnett, J.C., Jr.: A role for calcium in radiocontrast-induced reductions in renal hemodynamics Kidney Int. 27:465-468, 1985.

37. Dean, R.W., Andrew, J.H., Read, R.C.: The red cell factor in renal damage from angiographic media. J. Am. Med. Ass. 187:27-31, 1964.
38. Katzberg, R.W., Pabico, R.C., Morris, T.W., Hayakawa, K., McKenna, B.A., Panner, B.J., Ventura, J.A., Fisher, H.W.: Effects of contrast media on renal function and subcellular morphology in the dog. Invest. Radiol. 21:64-70, 1986.
39. Kleinknecht, D., Deloux, J., Hornberg, J.L.: Acute renal failure after intravenous urography: Detection of antibodies against contrast media. Clin. Nephrol. 2:116-119, 1974.
40. Lasser, E.C.: Etiology of Anaphylactoid Responses: The promise of nonionics. Invest. Radiol. 20 (Suppl):79-82, 1985.
41. Light, J.A., Perloff, L.J., Etheredge, E.E., Hill, G., Spees, E.K.: Adverse effects of meglumine diatrizoate on renal function in the early post-transplant period. Transplantation 20:404-409, 1975.
42. Heidemann, M., Claes, G., Nilson, A.E.: The risk of renal allograft rejection following angiography. Transplantation 21:289-293, 1976.
43. Lang, J.H., Lasser, E.C., Kolb, W.P.: Activation of serum complement by contrast media. Invest. Radiol. 11:303-308, 1976.
44. Kamdar, A., Weidmann, P., Makoff, D.L., Massry, S.G.: Acute renal failure following intravenous use of radiographic contrast dyes in patients with diabetes mellitus. Diabetes 26:643-649, 1977.
45. Fang, L.S.T., Sirota, R.A., Ebert, T.H., Lichtenstein, N.S.: Low fractional excretion of sodium with contrast media induced acute renal failure. Arch. Intern. Med. 140:531-533, 1980.
46. Ramirez, G., O'Neill, W.M., Lambert, R., Bloomer, A.: Cholesterol Embolization, a complication of angiography. Arch. Intern. Med. 138:1430-1432, 1978.
47. Smith, M.C., Ghose, M.K., Henry, A.R.: The clinical spectrum of renal cholesterol embolization. Am. J. Med. 71:174-180, 1981.
48. Almen, T.: Development of nonionic contrast media. Invest. Radiology 20 (Suppl):2-9, 1985.
49. Speck, V., Mutzel, W., Mannesmann, G., Pfeiffer, H., Siefert, H.M.: Pharmacology of noinoic dimers. Invest. Radiol. 15 (Suppl):317-322, 1980.

EFFECTS OF INTRAVENOUS INFUSION OF UROGRAPHIC CONTRAST AGENTS ON GLOMERULAR FILTRATION RATE, SERUM CONCENTRATION AND URINARY EXCRETION OF URIC ACID IN SUBJECTS WITH NORMAL RENAL FUNCTION

C. Jacobs, D. Nicolay, J. Grellet, Ph. Curet
and A. Jardin

Hôspital de La Pitié 83, Boulevard de l'Hôspital
75013 Paris, France

INTRODUCTION

The utilization of modern triiodinated radiocontrast agents for intravenous urography (IVU) is widely considered as a very safe procedure in patients free of currently well defined risk factors, amongst which the prominent ones are preexisting renal disease and diabetes mellitus complicated by deteriorated renal function (1,2,3). Whereas the incidence of nephrotoxicity accidents is extremely low in patients with no preexisting renal insufficiency, the risk of an acute, and sometimes definitive, deterioration of renal function following administration of radiocontrast agents has been evaluated as high as 90 % in insulin dependent diabetic patients with severe preexisting renal impairment (1).

The pathogenesis of the nephrotoxic accidents induced by contrast media remains uncompletely understood. Several separate mechanisms have been set forward, none of which is likely to account for all of the encountered clinical situations. A marked increase of uricosuria attributed to an enhanced tubular secretion of uric acid has been documented in patients with normal renal function following the administration of cholecystographic or cholangiographic agents (4,5). The uricosuric effect of these contrast materials has thus been postulated as a potential cause of nephrotoxicity through obstructive intra-tubular precipitation of uric acid, particularly in dehydrated patients. On the other hand, either no change, or only a moderate increase of urinary uric acid excretion was found after administration of the urographic contrast agent diatrizoate, rendering therefore less plausible a specific role of hyperuricosuria in the genesis of post urography deterioration of renal function (4,5). The purpose of this study is to assess the effect of three commonly used urographic contrast agents on serum uric acid concentration, urinary excretion of uric acid and creatinine clearance in subjects with normal renal function.

PATIENTS AND METHODS

The study was conducted in 30 hospitalized patients amongst whom 24 had undergone some type of urological operation within two weeks prior to IVU and 6 had been admitted for pre-operative work-up investigations. None of the patients had a history of diabetes or any illness suggestive of a previous derangement of urate metabolism, neither had they received any medication known to interfere with urate metabolism for at least 10 days prior to IVU. There were 19 males and 11 females whose age ranged between 18 and 78 years, their body weight ranged between 44 and 82 kgs. On the day preceding IVU, the patients' serum creatinine concentration did not exceed 133 μmoles per liter, and their serum uric acid concentration was no higher than 420 μmoles/l in males and 360 μmoles/l in females. They were given a standard hospital diet with no limitation in fluid intake during the three days of the study. The intravenous urography was performed around 8 o'clock in the morning, the patients being in a fasting state since midnight. The following contrast agents were injected intravenously as a 15 second bolus in three subgroups of each 10 randomly selected patients :

- sodium diatrizoate + meglumine : (RS 76)[1] : 1.5 ml/kg body weight
- sodium iothalamate : (MED 38)[2] : 1.5 ml/kg B.W.
- sodium diatrizoate : (SH 225)[3] : 1.85 ml/kg B.W.

The dose of iodine administered was thus set at 0.56 g/kg BW for all patients enrolled in the study ; it was only slightly higher than the one used routinely in the X-ray department for excretory urography in patients with normal renal function.

The serum concentrations and 24 hour urinary eliminations of urea, electrolytes, creatinine and urate were determined on the day prior to intravenous urography (D-1), day of investigation (D0) and the day after (D+1). The D0 blood samples were drawn about one hour after injection of the contrast agent.

Serum and urine urea, electrolytes and creatinine were measured with standard autoanalyzer techniques (Technicon[R]). Serum concentration and urinary output of uric acid were determined with the uricase method. Clearance calculations were made using Van Slyke's standard formula and statistical calculations with the Student's t test, the level of significance being set at 5 %.

RESULTS

The serum creatinine and uric acid concentrations as well as the daily urinary excretion of sodium, urea and uric acid recorded in the three subgroups of patients during the three days of data collection are indicated in table I. No significant difference in the serum concentrations of creatinine was evidenced in any of the three subgroups of subjects during the three days of investigation. The serum uric acid concentrations were not found significantly different on D0 and D+1 compared to baseline values in patients investigated with RS 76 and SH 225, whereas the D0 serum urate concentration was found lower than the baseline value in those who received MED 38 (270 $\pm$ 77 vs 282 $\pm$ 8 μmol/l, $p < 0.05$). A significantly higher urine volume on the day following IVU compared to the two preceding days was found only in patients investigated with RS 76 ($p < 0.05$). The 24 hour urinary sodium excretion was similar over the three days of the study in the patients who had received RS 76 and MED 38, but higher on D0 vs D-1 in those injected with SH 225 (146 $\pm$ 36 vs 115 $\pm$ 38 mmol, $p < 0.05$). The daily urinary urea excretion was found higher on D+1 compared to the two preceding days in the subgroup patients investigated with RS 76 ($p < 0.01$) and stable over the three days of urine collection in the two otners. The 24 hour urinary elimination of uric acid was found

1 - Radiosélectan 76 (Schering laboratories)
2 - Médiocontrix 38 (Guerbet laboratories)
3 - Urografine S (Schering laboratories)

Table I : Serum creatinine and urate concentrations, daily urinary excretion of sodium, urea and urate (mean ± SD) in patients undergoing intravenous urography.

	RS 76 (N = 10)			MED 38 (N = 10)			SH 225 (N = 10)		
	D-1	DO (IVU)	D+1	D-1	DO (IVU)	D+1	D-1	DO (IVU)	D+1
S. CREATININE (umol/l)	88±23	81±27	90±24	88±19	84±17	86±24	101±21	101±19	102±20
S. URATE (umol/l)	268±48	259±77	257±49	282±81	● 270±77	270±83	244±20	241±79	241±76
U. VOLUME (ml/24 H)	1975±826	1911±433	● 2221±707	2115±601	1964±796	2000±628	1965±739	1964±796	2000±624
U. NA/24 H (mmol)	111±47	133±72	142±50	120±36	127±50	126±54	115±38	● 146±36	139±55
U. UREA /24 H (mmol)	333±150	329±100	●●●● 363±150	330±117	330±117	342±115	367±100	417±107	383±132
U. URATE/24 H (umol)	3695±1320	4421±1952	3499±345	3415±1005	3885±1318	●● 3177±1238	4219±1136	5182±1880	●●● 3969±880

RS 76 : sodium diatrizoate + meglumine ; MED 38 : sodium iothalamate ; SH 225 : sodium diatrizoate ;
J0 vs J-1 : ● $p < 0.05$; J+1 vs J0 : ●● $p < 0.05$; ●●● $p < 0.01$; J+1 vs J-1 : ●●●● $p < 0.05$

Table II : Creatinine and urate clearances (mean ± SD) in patients undergoing intravenous urography.

	RS 76 (n = 10)			MED 38 (n = 10)			SH 225 (n = 10)		
	D-1	DO (IVU)	D+1	D-1	DO (IVU)	D+1	D-1	DO (IVU)	D+1
CL. CREATININE (ml/mn)	91 ± 20	97 ± 32	85 ± 24	94 ± 43	96 ± 36	95 ± 29	88 ± 33	88 ± 42	78 ± 25
CL. URATE (ml/mn)	10 ± 4	12 ± 4	10 ± 3	9 ± 3	11 ± 4 ●	9 ± 4	13 ± 5	16 ± 5	12 ± 4 ●●●
CL. URATE / CL. CREATININE x 100	11 ± 4	12 ± 3	12 ± 4	10 ± 4	11 ± 3	●● 9 ± 2	16 ± 6	21 ± 13	17 ± 7

RS 76 : sodium diatrizoate + meglumine ; MED 38 : sodium iothalamate ; SH 225 : sodium diatrizoate
J0 vs J-1 : ● $p < 0.05$; J+1 vs J0 : ●● $p < 0.05$; ●●● $p < 0.01$.

significantly lower on D+1 vs D0 (but not vs the baseline values) in the two subgroups of patients who received MED 38 and SH 225 ($p < 0.05$ and < 0.01, respectively). The average daily urinary elimination of urate (5182 μmoles) was found slightly higher on D0 than the upper normal range (5000 μmoles) in patients investigated with SH 225, with however wide individual variations.

No significant difference was observed in any of the three subgroups of patients regarding the creatinine clearance values on D0 and D+1 compared to their respective baseline levels (Table II). The uric acid clearance was found significantly higher on D0 vs D-1 in patients injected with MED 38 (11 ± 4 vs 9 ± 3 ml/mn, $p < 0.05$) and significantly lower on D+1 vs D0 in those who received SH 225 (12 ± 4 vs 16 ± 5 ml/mn, $p < 0.01$). The uric acid over creatinine clearance ratios were not found statistically different during the three days of the study in patients who received RS 76 and SH 225, whereas a significantly lower value was observed on D+1 vs D0 in those investigated with MED 38 (9 ± 2 vs 11 ± 3 ml/mn, $p < 0.05$) well in accordance with the lower urinary elimination of uric acid recorded in this group of patients on the same day.

DISCUSSION

According to several comprehensive reviews, the overall incidence of an acute deterioration of renal function (with or without oliguria) in patients with no preexisting renal disease does not exceed 0.6 % in those undergoing IVU and 2 % in those submitted to various angiographic procedures (1,2,3). The frequency of radiocontrast nephrotoxicity manifestations which occur in patients with clearly individualized risk factors (mainly preexisting renal insufficiency and diabetes mellitus with deterioration of renal function) remains a matter of debate, ranging, according to the published series, between zero and as high as 80 % of the populations submitted to intravascular administration of radiocontrast agents (1,6,7, 8,9,10). Several mechanisms have been proposed to enlight the pathogenesis of radiocontrast agent nephrotoxicity, none of which appears hitherto clearly unquestionable. A direct tubulotoxic effect of the iodinated contrast materials has been documented in experimental models but its specific role in man remains unproved (11). An acute alteration of the renal microcirculation mediated through the renin angiotensin system or due to an increased blood viscosity and/or erythrocyte aggregration induced by the very strong hypertonicity of the iodinated contrast agents has been advocated by some authors and denied by others (12,13). An intra tubular precipitation of Tamm-Horsfall protein has been documented in vitro and also in some patients with multiple myeloma (14) but its specific responsibility for the majority of cases of acute nephrotoxicity accidents remains to be demonstrated.

Neither hyperuricemia "per se" nor a basically elevated urinary elimination of uric acid are thus far considered as independent risk factors that can be accounted for in the genesis of contrast nephropathy accidents, whatever the underlying level of renal function (2). A marked increase of uricosuria has been reported following the administration of oral cholangiographic contrast agents, raising the possibility that some of the contrast nephropathy accidents might in fact be a manifestation of obstructive urate nephropathy (4,5). However, despite the uricosuric effect of these contrast media, no concomitant alteration of creatinine clearance was evidenced in the series of patients with normal renal function investigated by Postlethwaite and Kelley (5). As for the uricosuric effect of the urographic contrast agent diatrizoate, it was found very weak by these authors and even absent by Mudge (4).

The results observed in the present study do not demonstrate a clear uricosuric effect of three commonly used urographic contrast media in patients with normal renal function. No significant modification of the pre IVU creatinine clearance was recorded in any of the subgroups of patients within the 48 hours that followed the intravenous administration of the three contrast agents. The daily sodium and urea excretion remained also similar to the baseline pre IVU values in two of the three subgroups of patients. The serum uric acid concentration, urinary uric acid elimination, uric acid clearance and $\frac{\text{uric acid}}{\text{creatinine}}$ clearance ratio remained completely unchanged in the subgroup of patients who received sodium diatrizoate + meglumine. A significant decrease in serum uric acid concentration and concomitant increase of uric acid clearance was recorded on D0 only in patients who received sodium iothalamate. Patients investigated with sodium diatrizoate experienced a significant drop of urate elimination and uric acid clearance on D+1 vs D0, but these values returned in fact close to those recorded on the day preceding the IVU.

The significance of the findings presented in this paper should clearly be limited to the conditions under which the study was conducted, i.e. usual doses of triiodinated urographic contrast media administered intravenously to well hydrated subjects with normal renal function and no underlying systemic disease. The magnitude of the uricosuric effect induced by high doses of urographic or angiographic contrast media administered to patients with preexisting renal insufficiency and hyperuricemia has not been documented thus far by a prospective investigation protocol but the well known adverse effect of these procedures on the glomerular filtration rate in these categories of patients (15) certainly renders such a study rather hazardous.

In summary, the intravenous administration of usual doses of commonly used triiodinated urographic contrast agents to well hydrated subjects with normal renal function and no underlying systemic disease, does not cause any decrease of the endogenous creatinine clearance and is followed by only slight modifications of the serum concentration and 24 hour urinary elimination of urate. These findings plead against the role of an hyperuricosuric effect of intravenously administered contrast media in the genesis of post intravenous urography nephrotoxic accidents, at least in patients free of well defined preexisting risk factors.

REFERENCES

1. S. Harkonen and C. Kjellstrand, Contrast nephropathy, Am. J. Nephrol. 1:69 (1981).
2. G. H. Mudge, Nephrotoxicity of urographic radiocontrast drugs, Kidney Int. 18:540 (1980).
3. L. Byrd and R. L. Sherman, Radiocontrast induced acute renal failure. A clinical and pathophysiologic review, Medicine 58:270 (1979).
4. G. H. Mudge, Uricosuric action of cholecystographic agents : a possible factor in nephrotoxicity, N. Engl. J. Med. 284:929 (1971).
5. A. E. Postlethwaite and W. N. Kelley, Uricosuric effect of radiocontrast agents, Ann. Int. Med. 74:845 (1971).
6. S. Kumar, J. D. Hull, S. Lathi, A. J. Cohen and P. G. Pletka, Low incidence of renal failure after angiography, Arch. Int. Med. 141:1268 (1981).
7. B. C. Cramer, P. S. Parfrey, T. A. Hutchinson, D. Baran, D. M. Melanson R. E. Ethier and J. F. Seely, Renal function following infusion of radiographic contrast material. A prospective controlled study, Arch. Int. Med. 145:87 (1985).

8. B. E. Van Zee, W. E. Hoy, T. E. Talley and J. R. Jaenike, Renal injury associated with intravenous urography in non diabetic and diabetic patients, Ann. Int. Med. 89:51 (1978).
9. J. L. Teruel, R. Marcen, J. M. Onaindia, A. Serrano, C. Quereda and J. Ortuño, Renal function impairment caused by intravenous urography, Arch. Int. Med. 141:1271 (1981).
10. J. A. D'Elia, R. E. Gleason, M. Alday, C. Malarick, K. Godley, J. Warram, A. Kaldani and L. A. Weinrauch, Nephrotoxicity from angiographic contrast material, Am. J. Med. 72:719 (1982).
11. L. B. Talner and A. J. Davidson, Effect of contrast media on renal excretion of PAH , Invest. Radiol. 3:301 (1968).
12. S. M. Tadavarthy, W. Castaneda and K. Amplatz, Redistribution of renal blood flow caused by contrast media, Radiology 122:343 (1977).
13. P. Schiantarelli, F. Peroni, P. Turone and G. Rosati, Effects of iodinated contrast media on erythrocytes, Invest. Radiol. 8:199 (1973).
14. R. E. Berdon, R. H. Schwartz, J. Becker and D. H. Baker, Tamm-Horsfall proteinuria : its relationship to prolonged nephrogram in infants and children and to renal failure following intravenous urography in adults with multiple myeloma, Radiology 92:714 (1969).
15. N. Milman and P. Gottlieb, Renal function after high-dose urography in patients with chronic renal insufficiency, Clin. Nephrol. 7:250 (1977).

TUBULAR LESIONS SECONDARY TO CONVENTIONAL UROGRAPHY: A STUDY ON RENAL BIOPSIES BY LIGHT MICROSCOPY

Pasquale Stanziale, Giorgio Fuiano, Mario M. Balletta,
Anna Esposito, Aldo Foscaldi, Luigi Quaranta, and
Vittorio E. Andreucci

Chair of Nephrology
2^ Faculty of Medicine, Naples, Italy

INTRODUCTION

The contrast media generally used for radiologic examination may cause acute renal failure especially in patients with diabetes mellitus, myeloma and/or dehydration or salt depletion[1]. Some authors[2,3,4] have demonstrated that contrast media often cause tubular changes even when renal function is not impaired.

In order to validate this demonstration we have compared the histological changes observed in renal biopsies performed in patients a few days after conventional urography with those of renal biopsies performed in patients in whom no radiologic examination had been performed during the last three months.

METHODS

The study has been performed in 57 patients who underwent a renal biopsy for diagnostic purpose. Only 10 patients (group 1) had not performed any radiologic examination during the last three months: these patients underwent renal biopsy under echographic control. In 47 patients (group 2) an urography was performed with the infusion of contrast media (i.e. meglumine diatrizoate or iothalamate) no longer than five days before the renal biopsy. In particular the interval between urography and renal biopsy was: one day in 8 patients, two days in 4, three days in 9, four days in 8, five days in 18 (Table I).

Table I. Time interval between urography and renal biopsy. In brackets the number of biopsies with evidence of tubular changes.

Days	Cases
1	8 (6)
2	4 (2)
3	9 (2)
4	8 (0)
5	18 (1)

The dosage of contrast media were the following: meglumine diatrizoate 65%, 30-300 ml; iothalamate 66,8%, 30-250 ml; the doses were adjusted to body weight and renal function. Patients affected by systemic disease, metabolic disease or high grade hypertension and those in whom a tubulo-interstitial nephropathy was expected were excluded from this group.

The renal function before the urography and the renal biopsy was moderately reduced (creatinine clearance = 50-70 ml/min) only in 40% of the patients of group 1 and in 36% of the patients of group 2. In all patients creatinine clearance was also evaluated at least one time during the two days after the urography and again at least two times during the next eight days.

Clinical features of patients under study are shown in Table II:

Table II. Clinical features of patients before urography or echography (mean ± SD)

	N	Age	Serum Creatinine	Serum Albumin	Proteinuria
		years	mg/dl	g/dl	g/dl
Urography	47	28.9	1.4	2.7	4.9
SD		15.7	1.0	0.9	3.6
Echography	10	46.7*	1.9	3.0	5.0
		9.0	1.2	0.9	4.3

*$p < 0.005$ with unpaired t test.

Renal biopsy specimens were studied by light microscopy and by immunofluorescence. For light microscopy, two micron sections were stained by the following techniques: hematoxilin-eosin, Masson's thricrome, PAS, silver-metenamine, hematoxilin-Van Gieson.

RESULTS

Histological and immuno-histochemical examinations confirmed in all patients the clinical diagnosis of glomerulonephrites. The distribution of the histologic types of glomerulonephritis in the two groups is reported in Table III:

Table III. Distribution of the histological types of glomerulonephritis (GN) in group 1 (renal biopsies performed under echographic control) and in group 2 (renal biopsies performed soon after urography). In brackets the number of biopsies with evidence of tubular changes.

	Group 1	Group 2
Minimal Changes GN	0	3 (2)
Membranous GN	2	13 (2)
Membrano-proliferative GN	2	13 (4)
Focal sclerosis GN	1	4 (1)
Mesangial-proliferative GN	3	14 (2)
Amyloidosis	1	0
Sjögren's syndrome	1	0

Eleven biopsies of group 2 (23%) showed tubular changes with focal distribution, mainly a cellular cytoplasm vacuolization (fig 1).

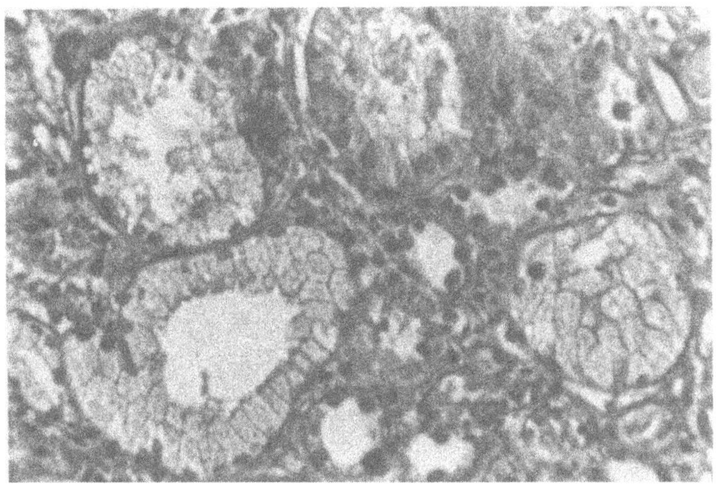

Figure 1

These changes were more extended and intense in proximal tubules in the biopsies performed between the third and the fifth day after urography. The entity and the site of these changes were not correlated with the level of renal function nor with the histological type of glomerulonephritis.

Four patients among those with tubular changes showed a small increase of serum creatinine (+ 25%) which returned to the basal values between four and seven days.

The patients with tubular changes showed clinical features which were not different from those of remaining patients of the same group (Table IV).

Table IV. Clinical data of patients with (A)or without (B)tubular damage after urography

	N	Age	Serum Creatinine	Serum Albumin	Proteinuria
		years	mg/dl	g/dl	g/l
A	11	33.6	1.2	2.2	5.6
± SD		19.3	0.7	0.9	3.5
B	36	27.8	1.5	2.8	4.7
± SD		14 1	1.1	0.9	3.7

No patients in group 1 showed tubular changes or serum creatinine increase after the renal biopsy.

DISCUSSION

The contrast media generally used in radiologic examinations are considered safe because of very low incidence of side effects. Nevertheless, Moreau et al[2] described tubular damage in 22% of the 211 renal biopsies performed after arteriography or urography with i.v. infusion of sodium diatrizoate or iotalamate. These changes were similar to those described by Allen[5] in experimental animals after i.v. infusion of hyperosmolar solution of sugar that he called "osmotic nephrosis". Moreau, however, included in his study patients with metabolic, systemic and tubulo-interstitial diseases; moreover, many renal biopsies were performed after an arteriography, which requires greater dosage of contrast media than urography.

In order to avoid these methodologic limitations, our cases were carefully selected and compared with a control group. Our findings confirm a high incidence of tubular changes (23%) also after urography. The pathogenetic relationship between i.v. infusion of contrast media and tubular damage observed in the renal biopsies is supported by the following observations: (a)no relation was found between tubular changes and renal function or bioptical diagnosis of glomerulonephrites; (b)no tubular changes were found in group 1 (patients who underwent a renal biopsy not preceded by administration of contrast media).

The site and the entity of tubular changes were related to the number of days between urography and renal biopsy. The more extended and intense damage observed in proximal tubules in the first 2 days after the urography may be accounted for by a greater sensitivity of proximal tubules. The slight severity of this tubular damage, however, would allow a rapid regression; this may explain the low grade of changes observed in proximal tubules in renal biopsies performed 3 to 5 days after urography. Distal tubules appear damaged later, but more intensively. Distal tubular lesions were, in fact, observed in biopsies performed between the third and the fifth day after urography. This late appearance of tubular changes could be due to a greater "resistance" of distal structures; the greater entity of changes may be accounted for by the greater concentration of contrast media in the distal tubules secondary to the isoosmotic reabsorption of glomerular filtrate along the proximal tubule.

Our results indicate that contrast media, even if used at relatively low dosage as in urographic examinations, may cause a tubular damage, even when renal function is not apparently impaired.

REFERENCES

1. V.E. Andreucci, Radiocontrast-induced ARF, in "Acute Renal Failure, Andreucci V.E.(ed), Martinus Nijhoff Publ., Boston (1984).
2. J.F. Moreau, D. Droz,J. Sabto, P. Jungers, D. Kleinknecht, N. Hinglais, J.R. Michel, Osmotic nephrosis induced by water-soluble triiodinated contrast media in man, Radiology, 115: 329 (1975).
3. A.B. Grunskin, O.H. Oetliker, N.M. Wolfish, N.L. Gootmann, J.Bernstein, C.M. Edelmann, Effects of angiography on renal function and histology in infants and piglets, Journal of Pediatrics, 76: 41 (1970).
4. S. Harkonen, C.Kijellstrand, Contrast nephropathy, Am J Nephrology, 1: 69 (1981).
5. A.C. Allen, "The Kidney. Medical and surgical disease", Grune and Stratton Publ., New York (1962).

DISEASE ENTITY ASSOCIATED WITH ACUTE RENAL FAILURE

THE HEPATORENAL SYNDROME (HRS)

Murray Epstein

Division of Nephrology
University of Miami School of Medicine and
Veterans Administration Medical Center
Miami, FL 33125

INTRODUCTION

Progressive oliguric renal failure commonly complicates the course of patients with advanced hepatic disease (1,2). While this condition has been designated by many names including "functional renal failure", and "the renal failure of cirrhosis", the more appealing albeit less specific term "hepatorenal syndrome" has been utilized commonly to describe this syndrome. For the purposes of this discussion, the hepatorenal syndrome may be defined as unexplained progressive renal failure occurring in patients with liver disease in the absence of clinical, laboratory, or anatomic evidence of other known causes of renal failure.

A. Clinical Features

A review of the clinical features of HRS reveals marked variability regarding both the clinical presentation and clinical course (1,2). In the United States, the HRS occurs usually in cirrhotic patients who are alcoholic, although cirrhosis is not a sine qua non for the development of HRS. HRS may complicate other liver diseases including acute hepatitis and hepatic malignancy (3,4,5). Renal failure may develop with great rapidity, often occurring in patients in whom normal serum creatinine levels have been previously documented within a few days of onset of HRS. Recently, Arieff (6) has suggested that the serum creatinine may be a poor index of renal function in patients with chronic liver disease, often masking markedly reduced GFR's. Implicit in such a formulation is the concept that HRS represents a progression in patients who already have markedly impaired renal function.

Numerous reports have emphasized the development of renal failure following events which reduce effective blood volume including abdominal paracentesis, vigorous diuretic therapy and gastrointestinal bleeding, although it can occur in the absence of an apparent precipitating event. In this context, several careful observers have recently noted that HRS patients seldom arrive in the hospital with preexisting renal failure. Rather, HRS seems to develop in the hospital, raising questions as to whether events in the hospital might precipitate this syndrome (1).

Virtually all HRS patients have ascites which is often tense and clinical stigmata of portal hypertension are usually present. The degree of jaundice is extremely variable. Although the majority of reports suggest that the HRS occurs in patients who manifest evidence of severe hepatocellular disease, it is quite apparent that the HRS can occur with minimal jaundice and with little evidence of severe hepatic dysfunction.

The majority of patients have a modest decrease in systemic blood pressure, but significant hypotension occurs usually as a terminal event. Most patients die within three weeks of onset of azotemia, although rare patients have survived for several months with mild azotemia (8).

HRS patients manifest a rather characteristic urine excretory pattern, voiding urine which is practically sodium-free and retaining the capacity to concentrate urine to a modest degree.

B. Pathogenesis

Several lines of evidence have lent strong support to the concept that the renal failure in HRS is functional in nature. Despite the severe derangement of renal function, pathologic abnormalities are minimal and inconsistent (1,2,7). Furthermore, tubular functional integrity is maintained during the renal failure as manifested by an unimpaired sodium reabsorptive capacity and concentrating ability. Finally, more direct evidence is derived from the demonstration that kidneys transplanted from patients with HRS are capable of resuming normal function in the recipient (9).

Despite extensive study, the precise pathogenesis of the HRS remains elusive. Since urinary diagnostic indices suggest intact renal tubular function in HRS, vascular rather than tubular events are felt to be important in the pathogenesis of the renal failure. According to this view, severe afferent arteriolar constriction diminishes glomerular plasma flow and glomerular capillary pressure sufficient to lower effective filtration. In this regard, many studies utilizing diverse hemodynamic techniques have all documented a significant reduction in renal perfusion (10-12). Since a similar reduction of renal perfusion is compatible with urine volumes exceeding one liter in many patients with chronic renal failure (13) it is unlikely that a reduction in mean blood flow per se is responsible for the encountered oliguria.

Our laboratory has applied the 133 Xe washout technique and selective renal arteriography to the study of the HRS and demonstrated a significant reduction in both mean renal blood flow as well as preferential reduction in cortical perfusion (10). In addition, Epstein and coworkers (10) carried out simultaneous renal arteriography to delineate further the nature of the hemodynamic abnormalities. Selective renal arteriograms disclosed marked beading and tortuosity of the interlobar and proximal arcuate arteries, and an absence of both distinct cortical nephrograms and of vascular filling of the cortical vessels. Postmortem angiography carried out on the kidneys of five patients studied previously during life disclosed a striking normalization of the vascular abnormalities with reversal of all the vascular abnormalities in the kidneys. The peripheral vasculature filled completely and the previously irregular vessels became smooth and regular. These findings provide additional strong evidence for the functional basis of the renal failure, operating through active renal vasoconstriction.

Although renal hypoperfusion with preferential renal cortical ischemia has been shown to underly the renal failure of HRS, the factors responsible for sustaining the reductions in cortical perfusion and the suppression of filtration in HRS have not been elucidated. Several major hypotheses have been implicated or suggested, including: a) the renin-angiotensin system; b) alterations in the endogenous release of renal prostaglandins; c) an increase in sympathetic nervous system activity; d) changes in the kallikrein-kinin system; and e) endotoxemia. These proposed mechanisms and their interrelationships are summarized schematically in Figure 1 and Table 1.

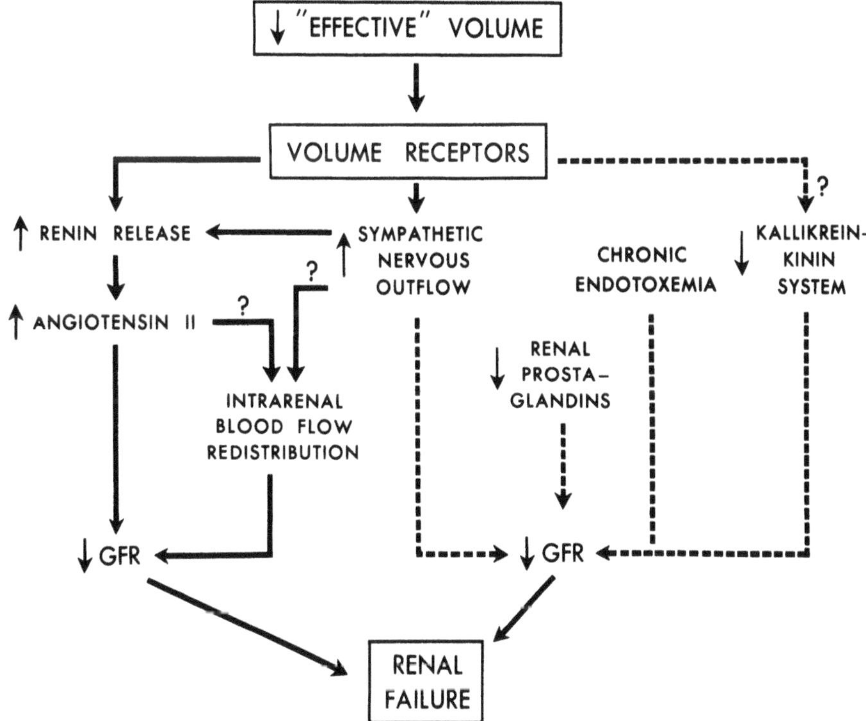

Fig. 1. Schematic representation of possible mechanisms whereby a diminished "effective" volume might modulate a number of hormonal effectors, eventuating in renal failure. The heavy arrows indicate pathways for which evidence is available. The dashed lines represent proposed pathways, the existence of which remains to be established. (Modified from Epstein, M., Ref. 2).

Table 1. Mechanisms Which May Participate In Mediating The Renal Failure Of Liver Disease

1. Activation of the renin-angiotensin system
2. Alteration in renal prostaglandins
3. Alterations in kallikrein-kinin system
4. Increase in sympathetic nervous system activity
5. Systemic endotoxemia
6. Glomerulopressin deficiency
7. Undefined humoral factors

Renin-Angiotensin System

Several lines of evidence have suggested a role for the renin-angiotensin axis in sustaining the vasoconstriction in HRS. Patients with decompensated cirrhosis with or without HRS frequently manifest marked elevations of PRA attributable to both decreased hepatic inactivation of renin and to increased renin secretion by the kidney (14,15). Often, the elevation of PRA occurs despite the presumed failure of hepatic synthesis of the alpha-2 globulin renin substrate. There are at least two alternative explanations for the persistence of high renin levels in cirrhosis. First, it is possible that the renal hypoperfusion is the primary event with a resultant activation of the renin-angiotensin in system. Alternatively, the activation of the renin-angiotensin system (perhaps in response to a diminished effective blood volume) may constitute the primary event. In light of compelling experimental evidence that angiotensin plays an important role in the control of the renal circulation (13), it is tempting to speculate that enhanced angiotensin levels contribute to the renal vasoconstriction and reduction in filtration rate of renal failure in cirrhosis.

Role of Renal Prostaglandins

It is probable that renal prostaglandins participate in mediating the renal failure of cirrhosis (16). Initially, this possibility was assessed by examining the renal hemodynamic response to the administration of exogenous prostaglandins (17). Unfortunately, the relevance of such studies in cirrhotic man is tenuous since recent studies suggest that any action of prostaglandins on the kidney must be as a local tissue hormone (18). Thus, any evaluation of the physiological role of prostaglandins on renal function necessitates an experimental design in which the endogenous production of the lipids is altered. Indeed, subsequent investigations of the role of prostaglandins on renal function have focused on comparisons before and after the administration of inhibitors of prostaglandin synthetase. Such studies have demonstrated that the administration of inhibitors of prostaglandin synthetase (both indomethacin and ibuprofen) resulted in a lowering of PRA and PA and marked decrements in GFR (19,20).

Thromboxanes and Renal Function in Cirrhosis

Studies conducted by Zipser et al (21) suggest that the <u>ratio</u> of the vasodilator prostaglandin E2 to the vasoconstrictor prostaglandin thromboxane A2 (TxA2) (i.e. E2/TxA2) rather than the absolute levels of PGE2 may modulate the renal vasonconstriction of the hepatorenal syndrome. Urinary excretion of PGE_2 and thromboxane B_2 (TxB_2) (the non-enzymatic metabolite of TxA2) were measured in 14 patients with HRS. It was observed that whereas PGE2 levels were decreased in comparison with those of healthy controls and patients with acute renal failure, TxB2 levels were markedly elevated. The authors interpreted their data to suggest that an imbalance of vasodilator and vasoconstrictor metabolites of arachidonic acid contributes to the pathogenesis of HRS. Additional studies are needed to confirm such alterations.

Of interest, there has been a recent attempt to modify the course of HRS by administration of selective inhibitors of thromboxane synthesis (22). Whereas nonspecific cyclooxygenase inhibitors, such as indomethacin and aspirin, reduce both thromboxane and prostaglandin synthesis to varying degrees in different biologic systems, selective inhibitors of thromboxane synthesis preserve or possibly increase the production of other metabolites of arachidonic acid, such as the potent vasodilator prostacyclin. Zipser et al (22) administered the thromboxane synthetase inhibitor, dazoxiben, to patients with alcoholic hepatitis and progressive azotemia. Although administration of dazoxiben reduce the urinary excretion of the thromboxane metabolite, thromboxane B2 (TxB2), by approximately 50%, PGE2 and 6-keto PGF1a were essentially unaltered. Despite reduction in thromboxane excretion, there was no consistent reversal of the progressive renal deterioration (22). Unfortunately, most of the patients had far advanced disease and may not have been capable of responding to therapeutic interventions. Additional studies with selective thromboxane inhibitors in patients with widely varying degrees of acute renal insufficiency will be required to establish definitively the role of thromboxane A2 as a major determinant of the renal vasoconstriction in HRS.

Kallikrein-Kinin System

The available evidence suggests that bradykinin and other kinins synthesized in the kidney may participate in the modulation of intrarenal blood flow and renal function. Measurements of plasma prekallikrein levels in patients with HRS disclosed undetectable levels in many such patients (23), raising the possibility that the decrease in prekallikrein levels results in diminished kinin formation. Since bradykinin has been suggested to be a physiological renal vasodilator, it is possible that failure of bradykinin formation may contribute to the renal cortical vasconstriction encountered in HRS.

Increase in Sympathetic Nervous System Activity

An increase in sympathetic nervous system activity might also contribute to the renal failure of cirrhosis. It is now well established that alteration of the input of cardiopulmonary receptors induces changes in renal sympathetic activity (24). Thus, a decrease in effective blood volume is sensed as a decrease in left atrial pressure (the sensor of the low pressure vascular system). This "unloads" the left atrial mechanoreceptors, wich in turn, discharge into afferent vagal fibers that have appropriate central nervous system representation. As a consequence, efferent renal sympathetic nerve activity is augmented (25). Such an increase in sympathetic tone would tend to produce renal vasconstriction and a decrease in GFR.

Despite such theoretical considerations, data bearing on the importance of alterations in the sympathetic nervous system in cirrhotic man are not conclusive. Early studies by Epstein et al (10) have raised the possibility that adrenergic activity may be enhanced in cirrhosis.

In the course of assessing intrarenal hemodynamics in cirrhotic patients, it was observed that the intrarenal infusion of the alpha adrenergic blocker, phentolamine, failed to increase renal blood flow significantly in cirrhotic patients (10). The failure of phentolamine to enhance renal perfusion was interpreted initially as indicating the absence of increased renal adrenergic tone. Caution is required in reaching such a conclusion, however, since a majority of patients who received an intrarenal infusion of phentolamine manifested transient hypotension with significant reductions in arterial blood pressure. Thus, concomitant alterations in systemic hemodynamics might have masked a phentolamine-induced enhancement of renal perfusion.

Additional support for increased efferent renal sympathetic nerve activity is derived from studies by Gatta et al (26). These investigators demonstrated that an injection into the renal artery of dihydroergocristine, an alpha adrenoceptor antagonist, produced a decrease in renal vascular resistance. Of note, the increases in urine flow rate and sodium excretion were small and insignificant.

During the past 5 years, several investigators have attempted to assess the activity of the sympathetic nervous system in cirrhotic man by measuring plasma catecholamine levels during basal conditions and following postural manipulations. My associates and I (27) and Bichet et al (28) and Henriksen et al (29) have recently reported that patients with advanced cirrhosis and ascites often (but not invariably) manifest elevated concentrations of plasma norepinephrine (NE). We have also assessed kinetically the relationship of plasma catecholamines to changes in renal function during a well-defined volume expansive maneuver i.e., head-out water immersion (30). In response to immersion, many of the patients manifested a striking augmentation of creatinine clearance (Ccr). Only 6 of 15 cirrhotic patients with ascites and/or edema manifested a suppression of NE levels.

An examination of the relationship between norepinephrine levels and renal function disclosed that the increments in Ccr during immersion varied independently of the immersion-induced alterations in plasma NE (as assessed by either basal norepinephrine levels or the extent of norepinephrine suppression) (27). Our findings suggest that the prominent etiologic role for renal vasoconstriction assigned to the sympathetic nervous system by some observers may be overinflated. Rather, it appears more likely that the derangements in renal function are attributable to a panoply of hormonal and neural mediators acting in concert.

In summary, it is apparent that the available data regarding the role of the sympathetic nervous system are suggestive but inconclusive. Clearly, more direct indices of autonomic activity are required to determine whether an increase in sympathetic activity, both in the kidney and in other areas, contributes to the renal failure of cirrhosis.

Endotoxins

It has been proposed that systemic endotoxemia may participate in the pathogenesis of the renal failure of cirrhosis (31). The increased endotoxin levels might result from incomplete hepatic inactivation and portal-systemic shunts of material of gastrointestinal origin in cirrhotic patients. Since several investigators have demonstrated a high frequency of positive Limulus amebocyte lysate (LAL) assays in cirrhotic patients with renal failure, but not in the absence of renal failure, it has been proposed that endotoxins might contribute to the pathogenesis of the renal failure.

Although endotoxemia is frequently observed in patients with chronic liver disease, its role in contributing to the development of renal failure is unclear. Attempts to correlate the occurrence of renal failure with the presence of endotoxemia are conflicting. On the one hand, Clemente et al (32) observed endotoxemia in nine of 22 patients with HRS, but not in cirrhotic patients with a normal GFR. On the other hand, Gatta et al (33) demonstrated that in patients with cirrhosis without overt renal failure, renal vasoconstriction did not seem to be related to endotoxemia.

Coratelli et al (34) have observed two patients before and after the development of HRS and demonstrated the appearance of endotoxemia coicident with the development of HRS.

Elsewhere in this symposium, Amerio and associates will report on their experience with the use of polyacrylonitrile dialyzing membranes in HRS patients and the clinical correlates following a decrease in LAL assay reactivity. The interesting hypothesis regarding the role of endotoxins awaits additional study and confirmation.

Glomerulopressin

Alvestrand and Bergstrom (35) proposed an intriguing and provocative hypothesis to explain the pathophysiology of HRS. They proposed that in normal individuals, the liver produces a hormone (termed glomerulopressin or GP) that is involved in the normal regulation of GFR. These investigators speculated that hepatic failure might result in decreased synthesis of all proteins, including GP. This could eventuate in the relatively unopposed action of vasoconstrictor substances including angiotensin II, norepinephrine, and vasoactive amines with a resultant decrease in GFR and the development of HRS.

Future Progress

Despite major advances, our understanding of the many ways whereby the liver affects normal renal processes is incomplete. The past two decades has witnessed much progress in the delineation of the intrarenal hemodynamic alterations which underly HRS. The numerous attempts at treating HRS empirically with vasodilators has not resulted in significant therapeutic innovations. It is apparent that any future breakthroughs in the definitive treatment of HRS will be predicated on greater clarification of mechanisms and delineation of mediators. Meaningful investigations of the pathogenesis of HRS must include the search for and characterization of vasoactive humoral factors capable of experimentally altering renal function and renal hemodynamics.

REFERENCES

1. S. Papper S, Hepatorenal Syndrome, in: "The Kidney in Liver Disease" M. Epstein, 2. ed Elsevier, New York, pp. 87 (1983).
2. M. Epstein, Hepatorenal syndrome, In: "Bockus Gastroenterology", 4th edition, edited by J.E. Berk, Saunders, Philadelphia, pp.3138 (1985).
3. M. Epstein, J.R. Oster, R.E. DeVelasco, Hepatorenal syndrome following hemihepatectomy. Clin. Nephrol. 5:128 (1976).
4. D.J. Ritt, G. Whelan, D.J. Werner, E.H. Eigenbrodt, S. Schenker,

B. Combes, Acute hepatic necrosis with stupor or coma. Medicine 48:151 (1969).

5. P. Vesin, A. Roberti, R.R. Viguie. Defaillance renale fonctionnell terminale chez des malades atteints de cancer du foie, primitif ou secondaire. Sem. Hop. Paris, 26:1216 (1965).
6. M.A. Papadakis, A.I. Arieff. Progressive deterioration of renal function in non-azotemic cirrhotic patients with ascites: A prospective study. Kidney Int. 27:149 (1985) (Abstract).
7. L. Shear, J. Kleinerman, G.J. Gabuzda, Renal failure in patients with cirrhosis of the liver. I. Clinical and pathologic characteristics. Am. J. Med. 39:184 (1965).
8. H. Goldstein, J.D. Boyle, Spontaneous recovery from the hepatorenal syndrome. Report of four cases. N. Engl. J. Med. 272:895 (1965).
9. M.H. Koppel, J.W. Cobrun, M.M. Mims, H. Goldstein, J.D. Boyle, M.E. Rubini, Transplantation of cadaveric kidneys from patients with hepatorenal syndrome. Evidence for the functional nature of renal failure in advanced liver disease. N. Engl. J. Med. 280:1367 (1969).
10. M. Epstein, D.P. Berk, N.K. Hollenberg, D.F. Admas, T.C. Chalmers, H.L. Abrams, J.P. Merrill, Renal failure in the patient with cirrhosis. The role of active vasoconstriction. Am. J. Med. 49:175 (1970).
11. M.C. Kew, R.R. Varma, H.S. Willimas, P.W. Brunt, K.J. Hourigan, S. Sherlock, Renal and intrarenal blood flow in cirrhosis of the liver. Lancet 2:504 (1971).
12. E.T. Schroeder, L. Shear, S.M. Sancetta, G.J. Gabuzda, Renal failure in patients with cirrhosis of the liver. III. Evaluation of intrarenal blood flow by para-amino-hippurate extraction and response to angiotensin. Am. J. Med. 43:887 (1967).
13. N.K. Hollenberg, M. Epstein, R.I. Basch, D.E. Oken, J.P. Merrill, Acute oliguric renal failure in man: Evidence for preferential renal cortical ischemia. Medicine, 47:455 (1968).
14. N.K. Hollenberg, Renin, angiotensin and the kidney: Assessment by pharmacological interruption of the renin-angiotensin system, In: The Kidney in Liver Disease, 2nd Edition, edited by M. Epstein, Elsevier, New York, pp.395 (1983).
15. E.T. Schroeder, R.H. Eich, H. Smulyan, A.B. Gould, G.J. Gabuzda, Plasma renin level in hepatic cirrhosis. Am. J. Med. 49:186 (1970).
16. M. Epstein, Renal prostaglandins and the control of renal function in liver disease. Am. J. Med. 80: (Suppl 1A)46-55 (1986).
17. A.I. Arieff, C.A. Chidsey, Renal function in cirrhosis and the effects of prostaglandin A1. Am. J. Med. 56:695 (1974).
18. J.C. McGiff, H.D. Itskovitz, Prostaglandins and the kidney. Circ. Res., 33:479 (1973).
19. T.D. Boyer, P. Zia, T.B. Reynolds, Effect of indomethacin and prostaglandin A1 on renal function and plasma renin activity in alcoholic liver disease. Gastroenterology 77:215 (1979).
20. R.D. Zipser, J.C. Hoefs, P.F. Speckart, P.K. Zia, R. Horton, Prostaglandins: modulators of renal function and pressor resistance in chronic liver disease. J. Clin. Endocrinol. Metab. 48:895 (1979).
21. R.D. Zipser, G.H. Radvan, K.J. Kronborg, et al. Urinary thromboxane B2 and prostaglandin E2 in the hepatorenal syndrome: Evidence for increased vasoconstrictor and decreased vasodilator factors. Gastroenterology 84:697 (1983).
22. R.D. Zipser, I. Kronborg, W. Rector, et al. Therapeutic trial of thromboxane synthesis inhibition in the hepatorenal syndrome. Gastroenterology 87:1228 (1984).
23. D.T. O'Connor, and R.A. Stone, The renal kallikrein-kinin system: Description and relationship to liver disease, in: The Kidney in Liver Disease, 2nd ed. M. Epstein, Elsevier, New York pp. 469

(1983).
24. M.D. Thames, Neural control of renal function: Contribution of cardiopulmonary baroreceptors to the control of the kidney. Fed. Proc. 37:1209 (1977).
25. G.F. DiBona, Renal neural activity in hepatorenal syndrome. Kidney Int. 25:841 (1984).
26. A. Gatta, C. Merkel, M. Grassetto, L. Milani, R. Zuin, A. Rual, Enhanced renal sympathetic tone in liver cirrhosis: evaluation by intrarenal administration of dihydroergocristine. Nephron 30:364 (1982).
27. M. Epstein, O. Larios, G. Johnson, Effects of water immersion on plasma catecholamines in decompensated cirrhosis. Implications for deranged sodium and water homeostasis. Mineral & Electrolyte Metab 11:25 (1985).
28. D.B. Bichet, V.J. VanPutten, R.W. Schrier, Potential role of increased sympathetic activity in impaired sodium and water excretion in cirrhosis. New. Engl. J. Med. 307:1552, (1982).
29. J.H. Henriksen, H. Ring-Larsen, I-L Kanstrup, N.J. Christensen., Splanchnic and renal elimination and release of catecholamines in cirrhosis. Evidence of enhanced sympathetic nervous activity in patients with decompensated cirrhosis. Gut. 25:1034 (1984).
30. M.Epstein, Renal effects of head-out water immersion in man. Implications for an understanding of volume homeostasis. Physiol. Rev. 58:529 (1978).
31. H. Liehr, and A.I. Jacob, Endotoxin and renal failure in liver disease, in: The Kidney in Liver Disease, 2nd ed. edited by M. Epstein, Elsevier, New York, pp.535 (1983).
32. C. Clemente, J. Bosch, J. Rodes, V. Arroyo, A. Mas, S. Maragall, Functional renal failure and haemorrhagic gastritis associated with endotoxaemia in cirrhosis. Gut 18:556 (1977).
33. A. Gatta, L. Milani, C. Merkel, R. Zuin, P. Amodio, L. Caregaro, A. Ruol, Lack of correlation between endotoxemia and renal hypoperfusion in cirrhotics without overt renal failure. Eur. J. Clin. Invest. 12:417 (1982).
34. P. Coratelli, G. Passavanti, I. Munno, D. Fumarola, A. Amerio, New trends in hepatorenal syndrome. Kidney Int. 28:S-143 (1985).
35. A. Alvestrand, J. Bergstrom, Glomerular hyperfiltration after protein ingestion, during glucagon infusion, and in insulin-dependent diabetes is induced by a liver hormone: Deficient production of this hormone in hepatic failure causes hepatorenal syndrome. Lancet 1:195 (1984).

ROLE OF ENDOTOXIN IN HEPATORENAL SYNDROME

Giuseppe Passavanti°, Pasquale Coratelli°, Irene Munno, Donato Fumarola and Alberto Amerio°

Institute of Nephrology° and Institute of Microbiology
University of Bari
Bari 70124, Italy

INTRODUCTION

It is known that patients affected by liver cirrhosis may develop functional renal failure induced by circulatory disorder of the kidney, likely due to active vasoconstriction with reduction of cortical perfusion (1), and characterized by reduced glomerular filtration rate with intact tubular function. In fact the urine sodium concentration in these patients is extremely low, usualy less than 10 milliequivalent per liter, and urine sediment is relatively unremarkable. This type of renal failure is called hepatorenal syndrome (HRS) and many factors have been considered in its pathogenesis, including activation of the renin - angiotensin system due to reduced "effective" blood volume (2,3,4), increase in sympathetic nervous system activity (5,6,7,8), alterations in the endogenous release of renal prostaglandins (9,10,11,12,13,14,15) and changes in the kallikrein-kinin system (16).

On the other hand, another factor to be considered in hepatorenal syndrome are endotoxins which may have vasoconstrictive effects on the renal circulation (17,18,19). The endototoxins are lipopolysaccharide components of the cell wall of gram-negative organisms. Bacterial endotoxins of intestinal origin, which may be found in portal blood (20,21), under normal conditions are considered to be detoxified by the liver. The hepatic clearance of endotoxins would appear to be largely a function of the Kupffer cells (22), although some evidence suggests that hepatocytes may also partecipate (23,24). Thus, conditions characterized by a reduced hepatic phagocytic activity (Kupffer cells), and/or the establishment of portal-systemic shunts which subtracts intestinal blood flow from the metabolic and filtering action of the liver, may permit endotoxins to enter the systemic circulation in the absence of a real gram-negative infection and play a role in the pathogenesis of renal failure in cirrhotic patients.

The availability of a sensitive assay to detect circulating endotoxins (25), the Limulus amebocyte lysate (LAL), has stimulated a series of studies designed to detect systemic endotoxaemia in liver disease associated with renal failure.

Thus, our study was performed in order to search clinical and experimental evidences which might support the pathogenetic role of the endotoxins in HRS.

PATIENTS AND METHODS

Fourty-three patients with advanced cirrhosis of the liver and ascites were studied.All had functional renal failure.Urine sodium concentration was not higher than 12 mmol/l,urine to plasma creatinine ratio was 32 and renal failure index 0.42. In none of the 43 patients the development of renal failure appeared secondary to abdominal paracentesis, vigorous diuretic therapy,and gastrointestinal bleeding. None of the patients with endotoxaemia had positive blood and/or urine cultures and none had other evidence of Gram negative infection. The endotoxaemia was therefore related to impaired hepatic clearance of toxins normally absorbed from the gastrointestinal tract.

Thirteen out of 43 patients with a clinical and biochemical pattern of progressive HRS were treated with hemodialysis using a plate dialyzer equipped with a polyacrylonitrile membrane in 9 and with a cuprophane membrane in 4 patients. In all patients submitted to dialytic treatment the LAL test was performed before the insertion of an arteriovenous shunt. In 7 cases of HRS submitted to dialytic treatment the LAL test was performed on pre-dialytic and post-dialytic plasma. Five out of these cases were dialyzed with polyacrylonitrile membrane and in others a cuprophane membrane was employed.

On the other hand, the in vitro study was designed to detect passage of Lipid A and Lypopolysaccaride (LPS) across the dialysis membrane using a previously described experimental procedure (26). In order to evaluate filtration of Lipid A across a cuprophane membrane 500 ml of blood volume were used, to which 1 mg of Salmonella Minnesota R 595 (Re) Lipid A was added, while in the case of a polyacrylonitrile membrane 1000 ml of blood volume were used, to which 2 mg of Salmonella typhimurium LPS were added.

The Limulus clotting activity was measured by LAL (Whittaker Microbiological Associates Bioproducts, Walkersville, Maryland USA). Blood samples collected in endotoxin free vials were centrifuged at 1500 rpm for 10 min and the platelet rich plasma (PRP) harvested. Then,200 µl of the PRP were dispensed in vials containing 200 µl of lysate. The negative control and positive control were respectively obtained by adding 200 µl of pyrogen-free water and 200 µl of E. coli 0111 BA LPS (1 ng/1 ml) to vials containing 200 µl of lysate. To remove possible inhibitors of the clotting activity able to produce false negative results, the procedure described by Cooperstock (27) was used:the PRP was diluted 1:3 in pyrogen-free water and heating at 100°C for 10 min. Then,all vials were incubated for 60 min at 37°C. In patients and experimental procedures endotoxin amount (ng/ml) was determined by diluting plasma in sterile endotoxin-free water in order to obtain a semiquantitative evaluation of the endotoxaemia. The test was scored as positive if a firm gel appeared that did not break when the vial was inverted 180°.

RESULTS

Out of 43 patients, 13 had a negative and 30 a positive LAL test. The 2 groups were similar as for age and presence of ascites. Creatinine clearance (Crcl) was 71.3 ± 2.5 ml/min (Mean ± S.E.M.) in LAL negative and 20.7 ± 3.3 in LAL positive patients.The mortality rate during the study which result of 30 days as average time was about 8% in LAL negative and about 77% in LAL positive patients (table I).

Results of LAL assay related to values of Crcl are indicated in figure 1.It shows that below 60 ml/min of Crcl all patients except one had a LAL positive reaction.

In 22 out of 30 LAL positive patients the LAL assay was determined on serial plasma dilutions in order to assess if there is relation between amount of circulating endotoxins and degree of renal failure (figure 2).Five patients with Crcl of 43.4 ± 5.66 ml/min (Mean ± S.E.M.) had a low LAL positivity (1:1), 6 patients with Crcl of 28.16 ± 8.51 had a higher LAL positivity (1:10) and finally 11 patients with Crcl of 6.74 ± 2.35 had a much higher LAL positivity (1:100). Furthermore, the percent mortality at time of study was 40% in the former and 66% in the latter reaching the 100% in the last group.

Table 1. Clinical and laboratory assessment in 43 patients at time of study.

	LAL ASSAY	
	NEGATIVE	POSITIVE
PATIENTS N°	13	30
AGE (YEARS) MEAN ± SEM	55 ± 3	58 ± 2
SEX M	3	20
SEX F	10	10
ASCITES	12 / 13	30/30
PLASMA CREATININE (mg/dl)	0.89 ± 0.04	3.31 ± 0.33
	$p<0.001$	
CLEARANCE CREATININE (ml/min)	71.3 ± 2.5	20.7 ± 3.3
	$p<0.001$	
MORTALITY %	7.69 (1/13)	76.66 (23/30)

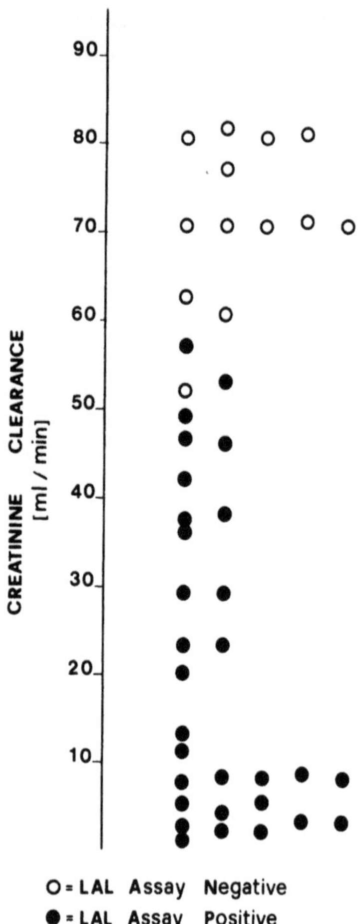

Fig. 1. Results of LAL assay related to values of creatinine clearance in 43 patients with HRS.

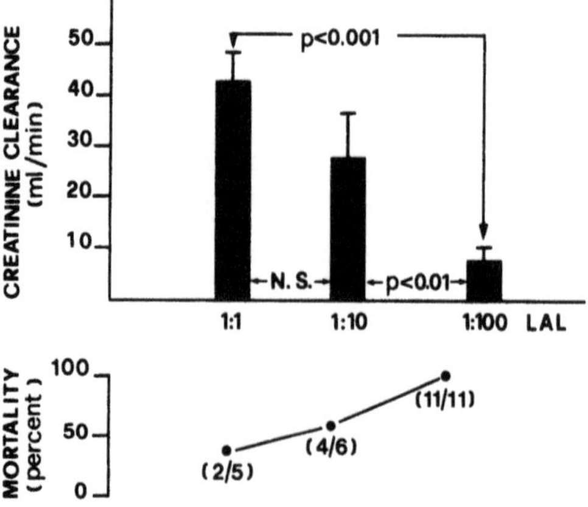

Fig. 2. Relationship of renal failure to plasma endotoxin levels in 22 patients. Solid bars represent creatinine clearance as Mean $\pm$ S.E.M.. The lower panel shows percent mortality at time of study.

In 3 patients during oral administration of bactericidal drug was demonstrated a progressive renal failure (figure 3). In patients n° 1 and n° 3 the progression of HRS was obtained within the first week and in patient n° 2 after two weeks of treatment. The progressive renal failure in these patients was characterized by appearance of endotoxaemia in patient n° 1 which was LAL negative before therapy and increase of circulating endotoxins in patients n° 2 and n° 3.

In 7 out of 13 progressive HRS cases treated with hemodialysis the LAL assay, evaluated on pre-dialytic and post-dialytic plasma using serial dilutions, showed a reduction of endotoxin plasma levels in all patients by comparing the LAL post-dialytic levels with the pre-dialytic ones (table 2). Among patients 1-4 only one dialysis was performed and in patient number 4 there was an increase of diuresis up to 600 ml/24 hours with recovery of renal function up to 20 ml/min.The others 3 patients were several times treated with hemodialysis and in two of them diuresis was recovered as well as renal function. In patient number 6 the diuresis increased up to 1000 ml/24 hours and the Crcl up to 23 ml/min, furthermore in patient number 7 the diuresis increased up to 1000 ml/24 hours and the Crcl up to 18 ml/min.

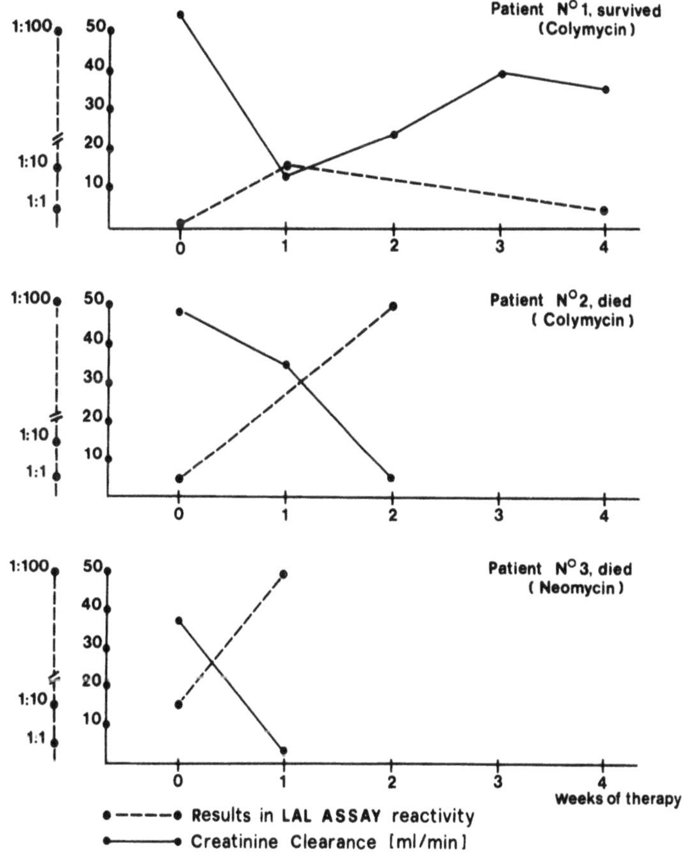

Fig. 3. Findings in 3 patients during oral bactericidal drug.

Table 2. LAL assay in 7 patients submitted to dialytic treatment.

Patient N°	Day N°	LAL Assay Before HD	LAL Assay After HD	Creatinine Clearance (ml/min)	Urine Output (ml/day)	Outcome	Cause of death
1	1	1 : 100	1 : 10	7.8	200	Died	Hepatic Coma
2	1	1 : 100	1 : 10	3	100	»	»
3	1	1 : 100	1 : 10	< 1	<50	»	Vascular Shock
4	1	1 : 10	1 : 1	20	600	»	Hepatic Coma
5	1	1 : 100	1 : 100	8	100		
	2	1 : 100	1 : 10		80		
	3	1 : 10	1 : 10		150		
	4	1 : 10	1 : 1		100	Died	Hepatic Coma
6	1	1 : 100	1 · 100	5	100		
	2	1 : 100	1 : 10		100		
	3	1 : 10	1 . 10		200		
	4	1 : 10	1 : 1	23	1000		
	5	Negative	Negative		800	Died	Pulmonary Oedema
7	1	1 : 100	1 : 100	2.7	100		
	2	1 : 100	1 : 10		200		
	3	1 : 10	1 : 1	18	1000	Died	Hepatic Coma

The first in vitro study (table 3) demonstrated no passage of LPS across dialyzing polyacrylonitrile membrane so that blood and hemofiltrate collections in the same time intervals (every 10 minutes) showed an unchanged LAL positivity in the plasma samples (1:200) and a persistent LAL negativity in the hemofiltrate.

Table 3. Absence of LPS filtration across polyacrylonitrile membrane: Experimental findings.

TIME, min.	LAL BLOOD VOLUME	LAL HEMOFILTRATE VOLUMES
10	1:200	NEGATIVE
20	1:200	"
30	1:200	"
40	1:200	"
50	1:200	"
60	1:200	"
70	1:200	"
80	1:200	"

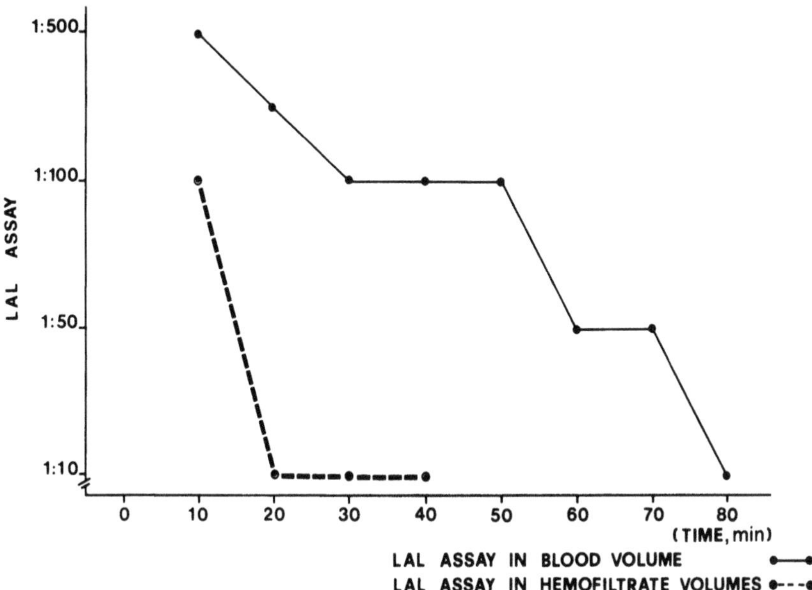

Fig. 4. Lipid A filtration across cuprophane membrane: Experimental findings.

Whereas the second in vitro study performed with Lipid A and dialyzing cuprophane membrane (figure 4) showed a progressive reduction of the endotoxaemia in blood volume. The LAL positivity decreased by starting values of 1:500 to 1:10 in the last plasma sample, while there was appearance of LAL positivity in hemofiltrate volume with values at first sample of 1:100 and then of 1:10 in others.

DISCUSSION

Our clinical evidences show that endotoxaemia may be responsible for the progression of HRS. This hypothesis is supported by the presence of circulating endotoxins in the patients with later phase of HRS and absence of endotoxaemia in others without progressive HRS.

The systemic endotoxaemia in hepatic cirrhosis has been already investigated by some authors. Wilkinson et al. (28) detected renal failure in 25 of 45 patients with liver cirrhosis and the Limulus assay gave positive results in 21 of the 25 patients with renal failure compared with only 2 of the 20 patients with normal renal function. Besides, the 21 patients with a positive Limulus reaction had significantly lower values for creatinine clearance than the 4 with a negative reaction. In a study of Clemente et al. (29) 22 of 43 patients with liver cirrhosis had renal failure and endotoxaemia was present in 8 of the 10 patients with progressive renal failure, but only in 1 of the 12 patients with steady renal failure. Furthermore, endotoxaemia was found in none of the 21 patients with normal renal function. Liehr et al. (30) demonstrated renal failure in 8 of 33 patients with liver cirrhosis and the Limulus assay gave positive results in 6 of the 8 patients with renal failure. Coratelli et al. (26) evaluated 23 patients with liver cirrhosis and renal failure. The Limulus assay gave positive results in 15 of the 23 patients. In addition, the 15 patients with a positive Limulus reaction had significantly lower values of creatinine clearance than the 8 patients with a negative reaction. On the other hand, Gatta et al. (31) demonstrated that in patients with cirrhosis, without overt renal failure, renal vasoconstriction did not appear to be related to endotoxaemia.

The pathogenetic role of endotoxin in the later phase of HRS rather than in the earlier stage, in terms of renal failure progression, results more evident trough the relationship demonstrated between endotoxin plasma levels and degree of renal failure. Furthermore, our data show that there should be also relation between endotoxaemia and prognosis. The mortality rate at time of study was higher in the LAL positive as to negative patients and was much more elevated in the LAL positive patients with higher endotoxin plasma levels. The prognosis of patients with liver cirrhosis and endotoxaemia was also evaluated by Tarao et al. (32). In their experience, death occurred within 6 months in 47;8% of the patients with a positive endotoxin test, whereas only 16,7% of those with a negative test died in the some period. Gaeta et al. (33) studied 104 patients with chronic liver disease and their results suggested that endotoxaemia may be indicative for a more advanced stage of the disease in these patients.

The findings obtained in patients during oral bactericidal drugs seem to confirm the relationship between endotoxaemia and renal failure progression in HRS. It is known that bactericidal drugs orally administered as a consequence of their bacterial lysis effect may increase the endotoxin intestinal pool. Thus, increased absorption of endotoxins, coupled with impaired hepatic clearance, might account for the endotoxaemia in our patients and for the progressive renal failure following oral administration of intestinal antibiotics, such as neomycin and colymycin.

The results with LAL assay in patients submitted to dialytic treatment demonstrate that the emodialysis may reduce the LAL assay plasma reactivity and suggest that a slight improvement of renal function is possible in some patient.

Nevertheless, in late HRS, hemodialysis, although effective in clearing the circulating endotoxins, is not effective in counteracting their systemic effects.

It has been demonstrated that endotoxins (lypopolysaccarides) with a molecular weight more than 100,000 daltons cannot pass across cellulose dialyzing membrane (34).

We obtained similar results using an high permeability membrane, the polyacrylonitrile. Endotoxins, however, could be fragmented and release smaller molecules which may pass across dialyzing membrane. It has been demonstrated that the Lipid A is a fragment representing the biologically active component of the lipopolysaccharide (35) and it is known to react with LAL (36). Thus, if such a fragment is produced naturally, native Lipid A would be easily dialyzed since its molecular weight is as small as 2000 daltons. This possibility is suggested by the endotoxin plasma levels reduction which might be related to Lipid A passage across dialyzing membrane. The results of the experimental study designed to determine if Lipid A may be able to filter across cuprophane membrane support our hypothesis and confirm our data on Lipid A hemofiltrability with polyacrylonitrile membrane (26).

Hemodialysis with cuprophane and polyacrilonitrile membrane is therefore able to remove Lipid A from the blood stream. However, all cases of dialyzed HRS had a severe prognosis: gastrointestinal bleeding, hypotension, and hepatic coma were the most frequent causes of death. Therefore in later phase of HRS, hemodialysis, although effective in order to reduce the endotoxaemia is not effective in order to counteract systemic effects of circulating endotoxins.

In conclusion, there is evidence that the development of endotoxaemia might be responsible for the progression of HRS.

Renal failure correlates with the degree of plasma levels of endotoxaemia, and a more severe prognosis is related to the higher amount of circulating endotoxins.

It has been demonstrated that, fallowing dialysis, LAL positivity decreases and since LPS do not filter because of their large molecular weight it is conceivable that Lipid A is the actual moiety which passes across membranes.

In fact, our experimental data confirm the passage of Lipid A through dialyzing filters and this suggests future studies to evaluate the efficacy of early dialysis in patients with HRS.

Acknowledgments

This research was supported by Ministero Pubblica Istruzione Grant 85/4478. The authors are indebted to Dr E. Jirillo for his help in the preparation of the manuscript.

REFERENCES

1. M.Epstein, Renal failure in the patient with cirrhosis, Am. J. of Med. 49:175 (1970).
2. S.M.Shasha, O.S.Better, C.Chamovitz, J.Doman, Y.Kishon, Hemodynamic studies in dogs with chronic bile duct ligation, Clin. Sci. 50: 533(1976).
3. E.T.Schroeder, G.H. Anderson, S.H. Goldman, D.H.P. Streeten, Effect of blockade of angiotensin II on blood pressure, renin and aldosterone in cirrhosis, Kidney Int. 9:511 (1976).
4. M. Epstein, R. Levinson,J. Sancho, E. Haber, R. Re, Characterization of the renin-aldosterone system in decompensated cirrhosis, Circ.Res. 41: 818 (1977).
5. E.J. Zambraski, C.F. Di Bona, G.J. Kaloyanides, Specifity of neural effect on renal tubular sodium reabsorption, Proc. Soc. Biol. Med. 151:543 (1976).
6. G.F.Di Bona, Neurogenic regulation of renal tubular sodium reabsorption, Am. J. Physiol. 233:F73 (1977).
7. O.S. Better, R.W. Schrier, Disturbed volume homeostasis in patients with cirrhosis of the liver, Kidney Int. 23:303 (1983).

8. G.F. Di Bona, Renal neural activity in hepatorenal syndrome, Kidney Int. 25:841 (1984).
9. M. Epstein, M. Lifschitz, D. Hoffman, J. Stein, Relationship between renal prostaglandin E and renal sodium handling during water immersion in normal man, Circ. Res. 45:71 (1979).
10. R.D. Zipser, J.C. Hoefs, P.F. Speckart, P.K. Zia, R. Horton, Prostaglandins: Modulators of renal function and pressor resistance in chronic liver disease, J. Clin. Endocrinol. Metab. 48:895 (1979).
11. H. J. Kramer, Humoral and hormonal factors in the pathogenesis of sodium retention in liver cirrhosis and the hepatorenal syndrome, in: "Hepatorenal Syndrome", edited by E. Bartoli and L. Chiandussi, Piccin, Padua, Italy, 1978, p. 311.
12. J.Kipnowshi, R.Dusing, H. J. Kramer, Hepatorenal syndrome, Klin. Wochenschr 59:415 (1981).
13. E.A. Lianos, N.Alavi, M.Tobin, R. Venuto, C.J.Bentzel, Angiotensin-induced sodium excretion patterns in cirrhosis: Role of renal prostaglandins, Kidney Int. 21:70 (1982).
14. G. Parelon, D. Mirouze, F. Michel, P. Crastes De Paulet, J. Chaintreuil, A. Crastes De Paulet, H. Michel, Prostaglandines urinaires dans le syndrome hépatorénal du cirrhotique: role du thromboxane A_2 et d'un déséquilibre des acides gras polynsaturés précurseurs, Gastroenterol. Clin. Biol. 9:290 (1985).
15. R.D. Zipser, G.H. Radvan, I.J. Kromborg, R. Duke, T.E. Little, Urinary thromboxane B_2 and prostaglandin E_2 in the hepatorenal syndrome: evidence for increased vasoconstrictor and decreased vasodilator factors, Gastroenterology 84:697 (1983).
16. P.Y. Wong, R.W. Colman, R.C. Talamo, B.M. Babior, Kallikrein-bradykinin system in chronic alcoholic liver disease,Ann. Intern. Med. 77: 205 (1972).
17. J.Y. Gillenwater, E.S. Dooley, E.D. Fröhlich, Effects of endotoxin on renal function and hemodinamics, Am. J. Physiol. 205 (2):293 (1963).
18. D. Cavanagh, P.S. Rao, D.M.C. Sutton, D.Bhagat, F. Bachmann, Pathophysiology of endotoxin shock in the primate, Am. J. Obstet. Gynecol. 108:705 (1970).
19. M.Grün, H.Liehr, H. Thiel, U.Rasenack: Effekt einer endotoxinämie auf die renale und intrarenale hämodynamic bei ratten mit und ohne portakavale anastomase, Z.Gastroenterologie 14:285 (1976).
20. H.Prytz, J.Holst-Christensen, B. Korner, H.Liehr, Portal venous and systemic endotoxaemia in patients without liver disease and systemic endotoxaemia in patients with cirrhosis, Scand.J. Gastroent.11:857 (1976).
21. D.R. Triger, T.D. Boyer, J.Levin: Portal and systemic bacteraemia and endotoxaemia in liver disease, Gut. 19:935 (1978).
22. J.P. Nolan, D.S. Camara, Endotoxin, sinusoidal cells and liver injury, in: "Progress in liver diseases", edited by H. Popper, F. Schaffner, New York, Grune and Stratton, 1982, p. 371.
23. G. Ramadori, U.Hopf, K.H.Meyer Zum Büschenfelde, Binding sites for endotoxic lipopolysaccharide on the plasma membrane of isolated rabbit hepatocytes, Acta Hepato-Gastroenterol. 26:368 (1979).
24. G.Ramadori, U.Hopf, G.Galanos, M. Freudenberg, K.H. Meyer Zum Büschenfelde, In vitro and in vivo reactivity of lipopolysaccarides and

lipid A with parenchymal and non-parenchymal liver cells in mice, in: "The reticuloendothelial system and the pathogenesis of liver disease", edited by H. Liehr and M. Grün, Amsterdam: Elsevier/North Holland, 1980, p. 285.

25. J.Levin, F.B. Bang, Clottable protein in Limulus: its localization and kinetics of its coagulation by endotoxin, Tromb.Haemost. 19:186 (1968).
26. P. Coratelli, G. Passavanti, I.Munno, D.Fumarola, A.Amerio, New trends in hepatorenal syndrome, Kidney Int. 28 (Supp 17):S143 (1985).
27. M.S. Cooperstock, R.P. Tucher, J.V. Baublis, Possible pathogenetic role of endotoxin in Reye's syndrome, Lancet 1:1272 (1975).
28. S.P. Wilkinson, H.Moodie, J.D. Stamatakis, V.V. Kakkar, R. Williams: Endotoxaemia and renal failure in cirrhosis and obstructive jaundice, Br.Med.J. 2:1415 (1976).
29. C.Clemente, J.Bosch, J.Rodés, V. Arroyo, A.Mas, S. Maragall, Functional renal failure and haemorrhagic gastritis associated with endotoxaemia in cirrhosis, Gut 18:556 (1977).
30. H.Liehr, M.Grün, D.Brunswig, T.Sautter, Endotoxinämia bei leberzirrhose, Z.Gastroenterologie 14:14 (1976).
31. A.Gatta, L.Milani,C. Merkel, R.Zuin, P.Amodio, L. Caregaro, A.Roul, Lack of correlation between endotoxemia and renal hypoperfusion in cirrhotics without overt renal failure, Eur. J. Clin. Invest. 12:417 (1982).
32. K. Tarao, T. Moroi, T. Ikeuchi, T. Suyama, O. Endo, K. Fukushima, Detection of endotoxin in plasma and ascitic fluid of patients with cirrhosis: its clinical significance, Gastroenterology 73:539 (1977).
33. G.B.Gaeta, P.Perna, L.E.Adinolfi, R.Utili,G. Ruggiero, Endotoxemia in a series of 104 patients with chronic liver diseases: prevalence and significance, Digestion 23:239 (1982).
34. J.J. Bernick, F.K. Port, M.S. Favero, D.G. Brown, Bacterial and endotoxin permeability of hemodialysis membranes, Kidney Int. 16:491 (1979).
35. O. Lüderitz, C. Galanos, V. Lehmann, M. Nurminen, E.T. Rietschel, G. Rosenfelder, M.Simon, O. Westphal, Lipid A: chemical structure and biological activity, J. Infect. Dis. 128 (Supp):S17 (1973).
36. C. Galanos, O. Lüderitz, E.T. Rietschel, O. Westphal, New aspects of the chemistry and biology of bacterial lipopolysaccharides with special reference to their Lipid A component, Int. Rev. Biochem. 14:239 (1977).

ACUTE RENAL FAILURE DUE TO OBSTRUCTIVE UROPATHY

Giuseppe Maschio

Institute of Nephrology
University Hospital
Verona, Italy

INTRODUCTION

Obstruction of the urinary tract is relatively frequent,with an incidence of approximately 4% in an autopsy series of over 32,000 cases (see Richie,1983).

Several factors may contribute to postrenal obstruction. They include congenital anomalies (ureteropelvic junction stricture,posterior urethral valves,urethral stenosis,ureterocoele,ectopic ureter),functional abnormalities (vesicoureteral reflux,neurogenic bladder,etc.),trauma (ureteral edema,stricture or injury,retroperitoneal hemorrage,intraureteral blood clots), inflammation (edema or stricture,prostatitis,pelvic inflammatory disease,retroperitoneal fibrosis,inflammatory bowel disease,genitourinary tuberculosis),tumors and masses intrinsic to urinary tract (carcinoma of bladder,urethra,ureter,or pelvis,nephrolithiasis,ureteral polyp),tumors and masses extrinsic to urinary tract (prostatic hypertrophy or carcinoma,cervical or endometrial carcinoma,ovarian tumors,retroperitoneal lymphoma or metastases,endometriosis).

The consequences of acute and chronic forms of urinary tract obstruction on renal hemodynamics and renal function have been extensively evaluated in experimental studies (see Badr et al.,1983; Buerkert and Klahr, 1983). Acute ureteral obstruction results in increased intraluminal ureteral pressure (from 0-5 up to 50 mmHg),increased ureteral wall tension ((from 0-1 up to 10×10^4 dynes/cm^2),increased proximal tubular pressure (from 0-10 up to 90 mmHg),and decreased GFR.

Chronic ureteral occlusion is followed by moderate rise in ureteral and proximal tubular pressures,increase in ureteral diameter and wall tension,pyelolymphatic and/or pyelovenous reflux,and decreased renal blood flow and GFR.

To summarize,obstruction to urinary outflow is followed by important changes of renal hemodynamics. After unilateral obstruction,an initial transient increase in renal blood flow may be observed,resulting from afferent arteriolar vasodilatation (a possible effect of locally acting prostaglandins). This vasodilatation is probably stimulated by acute increase in proximal tubular pressure. However,with the persistence of unilateral obstruction,renal blood flow decreases due to the effect of locally acting vasoconstrictor agents,like thomboxane (TxA2) and angiotensin II (A II). When obstruction is bilateral,a transient increase in renal blood flow may still be seen.

With chronic obstruction,however,both renal blood flow and GFR are persistently decreased. Then,through these pathogenetic events,associated with superimposed infection,obstructive uropathy (i.e.,structural changes in the urinary tract which impair urine outflow and rise proximal pressure) may result in obstructive nephropathy,which is the renal parenchymal damage secondary to an impedance to flow of urine or tubular fluid)(fig.1).

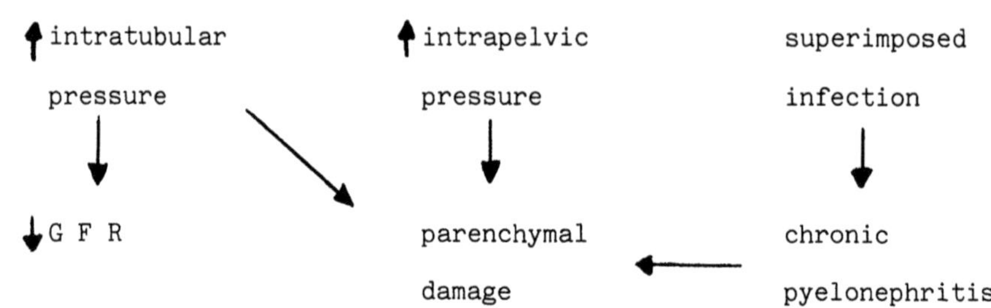

Fig. 1 : The pathogenetic mechanisms through which obstructive uropathy may result in obstructive nephropathy.

Chronic renal failure is relatively common in obstructive nephropathy, and results from pressure atrophy,ischemic atrophy,and pyelonephritis. This syndrome is usually associated with slowly progressive deterioration of renal function within years.

Acute renal failure (ARF) is less common and follows complete bilateral obstruction. It may present as oliguric (anuric) ARF,with abrupt decrease in renal function within a few days,or as non-oliguric ARF,with progressive deterioration of renal function within a few months.

Once again,most information on the pathogenesis of postobstructive ARF comes from animal studies. After 24 hours of bilateral ureteral obstraction in rats,single nephron GFR declines by 40% and remains depressed even after obstruction has been released,due to marked renal arteriolar vasoconstriction (Dal Canton et al.,1980). At least two vasoactive (vasoconstrictor) agents, A II and TxA2, have been implicated in this phenomenon. The role of intrarenal vasoactive hormones in obstructive nephropathy is summarized in Table 1.

In addition,recent experimental evidence suggests that the reduction of dietary protein intake may condition the renal response to acute obstruction,possibly by limiting the production and/or action of TxA2.

Table 1. THE ROLE OF INTRARENAL VASOACTIVE HORMONES IN POSTOBSTRUCTIVE ACUTE RENAL FAILURE.

1. The synthesis of PGE_2 and PGI_2 (vasodilators) and TxA_2 (vasoconstrictor) is increased in experimental hydronephrosis and after ureteral obstruction.

2. The activity of renin - angiotensin II is increased by ureteral obstruction. A II exerts vasoconstriction after release of obstruction.

3. Increased renal production and/or excretion of TxA_2 may be observed in several forms of acute renal injury.

4. The pharmacologic blockade of TxA_2 production (by administration of OKY-1581) significantly improves the depressed GFR seen after release of ureteral obstruction.

5. Dietary protein restriction may limit the production and/or the action of TxA_2,thus reducing the severity of renal dysfunction in postobstructive acute renal failure.

It is possible that the amount of ingested protein may also determine the severity of renal damage in other forms of ARF as well (Ichikawa et al.,1985).

The relationship between the duration of obstruction and the degree of recovery of renal function after release is not known in man. However,a permanent reduction of 50% GFR is to be expected. The renal blood flow is also decreased,and cortical blood flow is markedly reduced.

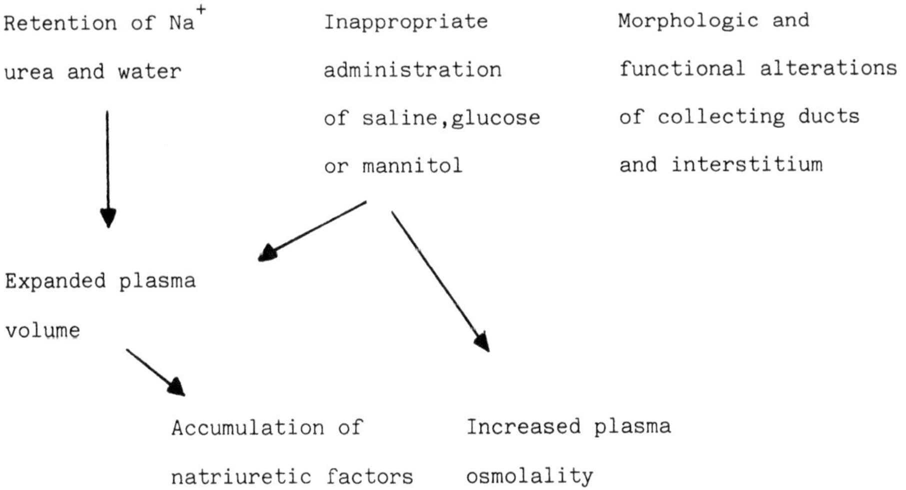

Fig. 2 : The pathogenesis of postobstructive diuresis,with increased excretion of sodium and water.

Obviously,the nature of the obstruting lesions,the site of obstruction, and the degree of the occlusion are all important determinants in the onset and evolution of clinical syndromes (Dal Canton and Andreucci,1984) (Table 2).

Table 2. OBSTRUCTIVE NEPHROPATHY : CLINICAL MANIFESTATIONS.

1. ALTERATIONS IN URINE OUTPUT : sequential occurrence of oliguria,or even anuria,and brisk polyuria.

2. PAIN,sometimes associated with renal enlargement.

3. INFECTION,recurrent and often resistant to therapy.

4. HYPERTENSION : usually multifactorial,may be volume-dependent,renin-dependent,or secondary to decreased synthesis of vasodepressor substances.

5. HYPEROSMOLAR SYNDROME : this rare syndrome occurs as a result of excessive excretion of "free water",i.e. water in excess of solutes.

6. POLYCYTHEMIA.

The diagnostic approach to patients with urinary tract obstruction is first based on history,physical examination,and laboratory studies. History may be of value when it shows evidence of urinary tract infection, stones,abnormalities in pattern of urine output,regular drug ingestion. At physical examination,a palpable mass in the flank area,or a suprapubic mass,is often found. Prostatic or gynecologic examination should be done. Laboratory studies include urinalysis,urine sediment (with special reference to the existence of red blood cells,white blood cells,bacteria, crystals),uriculture,and routine biochemistry with the evaluation of renal function.

The diagnosis should be confirmed with the aid of one of more of the following diagnostic methods:

a. Ultrasonography

b. Plain X-ray of the abdomen

c. Intravenous pyelography (with tomography)

d. Computerized tomography

e. Retrograde pyelography

f. Cystoscopy

g. Cystography.

Ultrasonography is the less invasive among the previously listed methods and should become routine in all patients presenting with ARF (Fig. 2).

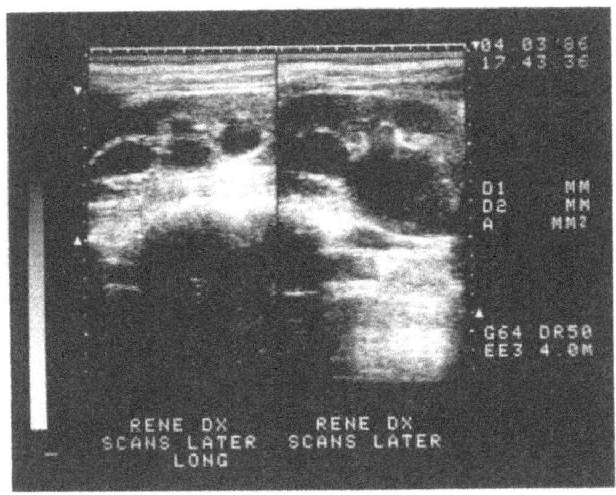

Fig.2 : Ultrasonography showing hydronephrosis of the right kidney due to ureteral obstruction.

REFERENCES

RICHIE J.P.: Clinical aspects of urinary tract obstruction. In Acute Renal Failure, ed. by BRENNER and LAZARUS, W.B. Saunders, 1983, p.499.

BADR K., ICHIKAWA I., BRENNER B.M.: Renal circulatory and nephron function in experimental obstruction of the urinary tract. In Acute Renal Failure, ed. by BRENNER and LAZARUS, W.B. Saunders, 1983, p.116.

BUERKERT J., KLAHR S.: Obstructive nephropathy. In Textbook of Nephrology, ed. by MASSRY and GLASSOCK, Williams Wilkins, 1983, p.6.237.

DAL CANTON A., CORRADI A., STANZIALE R., MARUCCIO G., MIGONE L.: Glomerular hemodynamics before and after release of 24-hour bilateral ureteral obstruction. Kidney Intern. 17: 491-496, 1980.

ICHIKAWA I., PURKERSON M.L., YATES J., KLAHR S.: Dietary protein intake conditions the degree of renal vasoconstriction in acute renal failure caused by ureteral obstruction. Am.J.Physiol. 249:F 54-61, 1985.

DAL CANTON A., ANDREUCCI V.E.: Acute obstructive renal failure (postrenal failure). In Acute Renal Failure. Pathophysiology, Prevention and Treatment, ed. by ANDREUCCI, Martinus Nijhoff, 1984, p.365.

HEMOLYTIC UREMIC SYNDROME

Antonio Vercellone, Piero Stratta, and Caterine Canavese

Department of Nephrology, S. Giovanni Molinette Hospital

Corso Bramante 88 - 10126 TORINO - Italia

THE HEMOLYTIC UREMIC SYNDROME

INTRODUCTION

The place to be accorded to the hemolytic-uremic syndrome (HUS) in the classification of acute renal failure (ARF) still poses considerable problems of an etiopathogenetic, anatomopathological and clinical nature. HUS is usually regarded as consisting of a symptomatological triad, namely microangiopathic hemolytic anemia, thrombocytopenia and ARF. First reported in children, it has since been demonstrated in adults.[1,2]
HUS is much more common in children. In some areas, it is the primary cause of ARF (65%) and follows glomerulonephritis and urological abnormalities as a cause of terminal uremia.[3] Endemic forms have been described in Argentina, South Africa, France, Holland and California. Epidemics, too, have been reported in association with infection by Shigella, Salmonella, verotoxin-producing E.coli and after drinking apple juice and cider. Other workers have described familial forms transmitted as dominant or recessive autosomic characters, recurrent and sporadic forms. The prodromic stage is usually marked by gastroenteric symptoms (abdominal pains, nausea, vomiting and frequently hematic diarrhea) or signs of involvement of the upper airways, but may well be entirely absent in familial, recurrent and sporadic forms, all of which usually have a more severe prognosis. Proteinuria, sometimes very marked, with micro- or macrohematuria, is observed within a clinical picture of malaise, asthenia, pallor and icterus. There is a rapid reduction of renal function with oligoanuria of varying length, often accompanied by arterial hypertension and signs of neurological impairment (stupor, convulsions, coma). A mortality rate of more than 50% has given way to levels of around 5% in the more recent series. Chronic renal failure is the probable outcome in 10-20% of cases, though in Argentina it is 50%. The prognosis is decidedly better in epidemic forms and when the patient is less than two years of age. In all series reduced mortality thanks to timely dialysis and better control of hypertension has naturally led to the observation of

Table 1. Primary and secondary HUS
(Department of Nephrology, Torino, 1972-1986)

HUS n 37	CHILDREN (n 16)	PRIMARY FORMS	Gastrointestinal prodromes	15
			Mumps	1
	ADULTS (n 21)	PRIMARY FORMS (n 5)	Pulmonary infections	2
			Post-partum	2
			Salmonella chronic carrier	1
		SECONDARY FORMS (n 16)	Preeclampsia-eclampsia	7
			Sclerodermas	5
			Malignant hypertension	1
			Biliary cirrhosis	1
			Evans syndrome	1
			Prostatic carcinoma	1

more cases of chronic renal failure (CRF).[1,3,4,5]
HUS is rarely epidemic or familial in the adult. It usually appears sporadically, often in the company of other diseases that complicate the task of diagnosis. Infectious prodromes are observed, but the usual background is marked by other events, including the taking of various drugs (estroprogestins, mitomycin, phenylbutazone and cyclosporin), radiation theray, pregnancy or post-partum, rejection of a kidney transplant, or systemic diseases (SLE, scleroderma , cryoglobulinemia, vasculitis and malignant hypertension). While HUS represents a relatively low percentage of cases of adult ARF (2% of the Morel-Maroger cases) the prognosis is much less promising. The mortality rate is still between 50 and 75% and residual chronic renal failure is described in 40- 70% of patients.[6,7]
Our series is in line with those in the literature. It consists of 37 cases, 16 in children and 21 in adults. Children HUS represents 29% of ARF observed from 1976 to 1986. In 15 cases there was the typical prodromic stage of gastroenteric symptomes; in one, HUS appeared after mumps. The mortality rate was 12,5%, and evolution on CRF was observed in 2 children (12,5%), respectively a recurrent form marked by severe hypertension, and a sporadic from in a 13 yr-old boy. Adult HUS represents 4% of ARF observed from 1972 to 1976. Primary forms, that is out of known existing pathologies, were observed only in 5 cases. The background to other forms was existing systemic disease (Table I). Ten patients died (47%) and chronic renal failure was observed in 33% in (7/21).

THE FEATURES CONSIDERED NECESSARY COMPONENTS OF THE SYNDROME

Microangiopathic hemolytic anemia

As already mentioned, HUS typically includes microangiopathic hemolytic anemia (MHA) as well as ARF. Thrombocytopenia ($< 140 \times 10^9/l$) is a less constant finding.

The term MHA is used to describe a set of factors pointing to Coombs--negative intravascular hemolysis: a rapid drop in hematocrit below 30% occurring in the absence of bleeding and associated with consumption of haptoglobin, reduced red cell life-span, increased indirect bilirubin and lactic DH, > 5% reticulocytosis, and, above all, the typical red cell deformation noted on the peripheral smear. Schistocytes (helmet, triangular and half-moon red cells), anisopoikilocytes, burr cells (echinocytes and acanthocytes) and micro- and macrocytes with signs of anisochromia are noted.

A closer look at the state of the art has now cast doubt on the definition of the hemolytic anemia as "microangiopathic" in the sense of interpreting red cell deformation as only secondary to passage into a microcirculation partially obstructed by fibrin thrombi. Critical reassessment of the assumption that red cell deformation is the result of mechanical damage caused by passage over fibrin matrixes in the microcirculation has been a much slow and arduous task, since the excellent papers of the Brain [8] have conditioned the literature to such an extent that no room seemed to be left for alternative suggestions. Several reasons can be put forward for the currently adoption of a different point of view:

1. The red cell deformations noted on the peripheral blood smear in HUS are much more varied and complicated than those of the schistocytes, which are all that Brain describe: actual "schistocytes" may indeed be the outcome of deformation on passage into the microcirculation. Burr cells, on the other hand, are certainly not attributable to mechanical microcirculatory injury, and are observed in such diseases as alcoholic cirrhosis, damage caused by contrast media and hyperalbuminemia.[9,10]
2. There are many proofs of a primary erythrocyte damage in HUS: structural changes in the phospholipid membrane, reduced superoxide-dismutase activity, reduced phosphatidyl ethanolamine content, morphological abnormalities on electron microscopy studies.[11,12]
3. Red cells directly damaged by various insults (toxic, peroxidative, pharmacological, metabolic) may undergo structural changes in the lipid mantle and the underlyng spectrin network that stiffen them to the point that they are unable to alter their shape when passing into the smaller vessels. These "dangerous red cells"[13] are capable of causing endothelial and rheological alterations in the absence of existing microcirculatory disturbances.[14]
4. There is a growing body of clinical observations of syndromes diagnosed as HUS owing to the presence of MHA+ARF that none the less lack a corresponding renal damage sufficient to substantiate the possibility of mechanical red cell deformation.[15]
5. Endotoxins involved in the pathogenesis of children HUS show a direct hemolytic activity.[12]
6. MHA and histological renal damage are dissociated in experimental models using different toxins. Shigella toxin leads to cortical necrosis without MHA.[16] Clostridium toxin leads to MHA+ARF without microvascular damage.[12] This could confirm that erythrocytic morphologic alterations can appear without the presence of an actual microcirculatory damage, and therefore there are not necessarily all secondary.

7. A hematological picture indistinguishable from that defined as typical of HUS is reported in neoplastic diseases in absence of microvascular deposits of fibrim, and is totally reversed by the removal of the primary carcinoma.[17]

From these observations it seems possible to conclude that at least some of the erythrocytic morphologic alterations seen in the blood smears of HUS can be traced to primary erythrocytic damage.

Acute renal failure

The central feature of the syndrome is ARF, though recent work has made it increasingly clear that renal damage occurs in the context of a systemic disease, with extrarenal involvement demonstrable in 80% of cases studied before the 10th day of illness but only in 32% of patients observed later during the acute hase. Microthrombosis necrosis and hemorrhage mainly involve colon, brain, heart, and, to a lesser extent, pancreas, adrenal glands, spleen and lungs. Even so, histopathological injury to the kidney is the typical and diffuse finding and may take several forms[18]

Clinical features of the renal injury are represented by increase of BUN, creatinine, phosphate, hydrogen ions, and a more prononced increase of uric acid out of proportion to the degree of renal failure. Urine volume may be normal, increased or reduced. Anuria accurs in 50% of cases. Hematuria, proteinuria and casts are common findings. Sometimes and actual nephrotic syndrome may be the presenting form.

The most striking feature of the renal pathological lesions in HUS is the wide variability, both qualitatively and quantitatively encountered in renal biopsies.

Three main patterns are described on light microscopy:

1) a glomerular picture characterized by endothelial cell swelling and double contour images. The capillary lumen may be congested and full of fragmented red cells. Equally typical is the observation of mesangial degradation with rarefaction and reticulation of the matrix (mesangiolysis), combined with aneurysmatic dilatation of some capillary loops (blood cysts). Actual intraluminal thrombosis is not a constant feature, but may be also diffuse. Mesangial widening, focal necrosis and sclerosis and mild mesangial proliferation are also sometimes reported.
2) Complete or patchy cortical necrosis is reported with the same frequence of the glomerular lesions.
3) A predominant arteriolar damage is also described, involving from smaller arterioles to larger vessels, with intimal proliferation responsible for an "onion peel" appearance, intraluminal thrombosis and fibrinoid necrosis.

There is not usually any immunofluorescence evidence of immune deposits. The most frequently described finding is material recognisable with antifibrinogen - like antibodies in the capillary wall mesangium and arteriolar lesions. Platelet deposits have also been described in these sites, as well as changes in the arrangement of fibronectin. Occasionally mesangial IgM deposits and C_3 are reported.

Better definition is obtained in the electron microscope, which shows in

Table II. Pathological findings in adult HUS
(Department of Nephrology, Torino, 1972-1986)

Pathological renal findings (13/21)		
THROMBOTIC MICROANGIOPATHY	5	: 1 Evans syndrome 1 Bacterial lung infection
(coupled with vascular lesions of existing disease)		3 Sclerodermas
CORTICAL NECROSIS	4	: 3 Preeclampsia-eclampsia 1 Chronic salmonella carrier
ARTERIOLAR INVOLVEMENT	2	: 1 Biliary cirrhosis 1 Bacterial lung infection
GLOMERULAR THROMBOSIS	1	: 1 Scleroderma
MESANGIAL WIDENING	1	: 1 Prostatic carcinoma

the damaged glomerul detachment of endothelium from the basement membrane, and a clear, widened subendothelial space with wrinkling and splitting of the basement membrane. In the subendothelial space there is accumulation of a voluminous deposit of translucent fluffy material with granular and fibrillar deposits of variable electron density, engulfing red cells and platelets. The same picture may be observed in the subendothelial space of damaged arterioles.

The term thrombotic microangiopathy (TMA) has been proposed[4] for the typical glomerular picture, namely swelling of endothelial cells with double contours, splitting of the basal membranes and fluffy translucent subendothelial deposits. Although this pattern is commun and characteristic, there are some reason against its adoption as an essential histological requisite for the diagnosis of HUS. First, TMA may be absent in patients with cortical necrosis who fulfil the diagnostic criteria for HUS, e.g. the early cases in children described by Gasser, the discoverer of HUS. Secondly, TMA does not appear in some experimental HUS models. Lastly, TMA is not a specific lesion because it is also found in diabetic kidney disease, focal glomerulosclerosis and in the renal damage associated with disease of the liver.[4,6]

It is probably that the wide variability, both qualitatively and quantitatively of the renal lesions observed in HUS accounts both for different interaction between the pathogenetic mechanisms involved, and for different times of observation in respect to the onset of disease. In adult forms furthermore, when often HUS is a secondary form superimposed existing disease, previons pathological lesions may explain more complex pictures.[19] In our series, histological evidence was collected from 13/21 adults (3 biopsies, 10 necropsies) (Table II).

Thrombocytopenia

A reduced platelet count (below 140 x $10^9/l$) is a frequent but not universal feature of HUS. Platelets are reduced by peripheral factors, as shown by normal or increased bone marrow activity and reduced life-span. Other findings include: signs of both platelet activation (increased plasma factor four and betathromboglobulin levels, and reduced intraplatelet serotonin content) and exhaustion (reduction of intragranular components, reduced aggregability, increased bleeding time). The mechanism whereby thrombocytopenia accurs is not fully understood, but the increased destruction of labelled platelet in spleen, liver, and, to a lesser extent kidneys, speaks against a primary consumption in microvascular thrombi. Platelet activation and exhaustion may be a consequence of endothelial damage, reduced prostacyclin activity and hemolysis by releasing serotonin, ADP and hemoglobin. In most cases, the platelet count returns to normal by 7 to 10 days after the onset, and the level to which the platelets fall has no prognostic values.
The pathogenetic role of platelet in HUS has not been clearly defined, but the observation of the prompt reversibility by platelet transfusion, in contrast with that observed in Thrombotic Thrombocytopenic Purpura (TTP), speaks against a crucial pathogenetic role.[20]

ETIOPATHOGENESIS

The concomitance of bacterial or viral infection is particularly noteworthy in children and strongly suggests an etiological connection, probably through the production of toxic factors, such as endotoxins and neuraminidases.[21,22]
Various theories have been put forward with regard to the pathogenetic mechanisms involved in HUS, though the position is far from being clear. Considerable progress has been made in recent years, however, to which clinical observations and the use of experimental models have both contributed. A closer look at the state of the art, too, has served to reduce to the rank of secondary mechanisms certain factors once regarded as of primary pathogenetic importance.[23,24]
Every epoch highlights different aspect, which are stressed in accordance with the point of view established by the paradigm of that period in which the discovery or interpretation is made. The 60s proposed the role of plasmatic coagulatory activation, but several elements speak against a primary responsability of the coagulation pathway in HUS.
First, signs of a systemic activation of the coagulation system are lacking, and, in particular, fibrinogen half-life is normal.
Secondly, both fibrin-like material deposition in the subendothelial spaces and microvascular thrombosis result as secondary features at the sites of endothelial damage. Furthermore, both thrombin and thromboplastin infusion are unable to develop HUS in experimental models. Lastly, heparin does not change the prognosis in controlled trials of children HUS. We may conclude that disseminated intravascular coagulation (DIC) is not a primary factor in the pathogenesis of HUS, and the changes suggestive of coagulation activation, when present, may result from rather than

cause the hemolytic anemia. This is true always in children HUS, while in adult HUS signs of DIC activation are sometimes reported, resulting from existing disease, mainly in HUS superimposed on preeclampsia-eclampsia with obstetric complications.[1-3,4,6,25]

The 70s underlined the relationship between platelets and endothelium.[26] It seems beyond dispute that the key lesion in HUS is that of the microvascular wall occasioned by a toxic insult. Damage to a structure so specialised in maintaining the circulating blood to wall ratio can obviously lead to functional disturbances of, for example, tissue fibrinolytic activator and factor VIII-vW synthesis and prostacyclin production. It may also lead to the secondary damages resulting in the exposure of the Thomsen-Friedenreich antigen.[15] Similar alterations such as prostacyclin imbalance, however, are observed in diseases whose only feature in common with HUS is predominant involvement of the microcirculation of various reasons (TTP, diabetes, crush syndrome, DIC, preeclampsia, Schönlein Henoch, hemolytic abortive syndrome, Bechet's disease).[27-31] In HUS, too, such alterations must be seen as secondary mechanisms that may amplify the injury. That they are devoid of a primary role is also suggested by their partial absence in infantile forms that more frequently proceed to complete regression. Here the less severe picture may explain (and be itself explained by) the non-initiation of such secondary mechanisms. Furthermore, the fact that some of these alterations persist in recurrent and familial forms of infantile HUS points to their secondary nature, since a substrate is formed for a particularly severe picture in response to a toxic insult comparable to that which causes minor, reversible injuries in most children. What we have said, of course, is primarily of theoretical interest with regard to the pathogenesis of HUS and in no way detracts from the importance of these alterations in the amplification and continuation of tissue damage. Indeed, they are often the only possible target for therapy, since the clinical overture is usually too late to allow action to be taken against the pathogenetic mechanisms upstream. It is clear, therefore, that every time microvascular damage occurs, irrespective of its cause, alterations in endothelial function involving maintenance of the fluid-wall equilibrium may be expected. Likewise, it is important to recognise such alterations so that promising situations can be discerned and appropriate treatment of the secondary mechanisms amplifying the damage devised.

The 80s stress the role of peroxidative damages and hemodynamic factors. In the past few years all we have familiarized with the concept of peroxidative damage and with the family of the oxygen free radicals. A free radical is any species with an odd electron. Oxygen toxic products arise from the univalent reduction of the oxygen, out of the respiratory mitochondrial chain. They include superoxide radical, hydrogen peroxide, hydroxyl radical and the singlet oxygen. All these oxygen toxic products are highly unstable, reactive, and cataclismic. They are potentially very dangerous for the cells, and the main mechanism of damage by which they lead to the explosion of the cell is represented by the peroxidation of polyunsaturated lipid layer of the all cellular structures, that is microsomes, nucleus, lysosomes, mitochondria, and cell wall. Their life is reduced to few microseconds by highly specialized enzymes capable of dismute them to water. This strong defence system is defined the "free radical scavenger" complex, and encompasses superoxide-dismutase, catalase, vitamin E, etc. A role fore the oxygen free radical as ultimate mediators of damage in many pathological processes as inflammation, aging, carcinomatous transformation, autoimmunity has been demonstrated, and therapeutical benifits by the use of free radical scavengers have been reported.[32,33]

There is much evidence for peroxidative damage in association with HUS. The cells of children with HUS lack superoxide-dismutase, which is their main enzyme defence against superoxide radicals, while administration of this enzyme significantly reduces renal damage in endotoxin-induced Sanarelli-Shwartzman reaction in the rabbit.[34] In infantile HUS, too, the uricemia is out of proportion to the degree of renal failure.[35] Since uric acid is the final step in the transformation of xanthine and hypoxanthine by xanthine oxidase, it may be a marker of enhanced activity of an enzyme complex known to be the biggest producer of free O_2 radicals. HUS can also occur in association with radiation therapy, wich is typically responsible for tissue damage mediated by membrane peroxidation mechanisms following the action of free oxygen radicals.[36] Lastly, HUS has been described in relation to the employment of drugs such as mitomycin,[37] whose toxicity displays the typical "oxygen enhancement" regarded as pathognomonic of injury caused by superoxide radicals. Vitamin E is one of the most potent antioxidants known. Eclampsia, endothelial damage, hemolytic anemia and Sanarelli-Shwartzman syndrome are all possible consequences of vitamin E deficiency, while its administration offers protection in experimental models of Shwartzman reaction and infantile HUS.[38,39]

Other observation point to a primary hemodynamic mechanism. In the first place a hemodynamic function has been fully demonstrated for the endotoxins associated with HUS.[12,16,22] Secondly, the fact that surgical sympathectomy, alpha-adrenergic blockade or chemical sympathectomy, which all impede vasospasm, also impede Shwartzman reaction, underscores the pathogenetic role of hemodynamic changes as a primary cause of renal damage. In addition, catecholamines may induce endothelial damage.[40-42] Lastly, glomerular morphology comparable with that of HUS (mesangiolysis, capillary aneurysms, engorgement with red cells) can be induced in the rat as what appears to be damage secondary to changes in intrarenal blood flow caused by prolonged ischaemia followed by no-reflow.[43]

Again, both the fact that children have a reduced defence system against the peroxidative damage, and that renal circulation in the child is marked by high cortical resistance, may offer explanation for a predisposing setting. This backgrounds could explain why peroxidative challenge or further vasospasm are responsible for an injury such as that of HUS, that is so much more frequent in children.

The current view of the pathogenesis of HUS thus envisages an insult capable of damaging both the microcirculation and the red cells separately. A series of observations suggest that this insult takes the form of peroxidative damage and hemodynamic alterations. A single noxa with two action could be advocated, acting in vivo and still now not definetively recognised, because experimental models are able to reproduce MHA or renal damage separately. Vasoactive agents, for example, such as the catecholamines, can directly cause endothelial damage and red cell lesions

leading to depressed flexibility and enhanced hemolysis. A hemodynamically active toxin may thus be simultaneously responsible for a primary red cell injury.
In this pathogenetic scheme, therefore, the severity of HUS, the extent of red cell injury and the relation between MHA and the renal lesion vary according to the combinations of either two insults, one hemodynamic, the other peroxidative, or the activity of a single noxa with two actions. Irreversible bilateral cortical necrosis is the likely outcome of intense and protracted vascular spasm and/or paralysis. Primary red cell injury explains not only "microangiopathic" morphological alteration, but also increased cateresis on the part of macrophages and possible fragmentation during the passage through spastic or paralysed glomerular capillaries. Red cell engorgement in these capillaries in HUS, in fact, may be secondary to slowing down of the circulation, itself caused by blockage of the flow by stiffened red cells, encouraged by local hemodynamic changes.[14] Stasis promotes the release of oxygen, resulting in its enhanced reduction by pathways other than that provided by the mitochondrial, and the establishment of secondary peroxidative damage. Moreover, the glomerular capillaries are supplied with an amply fenestrated, discontinuos endothelium to permit filtration. This may enhance stasis and hemoconcentration still further and explain the passage of plasma constituents into the subendothelial spaces. Stasis and the presence of altered red cells may activate phagocytosis on the part of local macrophages (mesangial and endothelial cells), thus causing greater peroxidative injury in the phagocytic "burst". Mesangiolysis could thus be seen as the final expression of peroxidative injury associated with hemodynamic alterations.[44] The presence of red cells and platelets in the subendothelial spaces, too, instead of being the expression of mural thrombi with supraendothelialisation, may be the consequence of phagocytic activation of local macrophages. Evidence in favour of this view can be seen in the frequent observation of demolished and fragmented red cells and platelets in the glomeruli in HUS.

DIFFERENTIAL DIAGNOSIS

The pathogenetic pattern we have described offers a series of distinctive features whereby HUS can be specifically classified and hence differentiated from similar syndromes with which it shares one or more symptoms.
The first point to be made is that the simple association of hemolytic anemia and ARF is not enough to substantiate a diagnosis of HUS. Were this so, the classification criteria would be even vaguer and confusion would increase. ARF, indeed, may be noted in other hemolytic abnormalities, such as those associated with incompatible transfusion, water hemolysis, nocturnal paroxysmal haemoglobinuria and red cell damage caused by solvents. From a pathogenetic point of view the difference is striking, because the kidney in this cases, contrary to that occurs in HUS, is only an innocent bystander of an hematological problem. In these cases the peripheral smear displays no evidence of red cell alteration, and renal damage is usually of the acute hemoglobinuric tubular necrosis type.[45]

In the second place, it is important to remember that the observation of a few peripheral schistocytes is not enough to sustain a diagnosis of HUS. This is a nonspecific and very common finding in a very large percentage of many diseases, such SLE, cryo, vasculitis, Schönlein-Henoch (60% in a review of 1400 personal cases)[46]. This type of finding probably corresponds to what was demonstrated by Brain, and is really evidence of red cell fragmentation within a microcirculation altered by a variety of processes. In these cases, kidney is the target of the pathogenetic damage, and red cell deformation can really be regarded as nothing more than an indirect, non specific indication of microangiopathy. Actual anemia, reticulocytosis and increase in LDH are usually absent, red cell alteration is confined to a few schistocytes and, what is more important, the clinical picture may help in the differential diagnosis.
From a pathogenetic point of view, HUS is likely **defined** by a double damage, both to red cells, and renal microcirculation. In clinical practice, however, it may be difficult to **make** differential diagnosis, mainly in the adult forms. Overlapping syndromes are frequent, and more specific diagnostic features are still lacking. A crucial diagnostic role is charged on the red cell alterations, which, however, may be a transient features.

TREATMENT

Dialysis is fundamental to improvement of the prognosis in HUS, not only because it permits survival during renal failure in the expectation of spontaneous regression, as is often the case in children, but also in the light of the recently formulated suggestion that it is able to remove substances such as endotoxins from the circulation..
At any events, there can be no doubt that earlier and more correct management of uremia and a better control of hypertension have led to a drastic improvement in survival.
Many forms of treatments have been proposed in keeping with differences of opinion concerning the pathogenesis of HUS. These have included corticosteroids and immunodepressor, heparin, systemic or local renal administration of fibrinolytic activators, and platelet antiaggregants. Sporadic successes have been reported, whereas controlled trials with heparin and urodinase in children have led to negative results. The successful employment of plasma infusion and plasma exchange in TTP has led to their being proposed for HUS as well. The rationale behind depletion management is that benefit will be obtained by the removal of toxic substances, such as endotoxins, viral or bacterial products, oxidants acting as mediators of the injury, intraplatelet or red cell release products and possible inhibitors of prostacyclin synthesis. Great significance is also attached to the possible use of plasma replacement for the introduction of missing factors.[47-49]
Examination of the reported cases leaves one with the impression that these protocols had no great influence on the outcome in cases involving children, where, as we have seen, the prognosis is generally good. In the adult, prompt regression of hematological alterations is certainly

Table III. Outcome of children HUS
(Department of Nephrology, Torino, 1976-1986)

CHILDREN HUS (n 16)				
		FULL RECOVERY	CRF	DEATH
Supportive care	8	6		2
Plasma therapy	8	6	2	

obtained, whereas the progress of renal function appears to be less affected. It is particularly difficult to find out any kind of relation between treatment and mortality, since in the adult this is too much influenced by systemic diseases, often altready present.

Our experience also shows that the prognosis is intrinsically good in infantile forms of HUS, in wich a total resolution was observed in 6/8 patients treated with supportive therapies alone, and in 6/8 treated with plasma therapies (Table III). In the adult, too, full recovery resulted in the same number of patients treated with supportive or plasma therapies. The mortality was higher in the patients treated with plasma therapies, probably because these treatment were adopted in the more complicated cases (Table IV). The effectiveness of any treatment, of course, will be influenced by the time elapsing between the initial injury and its adoption. The fact that secondary mechanisms are primarily being treated is also a cactor governing success.

Lastly, consideration must be given to the new possibilities of treating HUS suggested by recent explanations of its pathogenesis. Vitamin E is a candidate on account of its antioxidant and membrane stabilisation properties. Superoxide-dismutase, too, is a possible alternative. Both perhaps may be usefully associated with alphalytid blocking agents and (e.g. pentoxyphyllin) and drugs capable of improving red cell flexibility. Certainly, however, since HUS is not TTP, the parameter of therapeutical efficacy may not be only the normalization of hematological abnormalities, which are, in the former transient and reversible, and probably of different pathogenetic role that in the later.

Table IV. Outcome of adult HUS
(Department of Nephrology, Torino, 1972-1986)

ADULT HUS (n 21)				
		FULL RECOVERY	CRF	DEATH
Supportive care	10	2	5	3
Plasma therapy	11	2	2	7

REFERENCES

1. J.S.C. Fong, J.P. De Chadaverian, B.S. Kaplan, Hemolytic-uremic syndrome: current concepts and management. Ped Clin North Am 28: 835 (1982)
2. M.H. Goldstein, J. Churg, L. Strauss, hemolytic-uremic syndrome. Nephron 23: 263 (1979)
3. C.A. Gianantonio, Past and present of the hemolytic uremic syndrome in Argentina, in "Acute renal Disorders and renal emergencies, J. Strauss, ed., Martinus Nijhoff, Boston (1984)
4. R. Habib, M. Lévy, M.F. Gagnadoux, M. Broyer, Le prognostic dy syndrome hémolytique et urémique chez l'enfant, in "Actualité néphrologiques de l'Hôpital Necker", J-P. Grünfeld ed., Flammarion Médicine - Science, Paris (1981)
5. B.S. Kaplan, P.R. Goodyer, J.S. Fong, P.D. Thomson, The hemolytic-uremic syndrome: the most important cause of acute renal failure in infants and children in "Acute Renal disorders and renal emergencies", J. Strauss ed., Martinus Nijhoff, Boston (1984)
6. L. Morel-Maroger, Adult hemolytic-uremic syndrome. Kidney Int 18: 125 (1980)
7. R. Misiani, A.C. Appiani, A. Edefonti, E. Gatti, A. Bettinelli, M. Giani, E.C. Rossi, G. Remuzzi, G. Mecca: Haemolytic uraemic syndrome: therapeutic effect of plasma infusion. Br Med J 285: 1304 (1982)
8. M.C. Brain, J.V. Dacie, D.O'B. Hourihane, Microangiopathic hemolytic anemia: the possible rose of vascular lesions in pathogenesis, Brit J Haemat 8: 358 (1962)
9. E. Alhanaty, M.P. Sheetz, Control of the erythrocyte membrane: recovery from the effect of creting agents. J Cell Biol 91: 884 (1981)
10. M. Flamm, D. Schachter, Acanthocytosis and cholesterol enrichment decrease lipid fluidity of only the outer human erythrocyte membrane leaflet, Nature, Lond. 298: 290 (1982)
11. S. O'Regan, R.W. Chesney, B.S. Kaplan, K.N. Drummond, Red cell membrane phospholipid abnormalities in the hemolytic uremic syndrome, Clin Nephrol 15: 14 (1980)
12. R.P. Bolande, B.S. Kaplan, Experimental studies on the hemolytic-uremic syndrome. Nephron 39: 228 (1985)
13. J.A. Dormandy, Haemorheology and thrombosis, in "Advances in haemostasis and thrombosis", A. Cajozzo ed., Ciba-Geigy, Palermo (1983)
14. P. Stratta, Hemorheological approach to thrombotic microangiopathies, Nephron 40: 67 (1985)
15. A. Bohle, B. Grabenser, R. Fischer, E. Berg, H. Klust, On four cases of hemolytic-uremic syndrome without microangiopathy, Clin Nephrol, 24: 88 (1985)
16. T. Butler, H. Rahmon, K.A. Al-Mahmud, I. Moyenul, P. Bardhan, I. Kabin, M.M. Rahman, An animal model of haemolytic-uraemic syndrome in shigellosis: lipopolysaccharides of Shigella dysenteriae and S. flexnery produce leukocyte-mediated renal cortical necrosis in rabbit. Br J Exp Path 66: 7 (1985)
17. O. Ortega Marcos, F. Escuin, J.L. Miguel, P. Gomez-Fernandez, M. Perez Fontàn, R. Selgas, L.S. Sicilia, Hemolytic-uremic syndrome in a

patient with gastric adenocarcinoma: partial recovery of renal function after gastrectomy, Clin Nephrol 24: 265 (1985)

18. C.A. Gianantonio, Extrarenal manifestations of the hemolytic-uremic syndrome, In "Acute renal disorders and renal emergencies", J. Strauss ed. Martinus Nijhoff, Boston (1984)
19. R.H. Heptinstall, Microangiopathic hemolytic anemia, hemolytic-uremic syndrome, thrombotic thrombocytopenic purpura and scleroderma. In "Pathology of the Kidney", R.H. Heptinstall ed., Little Brown, New York (1974)
20. J.S.C. Fong, B.S. Kaplan, Thrombocytopenia in hemolytic-uremic syndrome, in "Acute renal disorder and renal emergencies", J. Strauss ed., Martinus Nijhoff, Boston (1984)
21. M.A. Karmali, M. Petric, C. Lim, P.C. Fleming, G.S. Arbus, H. Lior, The association between idiopathic hemolytic uremic syndrome and infection by verotoxin-producing Escherichia Coli.
22. P.E. Rose, J.A. Armour, C.E. Williams, F.GH. Hill, Verotoxin and neuraminidase induced platelet aggregating activity in plasma: their possible role in the pathogenesis of the haemolytic uraemic syndrome, J Clin Pathol 38: 438 (1985)
23. Editorial, Haemolytic uraemic syndrome, lancet ii: 1078 (1984)
24. G. Remuzzi, E.C. Rossi, The hemolytic uremic syndrome, Int J Art Organs, 8: 171 (1985)
25. A. Vercellone, P. Stratta, C. Canavese, La sindrome emolitico-uremico. Giornale It. Nefrologia 1: 73 (1984)
26. G. Remuzzi, R. Misiani, D. Marchesi, M. Livio, G. Mecca, G. De Gaetano, M.B. Donati, Haemolytic-uraemic syndrome: deficiency of plasma factor(s) regulating prostacyclin activity? Lancet 2: 871 (1978)
27. P. Stratta, C. Canavese, T. Bussolino, M.G. Mansueto, F. Gagliardi, A. Vercellone, Haemolytic abortive syndrome, Lancet i: 424 (1983)
28. R. Silberbauer, G. Schernethaner, H. Sinzinger, Decreased vascular prostacyclin in juvenile onset diabetes, New Engl J Med 300: 366 (1979)
29. P. Stratta, C. Canavese, F. Peiretti, P. Vallauri, A. Vercellone, Warning: platelet factor four, betathromboglobulin and thromboxane in donor's plasma units, Thromb Haemostas, 49: 51 (1983)
30. H. Sinzinger, W. Feigl, K. Silberbauer, prostacyclin generation in atherosclerotic arteries, Lancet ii: 469 (1979)
31. N. Hizli, G. Sahin, F. Sahin, E. Kansu, S. Duru, S. Karacadag, P. Batman, S. Dundar, T. Zileli, H. Telatar, Plasma prostacyclin levels in Behçet's disease, Lancet, i: 1454 (1985)
32. T.L. Dormandy, Am approach to free radicals, Lancet, ii: 1010 (1983)
33. B. Holliwell, M.C. Gutteridge, Oxygen toxycity, oxygen radicals, transitional metal and disease, Biochem J 219: 1 (1984)
34. T. Yoshikawa, M.Murakami, N. Yoshida, O. Seto, M. Kondo, Effects of superoxide dismutase and catalase on disseminated intravascular coagulation in rats, Thromb Haemostas (Stuttgart) 50: 869 (1983)
35. A.B. Gruskin, J.L. Naiman, M.S. Polinsky, M. Mellan, H.J. Baluarte, B.A. Kaiser, S.A. Perlmon, B.Z. Morgenstern, Uric acid perturbation in the hemolytic uremic syndrome, in "Acute renal disorders and renal emergencies", J. Strauss ed, Martinus Nijhoff, Boston (1984)

36. A.L. Tappel, Lipid peroxidation damage to cell components, Fed Proc 32: 1870 (1973)
37. V. Cattel, Mitomycin induced hemolytic uremic kidney, Am J Pathol 121: 88 (1985)
38. J. Nafstad, Endothelial damage and platelet thrombosis associated with PUFA-rich, vitamin E deficient diet fed to pig, Thromb Res 5: 251 (1974)
39. H.R. Powell, D.A. McCredie, C.M. Taylor, J.R. Burke, R.G. Walker, Vitamin E treatment of haemolytic uremic syndrome, Arch Dis Child 59: 401 (1984)
40. D.G. McKay, A.N. Whitaker, V. Cruse, Studies on catecholamine shock II. An Experimental model of microangiopathic hemolysis. Am J Path 56: 177 (1969)
41. L. Raij, W.F. Keane, A.F. Michael, Unilateral Shwartzman reaction: cortical necrosis in one kidney following in vivo perfusion with endotoxin. Kidney Int 12: 51 (1977)
42. P. Kincaid-Smith, Coagulation and renal disease, Kidney Int 2: 183 (1972)
43. H.L. Sheehan, J.C. Davis, Renal inschemia with failed reflow, J Pathol Bacteriol 78: 105 (1959)
44. T. Morita, J. Churg, Mesangiolysis, Kidney Int 24: 1 (1983)
45. P. Stratta, C. Canavese, L. Colla, A. Vercellone, Heomolysis, acute renal failure and haemolytic-uremic syndrome, Nephron 41: 119 (1985)
46. P. Stratta, Schizocytes en pathologie nephrologique. Néphrologie (in press)
47. G. Remuzzi, R. Misiani, D. Marchesi, M. Livio, G. Mecca, G. De Gaetano, M.B. Donati, Treatment of the hemolytic uremic syndrome with plasma, Clin Nephrol 12: 179 (1979)
48. P. Stratta, C. Canavese, F. Bussolino, A. Vercellone, Why is plasma infusion useful in hemolytic uremic syndrome? (letter) Clin Nephrol 22: 270 (1984)
49. B.S. Kaplan, P.D. Thomson, Current approaches to the management of hemolytic uremic syndrome, in "Acute renal disorders and renal emergencies" J. Strauss Ed., Martinus Nijhoff, Boston (1984)

LONG-TERM PROGNOSIS OF HAEMOLYTIC-URAEMIC SYNDROME IN CHILDREN

Rosanna Gusmano, Francesco Perfumo, Maria Rosa Ciardi, and Marcella Sarperi

Nephrology and Dialysis Department, G. Gaslini Institute Genoa, Italy

INTRODUCTION

Haemolytic-uraemic syndrome (HUS) is the most frequent cause of acute renal failure in children. Geographical surveys have demonstrated occurrence of HUS in both an epidemic and endemic manner (1) and familial occurrences have been reported (2). The clinical and histopathological features of HUS are well-known,while aetiology and physiopathology are not completely understood. The long-term evolution of renal function in children is incompletely documented. The recognition that HUS is not a conseq uence of a single clinico-pathologic entity may explain the conflicting results regarding prognosis.
In the present study we summarize our experience on the evolution of kidney function in children with HUS.

MATERIAL AND METHODS

Between January 1970 and August 1985 ninetytwo children affected by HUS were observed. The diagnosis of HUS was defined by the presence of the triad haemolytic anaemia,thrombocytopenia and acute renal failure. According to the criteria of Kaplan et al.(3,4) there were 77 severe and 15 mild cases. Clinical and biochemical data of this group of patients are presented in table 1.

The treatment varied during time: 47 patients received heparin therapy (5), 17 plasma infusions (10 ml/kg of plasma until the platelets' number was normalized) and 28 no "specific" therapy. All patients received antihypertensive and anticunvulsant therapy as needed.
Extrarenal epuration was instituted in 79 cases: 63 of them were treated by hemodialysis and the remaining 16 by peritoneal dialysis. The duration of dialysis ranged between 2 and 40 days in 77 children. In 2 patients the dialytic treatment (hemodialysis in one and continuous ambulatory peritoneal dialysis in the other) lasted for 24 and 10 months respectively before the patients could be treated by conservative measures.

Table 1.. Clinical and biochemical data at admission in 92 children affected by HUS (mean ± S.D).

PATIENTS	Number	92
	Sex M/F	50/42
	Age range (years)	0.1-14
	< 2 years (%)	51 (55.4)
	> 2 years (%)	41 (44.6)
PRODROMES	Gastroenteritis	75
	Fever	6
	Aspecific	7
	None	4
HAEMATOLOGY	Haemoglobin (g/dl)	5.8±1.2
	Platelets (x 10^3 $mm^3$7	53.9±33.5
RENAL FAILURE	Blood urea (mg/dl)	235.2±101.1
	Serum creatinine (mg/dl)	5.9±2.5
COMPLICATIONS	Arterial hypertension	41
	Convulsions	27
	Coma	4

The patients were evaluated 1,6 and 12 months after being discharged and subsequenly every year,when renal function was normal. The children with impaired renal function were observed at different intervals according to their clinical status.

Student's t-test and chi-square test were used for statistical analysis.

RESULTS

Short-term prognosis

During the acute phase of the illness there were 7 deaths (7.6% of the cases). The causes of the deaths were neurological complications in 6 patients and fungal pericarditis in the remaining one. When discharged 5 children were on chronic dialysis therapy, but subsequently 2 of them improved their renal function and dropped out from dialytic treatment. Three patients since being discharged have been lost to follow-up.

Long-term prognosis

The long-term evaluation of renal function deals with 79 children followed for a maximum of 11 years. The evolution of GFR,estimated as creatinine clearance,is shown in figure 1. The mean value of GFR (ml/m'/

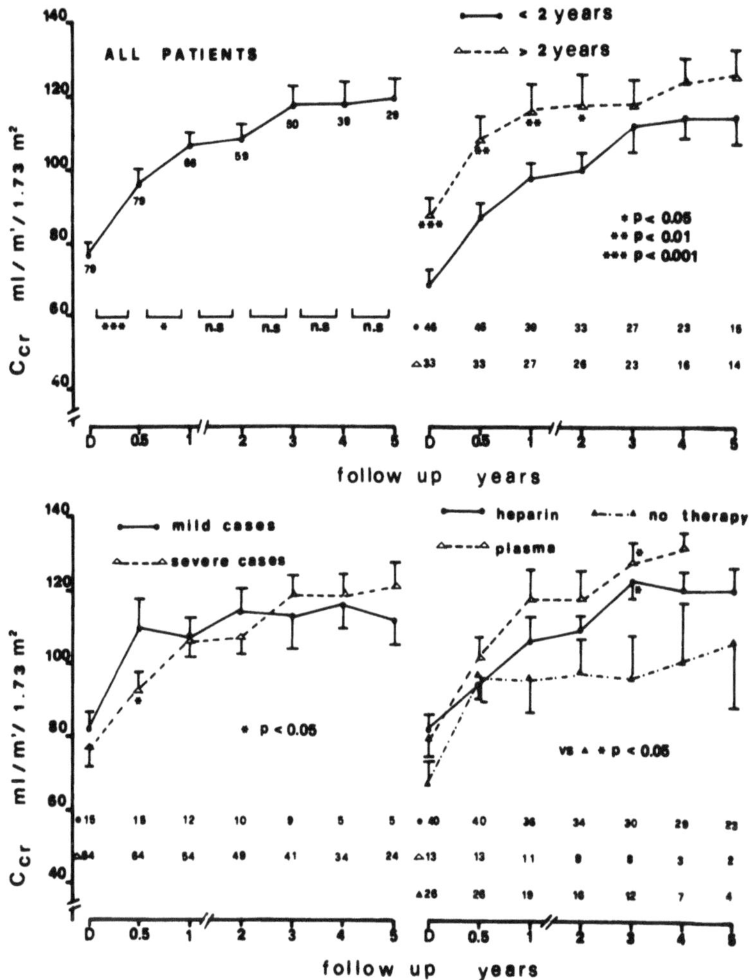

Figure 1. Long-term evolution of renal function evaluated as creatinine clearance (ml/min/1.73). D=discharge

1.73, mean±sem) was 76.8±3.1 at discharge and 96.6±3.4 after 6 months. Afterwards GFR increased and ranged between 105 and 120.

Figure 1 presents the evaluation of GFR with the patients subdivided into subgroups according to patients' age (< or > 2 years), to severity of the illness (mild and severe cases) and to treatment (heparin, plasma infusions or no therapy). The younger patients showed a lower creatinine clearance from the time of discharge to 2 years after the acute phase,but this might be the consequence of the maturation of the renal function,while the other subdivision into groups showed only an occasional statistically significant difference at a single time point.

In figure 2 the long-terme evolution of renal function in children with impaired GFR (< 70 ml/min/1.73) at the time of discharge is shown. It was possible to observe an improvement in all cases,and at 12 months after the discharge only 6 children out of 21 had a GFR below 70.

The urinary findings showed hematuria and proteinuria in all cases

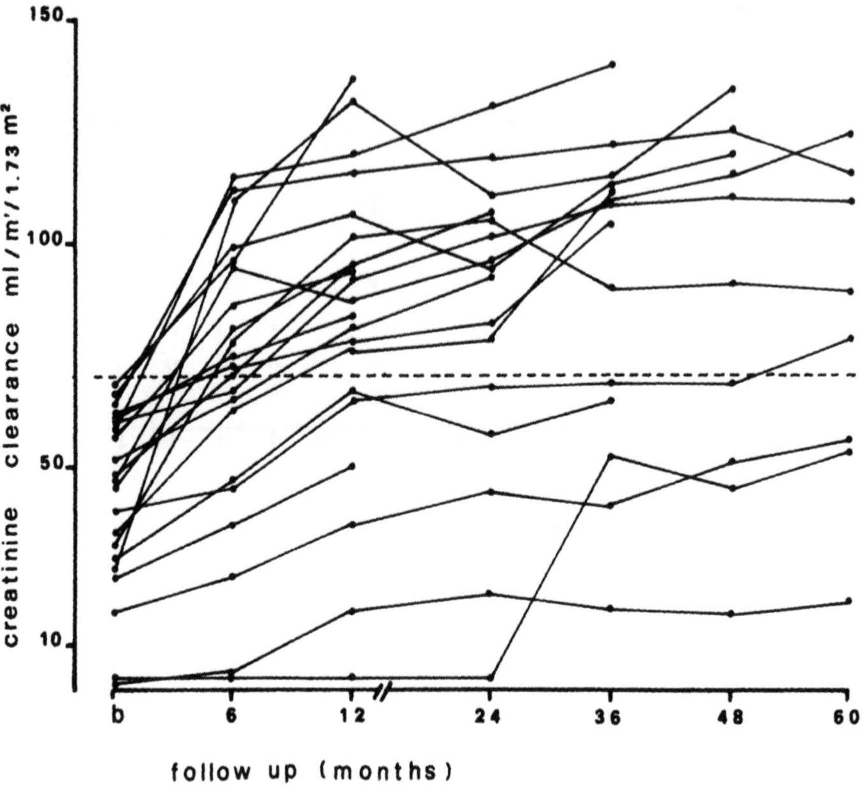

Figure 2. Long-term evolution of renal function in 21 children with impaired GFR (creatinine clearance < 70 ml/min/1.73) at the time of discharge (D).

at admission,but urinary abnormalities persisted only in 3 patients after 1 year.

In search of prognostic indicators (table 2) we sudivided the patients into group A (73 children with complete recovery of renal function within 1 year from the acute phase) and group B (16 patients: 7 died, 3 on chronic dialysis and 6 with chronic renal failure). We found a significant difference only for the presence of prodromal gastroenteritis,while no significant difference was observed for age or for the presence of con-

Table 2. Prognostic indicators at admission

	Group A	Group B	p
Age < 2 years	42/73	8/16	NS
Gastroenteritis	60/73	8/16	<0.05
Convulsions	19/73	8/16	NS
Hypertension	33/73	8/16	NS

vulsions or arterial hypertension.

COMMENT

HUS is predominantly a disease of infants and young children, but in consideration of the heterogeneity of the clinical and laboratory findings HUS is probably not a single disease entity. Considerable controversy exists concerning the aetiology, pathogenesis and treatment of patients with HUS. In addition data on long-term prognosis are scanty, thus present knowledge is uncertain (6).

It is apparent that with early recognition of renal impairment and the availability of dialytic techniques the acute mortality rate has been lowered. The other treatments, such as heparin (3,5,7,8), fibrinolytic therapy (9,10), platelets-deaggregating agents (11,12) and plasma (13), that have been employed, remain to be evaluated in order to determine the effects on both acute survival and long-term prognosis.

Several reports have been published on the prognosis of infants and children with HUS. The acute mortality rate of 7.6% of our series is of the same magnitude in most series (14,15,16), but it is noteworthy that in no patient did progressive disease follow the acute phase as previously reported (7); indeed our data agree with a subsequent report (16).. The fact that no secondary deterioration of renal function has occurred is of great practical importance.

In our experience there was no difference in long-term evolution of GFR when patients were subdivided into different subgroups according to age, severity of the disease or modality of treatment. This last assumption, although not derived from controlled trials, must be underlined and confirms the conflicting results regarding efficacy of different forms of therapy.

Another point to stress from our study is the observation that long-term evolution of renal function may be predicted from the results observed during the first year after the acute phase: all the patients with complete recovery of renal function reached normal GFR within 1 year of discharge.

REFERENCES

1) M.Levin and T.M.Barratt, Haemolytic-uraemic syndrome. Arch.Dis.Child 59:397 (1984).
2) B.S.Kaplan, R.W.Chesney and K.N.Drummond, Haemolyticuraemic syndrome in families. New Engl.J.Med., 292:1090 (1975).
3) B.S.Kaplan, J.Katz, S.Krawitz and A.Lurie, An analysis of the results of therapy in 67 cases of the hemolytic-uremic syndrome. J.Pediatr., 78:420 (1975).
4) B.S.Kaplan, P.D.Thomson and J.P.de Chadarevian, The hemolytic-uremic syndrome. Pediatr.Clin.N.Am., 23:761 (1976).
5) R.Gusmano, F.Perfumo, G.C.Basile and L.Formicucci, Risultati della terepia anticoagulante e dialitica nella sindrome emolitico-uremica dell'infanzia. Min.Nefrol., 23:286 (1976)

6) R.S.Trompeter,R.Schwartz ,C.Chantler et al.,Haemolytic-uraemic syndrome: an analysis of prognostic features. Arch.Dis.Child.,58:101 (1983).

7) C.A.Gianantonio,M.Vitacco,F.Mendilaharzu et al.,The hemolytic-uremic syndrome. Nephron,11:174 (1973).

8) W.Proesmans and R.Eeckels, Has heparin changed the prognosis of the hemolytic-uremic syndrome ? ,Clin.Nephrol.,2:169 (1974).

9) H.R.Powell and H.Ekert, Streptokinase and antithrombotic therapy in the hemolytic-uremic syndrome. J.Pediatr.,84:345 (1974).

10) C.Loirat,F.Beaufils,E.Sonsino et al., Traitement du syndrome hémolitique et urémique de l'enfant par l'urokinase.Essai controllé coopératif. Arch.Fr.Pédiatr.,48:15 (1984).

11) G.B.Arenson and C.S.August, Preliminary report. Treatment of the hemolytic-uremic syndrome with aspirin and dipyridamole. J.Pediatr., 86:957 (1975)

12) C.A.Thorsen,E.C.Rossi,D.Green and F.A.Carone, The treatment of the hemolytic-uremic syndrome with inhibitors of platelet function. Am.J.Med.,66:711 (1979).

13) G.Remuzzi,R.Misiani,D.Marchesi et al., Treatment of the hemolytic-uremic syndrome with plasma. Clin.Nephrol.,12:279 (1979).

14) M.Ekberg,L.Holmberg and T.Denneberg, Hemolytic-uremic syndrome results of treatment with hemodialysis. Acta Paediatr.Scand.,66:693 (1977).

15) R.A.Donckerwolcke,H.Tidens and R.Kuijten, Haemolytic-uraemic syndrome. Paediatrician, 8:378 (1979).

16) P.Binda ki Muaka,W.Proesmans and R.Eeckels, The hemolytic-uremic syndrome in childhood:a study of the long-term prognosis. Eur.J. Pediatr.,136:237 (1981).

POST-TRANSPLANT ACUTE RENAL FAILURE

Jean-Louis Touraine, Jane-Luce Garnier
Alain Mercatello, Denise Mongin-Long, Jean-Louis Faure, Felix Cantarovich, and Jules Traeger

Transplantation Unit, Pavillion P, INSERM U80
Place d'Arsonal, 69374 Lyon Cedex 08, France

INTRODUCTION

Acute renal failure (ARF) is still a frequent event in the immediate post-transplant period. In itself, it has usually no dramatic consequence since, following a period of 2 to 3 weeks when dialysis is frequently required, renal function develops up to a normal degree in most cases. However, ARF over these initial weeks may mask some of the clinical manifestations of other post-transplant complications, especially rejection crises, and delay their treatment.

In this paper, we try to identify the major risk factors associated with the development of ARF immediately after transplantation, based on our experience with 1100 kidney transplants, a majority of which having involved cadaver donors. The more precise analysis of some individual factors and some potential prophylactic measures have been carried out in more limited series of patients over the last few years.

CAUSES OF ARF

Four main etiologies of ARF can be encountered in the early post-transplant period.

Hyperacute Rejection

This complication is now very rare, thanks to the systematic practice of sensitive cross-matches between donor cells and recipient sera. Patients with pre-formed antibodies against ABO or HLA antigens of the donor are not transplanted with the corresponding organs. When the cross-match is positive, due to auto-antilymphocyte antibodies, and if anti-HLA antibodies can be demonstrated to be absent, the transplant can be carried out without special risk of hyperacute rejection. Anti-B-cell antibodies are not either a contra-indication.

The frequency of this complication may slightly rise, due to the desire of transplanting hyper-immunized patients with kidneys from donors against whom they had, in the past, developed some degree of sensitization. This method is currently under investigation and it will be seen whether such transplants can be carried out, with special care, in the absence of severe rejection.

The clinical manifestations of hyperacute rejection include abrupt swelling of the transplant, associated with fever, intra-vascular coagulation and it frequently leads to cortical necrosis.

Vascular Occlusion

This complication is also becoming rarer and rarer. Arterial thrombosis was classically said to occur in 2 to 8 % of cases (1,2),venous thrombosis in less than 1 % (2). At the present time, the frequency of these complications is much lower due to improved surgical technics. The diagnosis of this type of ARF can be made by radionuclide scanning or by angiography. When identified early, a surgical repair is possible, with good functional results.

Ureteric Obstruction or Leakage.

ARF of urologic origin accounts for 2 to 8 % of oliguria following renal transplantation (1). They include ureteric leakage which frequently needs surgery, or obstruction (ureteric stenosis, compression, or clots). The diagnosis is provided by ultrasound investigation or radionuclide scanning.

Acute Tubular Necrosis

This complication is by far the most common cause of ARF in the immediate post-transplant period. The frequency of acute tubular necrosis (ATN) varies among centers, between 10 and 50 % in cadaver kidney transplants and between 1 and 7 % in living donor kidney transplants.

This complication appears to be of multi-factorial origin, related in particular with prolonged ischemia and hemodynamic factors both in donors and recipients.

FACTORS INVOLVED IN ATN

It is not always easy to identify the very cause of ATN in an individual patient. The factors may be numerous and intricated. However, it is important to know the main etiologies of ATN in the post-transplant period, in order to develop prophylactic measures. Based on pathophysiology, it is possible to classify these causes in pre-renal, intra-renal and post-renal factors (3).

Hypovolemia and hemodynamic instability due to agonal state may occur in the donor. Hypovolemia is also frequent in the recipient ; it may be secondary to vigorous dialysis immediately before surgery, blood loss, salt and water depletion, etc. A rise in plasma oncotic pressure, an augmented renin release and an increased conversion of angiotensin I, into angiotensin II result in reduction of glomerular filtration rate.

Prolonged cold ischemia and, even more important, warm ischemia can result in ATN. The evidence for the role of ischemia is demonstrated by the significant difference between frequency of ATN in recipients of cadaver organs and of living related transplants.

Increased occurrence of ATN has also been associated with poor renal function at the time of removal from the donor and graft failure has been shown to be more frequent when serum creatinine of the donor was above 2 mg/dl (4). The cause of death of the donor did not seem to influence graft outcome (4). The age of the donor, over 45 or when it is in the pediatric group, has been shown to increase the risk of ATN ; the best results have been obtained with organs removed from twenty to thirty year old donors (4). Immediately after the transplant, the kidney seems to be very vulnerable to the usual factors responsible for ATN : a moderate depletion in water or sodium, an usual dose of potentially nephrotoxic antibiotics or other compounds such as cyclosporine can delay restoration of a normal renal function.

In this same period, the use of large quantities of radiographic contrast agents has the same potential dangers as in all cases of renal failure.

Surgery itself may play a part in ATN : warm ischemia above 30 and even more 40 minutes explains some cases of ATN (3). The conditions of removal of the kidney and dissection of vessels may also play a role, possibly through vasoactive influences. The mode of anesthesia, which may modify hemodynamic parameters, has sometimes been implicated in a few case of ATN .

Any urologic complication in the immediate post-transplant period can also increase the probability of ATN in relatively fragile transplants.

In a recent analysis of 55 sequential cadaver kidney transplants in our institution, 17 patients required hemodialysis in the post-transplant period. When the patients who developed ATN were compared to the others, the only significant difference that we could identify was the increased value of systolic blood pressure in the group of patients who did not develop ATN (Table 1). Whether blood pressure itself or the requirement for antihypertensive compounds in most of hypertensive patients was responsible for resistance to ATN is not known. The two groups of patients (with or without ATN) remained significantly different in terms of mean blood pressure all over the first week after transplantation.

Table 1. HEMODYNAMIC PARAMETERS DURING SURGERY

Parameters	NTA -	NTA +	
Duration of surgery	132 ± 36 min	125 ± 19 min	N.S.
Systolic blood pressure (mmHg)	155 ± 32	138 ± 30	p<0.05
Central venous pressure (cmH2O)	11 ± 3	11 ± 2	N.S
Need for volemia expansion (% of patients)	34%	59%	N.S

Another factor that was apparent in a larger series of patients that we analysed previously was the influence of anti-lymphocyte globulins (ALG). All patients had, at that time, azathioprine and 1 mg/kg/day of steroids. By randomization, half of the patients also received ALG ; these patients had a significantly lower incidence of acute renal failure requiring hemodialysis in the early phase after surgery (Table 2).

Table 2. PERCENTAGE OF PATIENTS REQUIRING HEMODIALYSIS (Day 0 - Day 15)

Treatment	HD +	HD -
ALG -	35 %	65 %
ALG +	13 %	87 %

p<0.002

HD = hemodialysis - ALG = Antilymphocyte globulins

PROPHYLACTIC MEASURES

Prophylaxis of ATN obviously involved prevention of the above-mentioned factors. The control of volemia and hemodynamic state, the avoidance of nephrotoxic treatment, the efforts to shorten ischemia and the well-controlled use of diuretics such as furosemide or mannitol (in sufficient but not excessive amounts) are among these measures. In addition, several attempts have been carried out to further reduce the frequency of ATN. Expansion of volemia, up to the limit of tolerance, using a very careful monitoring has reduced the need for hemodialysis from 26% to 3.2% in one study (5). In a series of 272 patients analysed between 1979 and 1983, we have also been able to decrease the frequency of hemodialysis from 21% to 4.2% by a careful fluid expansion protocol, carried out during and after surgery, and combined with administration of adjusted doses of furosemide and mannitol.

Various molecules have been tried to improve kidney vascularization. Up to now, few studies have demonstrated a significant benefit of any single treatment. When we compared the effect of dopamine plus furosemide versus furosemide alone, the frequency of ATN did not appear to be significantly different : in patients receiving dopamine, the requirement for hemo-dialysis was observed in 28% of cases and in the patients without dopamine it was found in 23.5%. Great hopes presently reside in the potentially beneficial use of calcium channel blockers. In one study, the administration of 20 mg of verapamil to 20 renal donors led to better urine output and serum creatinine on the first day after transplantation (6).

MANAGEMENT OF THE TRANSPLANT PATIENT WITH ATN

The diagnosis of ATN can be assessed by non-invasive means, such as radionuclide scanning. The main difficulty is represented by the loss of major clinical manifestations of rejection : the usual criterion of renal function deterioration is missing ; fever and graft tanderness remain useful indicators. Sequential cytologies after fine needle aspiration are very valuable. Immunological monitoring may sometimes provide suggestive evidence of a rejection crisis. In doubtful cases, as well as in patients without any recovery of urine output after two or three weeks, needle biopsy seems to be justified to demonstrate histological manifestations of rejection, cortical necrosis, abnormally prolonged tubular necrosis or any other complication.

During this period of ATN, eviction of nephrotoxic agents, such as antibiotics or radiographic contrast agents in large amounts, is preferable. Whether or not cyclosporine can be given to the patient is still a matter for debate (1). The incidence of ATN has been shown to be higher in cyclosporine-treated patients, with a longer time for recovery (7).

CONCLUSION

The occurrence of ATN does not seem to be very significantly detrimental for future renal function (3). The long-term transplant survival is either somewhat reduced or not significantly different in patients with initial ATN as compared to patients with an immediately good renal function, depending on the studies (4,8). In any case, occurrence of oliguria in the post-transplant period adds some difficulties in the monitoring of the patients, may favour some complications and renders the diagnosis of rejection crisis more difficult. Efforts to prevent ATN are therefore important. Since this complication appears to be caused by a number of factors, it would appear reasonable to prevent as much as possible all these etiological factors. This approach, added to the simultaneous use of pharmacological agents improving resistance of tubular cells to ischemia and augmenting kidney vascularization will probably reduce the incidence of ATN in transplant patients.

REFERENCES

1. Robinson B.H.B., Acute renal failure following renal transplantation. In : V.E. Andreucci (Ed) : Acute renal failure. Martinus Nijhoff Pub., Boston, 387-402,1984.
2. Jordan M.L., Cook G.T., Cardella C.J. Ten years of experience with vascular complications in renal transplantation. J. Urology, 128, 689-692, 1982.
3. Goldszer R.C., Strom T.B., Tilney N.L. Acute renal failure associated with renal transplantation in Brenner Ed. Acute renal failure, Saunders Pub., Philadelphia, London, Toronto, Mexico City, Rio de Janeiro,Sydney, Tokyo, 555-566, 1983.
4. San Filippo F., Vaughn W.K, Spees E.K., Lucas B.A. The detrimental effects of delayed graft function in cadaver donor renal transplantation. Transplantation, 38, 643-648, 1984.
5. Luciani J., Frantz Ph., Conrad A., Chareire M.F., Rottenbourg J., Küss R. Reprise immédiate de la fonction rénale après transplantation. Néphrologie, 2, 120-124, 1981.
6. Duggan K.A., Mac Donald G.J., Charlesworth J.A., Pussell B.A.. Verapamil prevents post-transplant oliguric renal failure. Clin. Nephrolology, 24, 289-291, 1985.
7. Canadian multicentre transplant study group. A randomized trial of cyclosporine A in cadaveric renal transplantation. N. Engl. J. Med., 309, 809-815, 1983.
8. Brophy D., Najarian J.S., Kjellstrand C.M. Acute tubular necrosis after renal transplantation, 29, 245-248, 1980.

POST TRAUMATIC ACUTE RENAL FAILURE

Joseph M. Letteri

Division of Renal Diseases
Nassau County Medical Center, East Meadow, N.Y. 11554 and
S.U.N.Y. at Stony Brook, N.Y. 11790

Early references to trauma related acute renal failure were all associated with injury of a crushing type. During the Messina earthquake in 1909, victims crushed by falling masonry almost uniformly died (1). Traumatic uremia was largely overlooked during the First World War despite the high incidence of crushing injuries of trench warfare. Bywaters and Beall in 1941 described the clinical picture of crushing and acute renal failure (2) amongst air-raid casualties during the London blitz.

Depicted here is their description of the syndrome.

"The patient has been buried for several hours with pressure on a limb. On admission he looks in good condition except for swelling of the limb, some local anesthesia and whealing. The hemoglobin, however, is raised, and a few hours later, despite vasoconstriction, made manifest by pallor, coldness and sweating, the blood pressure falls. This is restored to preshock level by (often multiple) transfusions of serum, plasma or occasionally blood. Anxiety may now arise concerning the circulation in the injured limb, which may show diminution of arterial pulsation distally accompanied by all the changes of incipient gangrene. Signs of renal damage soon appear, and progress even though the crushed limb may be amputated. The urinary output, initially small, owing perhaps to the severity of the shock diminishes further. The urine contains albumin, and many dark brown or black granular casts. These later decrease in number. The patient is alternatively drowsy and anxiously aware of the severity of his illness. Slight generalized edema, thirst, and incessant vomiting develop and the blood pressure often remains slightly raised. The blood urea and potassium, raised at an early stage become progressively higher and death occurs comparatively suddenly, frequently within a week. Necropsy reveals necrosis of muscle and in the renal tubules, degenerative changes and casts containing brown pigment."

Bywaters and Beall noted severe degenerative changes in the proximal convoluted tubules and in the more distal part of the nephron brown pigmented casts. The urine, in these patients, was not concentrated. Urine/plasma urea ratios averaged 1.68 on the third oliguric day while the urinary chlroide averaged 489 mg per 100 ml or 14mEq/L over the course of renal failure.

Post traumatic renal failure is a major problem in military medicine. In World War II 40 per cent of one group of severely wounded patients developed acute post-traumatic renal insufficiency with a case fatality rate of 91 per cent among the severely oliguric. Teschan _et al_ (3) during the Korean War estimated an incidence of acute renal failure approximating 0.5 per cent of all acutely wounded patients. This underestimates the problem. Approximately 20 per cent of soldiers hit in action in Korea were killed instantly or died before they reached forward hospitals. Of the casualties who reached forward hospitals alive, approximately 98 per cent survived their wounds. Most of these had relatively minor wounds with uncomplicated convalescence. It is the smaller number of severely wounded that renal failure constitutes an important cause of death. For example, in Italy during World War II, at least 40 per cent of a group of very severely wounded casualties at one forward hospital developed acute renal failure.

During the Korean, Vietnam and Middle East War the incidence of acute renal failure was estimated as high as 0.5 to 4.7 per cent of battle casualties with multiple injuries involving the abdomen, thigh and leg and head and cervical spine (4-5). Despite the institution of aggressive surgical and advanced medical care, similar observations have been noted with civilian trauamtized patients and the mortality of acute renal failure in the post traumatic patient remains excessive and approaches 60 per cent.

PATHOGENESIS OF POST TRAUMATIC RENAL FAILURE

The variable incidence of renal failure following severe injury indicates that the acute renal failure is of diverse etiology. Minami (1) in 1923 described the most complete pre World War II experience with acute renal failure and was the first to hypothesize that intrarenal obstruction was the cause of acute renal failure because of the widespread presence of pigmented casts in the tubules of patients dying with this syndrome. He suggested that myohemoglobinuria was involved in producing the renal abnormalities.

It seems likely that as in other conditions associated with acute renal failure, the pathogenesis of the decline in renal function, particularly the low glomerular filtration rate is multifactorial.

Some of the potential factors which could contribute to the decline in glomerlular filtration rate and the subsequent lack of adequate excretion of metabolic end products included a decrease in effective surface area of the glomerular capillary as well as a decrease in renal blood flow. At some point after the initiating event, tubular factors may result in an increase in intra-tubular hydraulic forces exceeding filtration pressure. In addition, damage to the tubule cells could result in passive back diffusion of filtrate into the renal capillaries or lymph. As suggested by Minami, in post traumtic renal failure myoglobinuria is not uncommon. The potential nephrotoxicity of myoglobin, hemoglobin and their derivatives have been evaluated in a number of studies. In general, these studies have indicated these pigments are relatively non toxic to renal tissue. Moreover, other substances may be released from damaged muscle tissue which induce renal injury (6).

Myoglobin, with a molecular weight of 17,000 Daltons, when released into the circulation is bound to a plasma protein, an alpha-2 globulin. About 50 per cent of the plasma myoglobin is bound to the protein at myoglobin concentrations less than 23 mg/dl (7). The renal threshold for myoglobin appears to be between 0.5 to 1.5 mg/dl.

Myoglobin appears in the urine at concentrations exceeding this threshold. At plasma concentration between 1.5 and 23 mg/dl, approximately 50 per cent of the circulating myoglobin is filtered. The renal tubule resorbs myoglobin by endocytosis. Before the urine becomes discolored by myoglobin, the urine concentration of myoglobin must exceed 100 mg/dl. Myoglobinuria is thus dependent on the plasma concentration exceeding the renal threshold.

Myoglobin is not nephrotoxic itself. Aciduria appears to be a prerequisite for myoglobin nephrotoxicity which is potentiated by dehydration. At or below a urine pH of 5.6, myoglobin is converted to ferrihemate which is toxic to the kidney, the vascular and reticular-endothelial system (8-12). In the presence of enhanced uric acid production and excretion commonly associated with trauma, ferrihemate and uric acid may precipitate in concentrated acid urine and contribute to the impairment of renal function. The effect of myoglobin on renal hemodynamics remains controversial.

Crush injury is associated with hypovolemia as described by Bywaters originally and can lead to shock. Hypotension with hemoconcentration resulting in decreased effective circulating volume is secondary to a loss of fluids and electrolytes from the vascular system into damaged muscles and tissues. This initial event, hypovolemia, results in renal ischemia which is potentially reversible by massive expansion of intra-vascular volume. The lower incidence of acute renal failure following civilian trauma is probably related to the rapid replacement of intra vascular volume after early transfer of the patient to hospitals and trauma centers. If not corrected, the hypotensive episode may exacerbate the renal effects of myoglobin released from damaged muscle, thereby resulting in acute pigment related renal failure. Neurogenic factors initiated by the injury as well as release of vasoactive peptides are believed to result in renal vasoconstriction which could enhance the toxicity of myoglobin in crush injury.

Experimental Models of Pigment Nephropathy

The most widely applied models of myoglobinuric acute renal failure are produced by intravenous infusion of methemogloblin or by intramuscular injection of hypertonic glycerol solution (13-16).

Intramuscular glycerol causes muscle cell necrosis with local fluid accumulation. The transfer of fluids and electrolytes into the injured tissues result in decreased renal blood flow and an increase in renal vascular resistance in rats (17). The decline in renal blood flow is rapid, within 10 minutes, and associated with redistribution of blood flow within the kidney. The outer cortex of the kidney is more ischemic than the inner cortex and medulla (18-21). The decrease in renal blood flow is patchy in distribution and not affecting all nephrons. This initial decline in renal blood flow is partially restored by acute volume expansion. It thus appears likely that in the model of myohemoglobin acute renal failure, the decrease in renal blood flow in the initiating phase of the syndrome is responsible for the decrease in glomerular filtration rate. During the maintenance phase of glycerol induced acute renal failure, normal and persistently low renal blood flows have been observed (13-17). With volume expansion during maintenance acute renal failure, renal blood flow is restored to normal but glomerular filtration rate is not necessarily restored or improved. Thus, during the maintenance phase of glycerol induced acute renal failure, the decrease in glomerular filtration rate is not a consequence of the fall in renal blood flow once acute renal failure is established.

The formation of pigmented casts in the tubule is mediated by the interaction of myoglobin with the anionic Tamm-Horsfall protein. Myoglobin with a high isoelectric point (6.8) in acid urine would have a high propensity to form casts with the naturally occuring Tamm-Horsfall protein. Early in the study of glycerol induced acute renal failure, increased intratubular hydraulic pressure was believed to be the factor responsible for the decrease in filtration rate (22). Low intratubular hydraulic pressures have been measured within the first four hours of glycerol induced acute renal failure (23). With methemoglobin administration, proximal hydraulic pressures are increased within three hours when surface nephrons contain casts obstructing the tubular lumens (15). Normal or elevated intratubular pressures have been measured during the maintenance phase of acute renal failure induced by glycerol injection (24). Thus it is not clear whether tubular obstruction by casts is the primary mechanism for the decrease in filtration rate. Back leak of filtrate is not supported by the studies of Jaenike (14). Tubular fluid to plasma inulin ratios in normal rats did not differ from values obtained in methemoglobin infused rats indicating that the tubular permeability of sampled nephrons was not altered in acute renal failure induced by this model. Others have demonstrated that recovery of markers of tubular permeability injected into proximal tubules of methemoglobin damaged nephrons is associated with only a decrease in the recovery of the markers from more distal sites of the nephron (25). Thus the reduction of glomerular filtration during the maintenance phase of myoglobinuric acute renal failure cannot be readily explained by the experiments performed to date and is probably not related to intra tubular obstruction or back leak of filtrate by increased tubular permeability.

Clinical Characteristics of Traumatic Renal Failure

Acute renal failure associated with severe trauma is clinically characterized by a hypercatabolic course: intense negative nitgrogen balance, wasting and poor wound healing. Daily increments in blood urea nitrogen often exceed 50 mg/dl/day. The serum creatinine increases out of proportion to the urea nitrogen levels. Hyperkalemia and hyperphosphatemia ensue because of release of potassium and phosphorus from injured tissues. Profound metabolic acidosis and hyperuricemia and enhanced uric acid excretion secondary to enhanced catabolism of purine precursors are common features of this clinical syndrome. Severe hypocalcemia is often encountered in the oliguric phase while hypercalcemia is noted sometimes in the diuretic phase of those patients with severe muscle injury.

Metabloic Consequences of Post Traumatic Renal Failure

In traumatized patients cellular protein is lost in the absence or presence of renal impairment. The magnitude of the urea nitrogen excretion generally parallels the extent of the injury. Multiple trauma, peritonitis and burns are associated with losses of nitrogen, sometimes exceeding 10 grams/day. The excretion of nitrogen reflects increased degradation of skeletal muscle protein. Decreased lean body mass is observed. Total nitrogen turnover is markedly increased and both protein degradation and synthesis are elevated but degradation exceeds snythesis causing nitgrogen balance to become negative. The release of amino acids from the muscle is increased and are taken up by the liver and converted to glucose, acute phase proteins and urea.

The mechanisms responsible for the accelerated catabolism in traumatized patients with and without renal failure are poorly understood. Interleukin-1, a peptide released from monocytic phagocytes has been implicated in the genesis of increased muscle breakdown of acute trauma (26). Interleukin-1 induces vascular endothelial cells to release prostaglandins which could contribute to the muscle breakdown. Circulating proteases have been implicated by Horl et al in the catabolic response of traumatized patients (27-28). Recently, Mitch and co-workers in rat noted that metabolic acidosis stimulates muscle protein degradation in a glucocorticoid dependent mechanism (29).

Hypocalcemia associated with severe hyperphosphatemia is often encountered in pigment nephropathy associated with muscle injury. Hyperphosphatemia results from release of phosphate from injured skeletal muscle and may be one of the factors resulting in severe hypocalcemia. The chemical reaction of phosphorous with calcium in blood in poorly understood but eventually results in deposition of calcium phosphate in tissues. Meroney and associates noted that serum calcium was unusually low in patients with traumatic acute renal failure. In dogs with experimental muscle trauma, radioactive calcium 47 is deposited in the injured skeletal muscles at a faster rate than in normal animals (30). Thus, a translocation of calcium into injured muscle in the traumatized patient occurs. Llach and co-workers suggest that in muscle injury, muscle stores of $1,25(OH)_2D_3$ are released which enhances phosphorous release and hyperphosphatemia (31). The resulting hyperphosphatemia suppresses renal production of $1,25(OH)_2D_3$ and increases parathyroid hormone secretion. The depression of $1,25(OH)_2D_3$ synthesis facilitates calcium entry into cells. PTH enhances calcium uptake into the cytosol by its presumed ionophoric properties. Enhanced cytosolic calcium may enhance cellular necrosis by consequent activation of proteolytic enzymes. During the diuretic phase of pigment nephropathy associated with muscle injury, hypercalcemia is not common and probably results from calcium mobilization from deposits in injured tissues and from persistently elevated levels of parathyroid hormone.

The Efficacy of Therapy in Acute Renal Failure Associated with Trauma

The efficacy of therapy of post-traumatic renal failure is difficult to assess. Since the majority of battle and civilian casualties do not develop renal failure, it is likely that aggressive restoration of intravascular volume and transfer to sophisticated trauma centers are important in prevention of acute renal failure. Based on the experimental model of glycerol induced acute myoglobinuric renal failure, restoration of intravascular volume aborts the decline in renal blood flow and glomerular filtration rate during the initiating phase and application of this modality of treatment to the clinical setting of the acute traumatized patients is clearly mandatory. Once established, acute myoglobinuric renal failure appears not to be influenced by volume expansion. Induction of a diuresis with mannitol and alkalization of the urine to prevent pigment cast formation has been recommended but is problematic and controversial. Although reports have supported the value of mannitol and bicarbonate infusions, these observations have not been validated by a controlled trial (32). The risks of congestive heart failure from infusions of sodium bicarbonate and mannitol must be balanced against the unproven potential benefit of these agents in the clinical setting of pigment induced acute renal failure.

The mortality of patients with post-traumatic renal failure, even in the civilian setting, remains high. It is apparent that early dialysis reduces mortality. The overall mortality during the Korean War of patients with post traumatic renal failure treated with hemodialysis was 65 per cent, significantly lower than the mortality noted in battle casualties with acute renal failure during World War II when no hemodialysis was in use. During the Vietnam War, mortality remained high approximating 65 per cent despite availability of dialysis. Early dialysis appears to affect mortality and decreases morbidity. Kleinknecht (33) and co-workers noted that in a restrospective study that initiation of dialysis and institution of the frequency of dialysis to maintain blood urea nitrogen below 100 mg/dl was associated with significantly decreased mortality as compared to patients whose blood urea nitrogen was in excess of 175 mg/dl. The improvement in morbidity and mortality was due to a decreased incidence of septicemia and gastrointestinal bleeding.

Conger, in a prospective study of 18 post war trauma patients with acute renal failure with similar degrees of trauma, noted decreased mortality with early and frequent dialysis to maintain blood urea nitrogen and creatinine at 50 and 3.5 mg/dl respectively (34). The overall mortality was 37 per cent in the low blood urea nitrogen/creatinine group as compared to a mortality of 80 per cent in a group with a mean blood urea nitrogen of 120 per cent and a creatinine of 9.7 mg/dl. The improved mortality was due to a decrease in the frequency of septic episodes and hemorrhage in the low blood urea nitrogen/creatinine group.

Despite this study and other retrospective studies, it is difficult to assess these observations on survival data. Most studies compared survival data before the advent of frequent dialysis to contemporary periods. Other factors other than frequency and timing of dialysis such as improvement in surgical and overall medical care, newer antibiotics and drugs, and hyyperalimentation may have contributed to the apparent decline in morbidity and mortality than early or frequent hemodialysis.

The use of oral or parenteral nutrition in certain patients is undoubtedly beneficial and prevents muscle wasting and diminishes the metabolic consequences of renal insufficiency. Abel and co-workers (35) noted in a double blind trial that patients receiving glucose and essential amino acids with hyperçatabolic acute renal failure had a better chance of survival of an episode of acute renal failure than patients given glucose alone. Eventual survival in hospital discharge also improved. However, other studies using parenteral nutrition with glucose and amino acids have reported no increase in survival (36-39). It is likely that the overall mortality rate of post traumatic hypercatabolic renal failure is due in part to factors other than acute renal failure which are known to be associated with a poor prognosis. Advanced age, recent surgery, sepsis, peritonitis and gastrointestinal hemorrhage are major factors in determining the outcome of the patient. Thus, despite advances in dialysis techniques, parenteral nutrition, enhanced overall medical care and improved surgical techniques, the mortality from post traumatic renal failure appears to be determined not by the degree of renal failure, but by the basic problem initiating the disease.

References

1. S. Minami: Uber Nierenveranderungen nach verschuttung, Arch. Pathol. Anat. 245:247 (1923).
2. E. G. L. Bywaters and D. Beall: Crush injuries with impairment of renal function, Brit. Med. J. 1:427 (1941).
3. P. E. Teschan, C. R. Baxter, T. F. O'Brien, J. V. Freyhof and W. H. Hall: Prophylactic hemodialysis in the treatment of acute renal failure. Ann. Intern. Med. 53:991 (1960).
4. D. Whelton and J. V. Donadio, Jr.: Post-traumatic acute renal failure in Vietnam. Johns Hopkins Med. J. 124:95 (1969).

5. R. S. Barsoum, Z. E. B. Rihan, O. K. Bagligh, A. Hozayen, E. G. El-Ghoneimi, M. F. Ramzy and A.S. Ibrahuim: Acute renal failure in the 1973 Middle East War - experience of a special ized base hospital: effect of site of innury. J. Trauma 20:303-307 (1980).
6. Y. Blachar, J. S. C. Fong, J. P. DeChadarevian and K. N. Drummond: Muscle extract infusion in rabbits: a new experimental model of the crush syndrome. Arc. Res. 49:114-124 (1981).
7. M. S. Wheby, O. Barrett and W. H. Crosby: Serum protein binding of myoglobin, hemoglobin and hematin. Blood 16:1579 (1960).
8. S. R. Braun, F. R. Weiss, A. I. Keller, J.R. Ciccone and H. G. Preuss: Evaluation of the renal toxicity of heme proteins and their derivatives: a role in the genesis of acute tubule necrosis. J. Exp. Med. 131:443 (1970).
9. W. A. D. Anderson, D. B. Morrison and E. F. Williams: Pathologic changes following injections of ferrihemate (hematin) in dogs. Arch. Path. 33:589 (1942).
10. A. C. Corcoran and I. H. Page: Renal damage from ferroheme pigments, myoglobin, hemoglobin, hematin. Texas Reports of Biol. Med. 3:528 (1945).
11. R. J. Bing: The effect of hemoglobin and related pigments on renal function of the normal and acidotic dog. Bull. Johns Hopkins Hosp. 74:161 (1944).
12. E. G. L. Bywaters and J. K. Stead: The production of renal failure following injection of solutions containing myohemoglobin. Quart. J. Exp. Physiol. 33:53 (1946)
13. T. Suzuki and F. K. Mostofi: Electron microscopic studies of acute tubular necrosis. Early changes in the rat kidney after subcutaneous injection of glycerin. Lab. Invest. 28:8 (1970).
14. J. R. Jaenike: Micropuncture study of methemoglobin-induced acute renal failure in the rat. J. Lab. Clin. Med. 73:459 (1969).
15. A. Ruiz-Guinazu, J. B. Coelho and R. Paz: Methemoglobin-induced acute renal failure in the rat. In vivo observation, histology and micropuncture of intratubular and post glomerular vascular pressures. Nephron 4:257 (1967).
16. E. S. Finckh: Experimental acute tubular necrosis following sub-cutaneous injection of glycerol. J. Pathol. Bacteriol. 73:69 (1957).
17. G. Ayer, A. Grandchamp and B. Truniger: Intrarenal hemodynamics in glycerol-induced myohemoglobinuric acutre renal failure in the rat. Circ. Res. 29:128 (1971).
18. T. W. Kurtz, R. M. Maletz and C. H. Hsu: Renal Cortical blood flow in glycerol-induced acute renal failure in the rat. Circ. Res. 38:30 (1976).
19. M. F. Chedru, R. Baethke and D. E. Oken: Renal cortical blood flow and glomerular filtration in myohemoglobinuric acute renal failure. Kidney Int. 1:232 (1972).
20. S. Churchill, M.D. Zarlengo, J. F. Carvalho, M. N. Gottlieb and D. E. Oken: Normal renal cortical blood flow in experimental acute renal failure. Kidney Int. 11:246 (1977).
21. C. H. Hsu, T. W. Kurtz and T. P. Waldinger: Cardiac output and renal blood flow in glycerol induced acute renal failure in the rat. Circ. Res. 40:178 (1977).
22. D. E. Oken, M. L. Arce and D. R. Wilson: Glycerol induced hemo globinuric acute renal failure in the rat I. Micropuncture study of the development off oliguria. J. Clin. Invest. 45:724 (1966).
23. G. O'Conner, J. Bardgette, M. Lifschitz, J. Reineck and J. Stein: Sequential studies on the pathophysiology of

glycerol induced acute renal failure in the rat. Kidney Int. 12:531 (1977).

24. J. Mason, C. Olbricht, T. Takabatake and K. Thuran: The early phase of experimental acute renal failure. I. Intratubular pressure and obstruction. Pflugers Arch. 373:251 (1977).
25. C. Olbricht, J. Mason, T. Takabatake and K. Thuran: The early phase of experimental acute renal failure. II. Tubular leakage and reliability of glomerular markers. Pflugers Arch. 373:251 (1977).
26. G. H. A. Clowes, Jr., B. C. George, C. A. Villee, Jr. and C. A. Saravis: Muscle proteolysis induced by a circulating peptide in patients with sepsis or trauma. N. Eng. J. Med. 308:545-552 (1983).
27. W. H. Horl and A. Heidland: Enhanced proteolytic activity. A use of protein catabolism in acute renal failure. Am. J. Clin. Nutr. 33:1423 (1980).
28. W. H. Horl, C. Gantert, I. O. Auer and A. Heidland: In vitro inhibition of protein catabolism by $alpha_2$-macroglobulin in plasma from a patient with post-traumatic acute renal failure. Am. J. Nephrol. 2:32 (1982).
29. R. C. May, R. A. Kelly and W. E. Mitch: Metabolic acidosis stimulates protein degradation in rat muscle by a glucocorticoid-dependent mechanism. J. Clin. Invest. 77:614 (1986).
30. W. H. Meroney, G. K. Arney, W. E. Segar and H. H. Balch: The acute calcification of damaged muscle, with particular reference to acute post-traumatic renal insufficiency. J. Clin. Invest. 36:825-832 (1957).
31. F. Llach, A. J. Felsenfeld and M. R. Haussler: The pathophysiology of altered calcium metabolism in rhabdomyolysis-induced acute renal failure. N. Eng. J. Med. 305:117 (1981).
32. J. F. Eneas, P. Y. Schoenfeld and M.H. Humphreys: The effect of infusion of mannitol-sodium bicarbonate on the clinical course of myoglobinuria. Arch. Intern. Med. 139:801 (1979).
33. K. Kleinknecht, P. Jungers, J. Chanard, C. Barbanel and D. Ganeval: Uremic and non-uremic complications in acute renal failure: evaluation of early and frequent dialysis on prognosis. Kidney Int. 1:190 (1972).
34. J. D. Conger: A controlled evaluation of prophylactic dialysis in post-traumatic acute renal failure. J. Trauma. 15:1056 (1975).
35. R. M. Abel, C. H. Beck, Jr., W. M. Abbott, J. A. Ryan and G. O. Barnett: Improved survival from acute renal failure after treatment with intravenous essential L-amino acids and glucose. New Engl. J. Med. 288:695 (1973).
36. S. M. Baek, G. G. Makaboli, C. W. Bryan-Brown, J. Kusek and W. C. Shoemaker: The influence of parenteral nutrition on the course of acute renal failure. Surg. Gynecol. Obstet. 141:405 (1975).
37. C. D. Leonard, R. G. Luke and R. R. Siegel: Parenteral essential amino acids in acute renal failure. Urology 6:154 (1975).
38. H. Freund, S. Harmian and J. E. Fischer: Comparative studies of parenteral nutrition in renal failure using essential and non-essential amino acid containing solutions. Surg. Gynecol. Obstet. 151:652 (1980).
39. E. I. Feinstein, M. J. Blumenkrantz, M. Healy, A. Koffler, H. Silberman, S. G. Massry, and J. D. Kopple: Clinical and metabolic responses to parenteral nutrition in acute renal failure. Medicine 6:124 (1981).

MYELOMA AND ACUTE RENAL FAILURE

M. Olmer, Y. Berland, and G. Shutz

Service de Nephrologis, Hopital de la Conception

13005 Marseille, France

INTRODUCTION

Renal Failure is a frequent complication of multiple myeloma (1-6). In most cases it takes months or years for the progression of renal disease (7-8). However, patients with multiple myeloma may also develop acute renal failure.

Unfortunately, only few studies have been reported concerning the development of acute renal failure in patients with multiple myeloma (6,8,12) and most of them concern small number of patients.

The goal of this paper is to report our experience with 23 patients with multiple myeloma who presented with acute renal failure.

I - PATIENTS

Between 1972 and 1985, 23 patients with acute renal failure related to multiple myeloma were admitted in our intensive care unit. Diagnosis of myeloma was based on a medullary plasmocytosis above 10%, a monoclonal globulin peak in blood and/or urines.

The diagnosis of acute renal failure was based on a rapid and recent rise in serum creatinine. Immediately after their hospital admission, patients were rehydrated and given alkali therapy. Only those who maintained a creatininemia above 200 μmol/ℓ were included in this study.

When diuresis was lower than 600 ml/day the acute renal failure was considered when serum calcium exceeded 2.75 mmol/1.

All the patients who after the first month survived were treated with corticosteroids alone or in combination with other chemotherapeutic agents.

Mean age for these 23 patients was 60 years (from 46 to 83 years); 7 were women and 16 men.

Two different groups of patients were included in this study:
- Group I concerns 12 patients in whom myeloma was previously known for an average duration of 33.6 months (2 to 156 months). Most of them were treated with chemotherapy.

- Group II, includes 11 patients in whom the diagnosis of multiple myeloma was unknown before the acute renal failure.

Nine patients had light chains myeloma, 9 IgA myeloma and 5 IgG myeloma. In 20 of them light chains had been concurrently identified in blood and in urines: 10 patients had lambda chain and 10 had kappa chain in the urines.

Serum total protein exceeded 90 g/1 in 6 patients, proteinuria varied between 0.4 and 6 g/1. Oliguric was present in 12 patients. Dehydration was present in 12 patients when admitted in our unit. A severe infection was evident in 10 patients and serum calcium was above 2.75 mmol/1 in 6 patients.

One patient had received contrast agents just before the admission; 2 patients had received aminoglycosides and 2 had received a non steroid anti-inflammatory drugs a few days prior to admission.

II - RESULTS

TABLE

MULTIPLE MYELOMA AND ACUTE RENAL FAILURE = OUTCOME OF DIALYSED PATIENTS

DIALYSED PATIENTS : 17

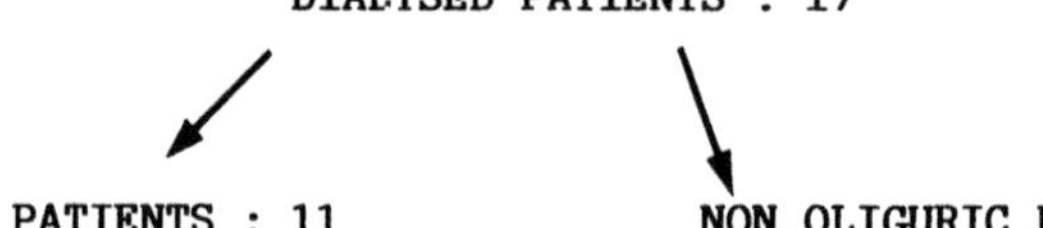

OLIGURIC PATIENTS : 11	**NON OLIGURIC PATIENTS : 6**
.recovery of diuresis : 3	**.Recovery of renal function : 1**
.chronic hemodialysis : 11	**.Chronic hemodialysis : 5**

TABLE 2

MULTIPLE MYELOMA AND ACUTE RENAL FAILURE = OUTCOME OF NON DIALYSED PATIENTS.

NON DIALYSED PATIENTS : 6
(S. creatinine : 380-1185 μ mol/1)

.improvement of renal function
(380 μ mol/1) : 1

.stable renal function : 2
(S. creatinine : 400 and 800 μ mol/1)

.Death < 15 days : 2

Among patients of Group I, one had hypercalcemia, two had light chains myeloma and five had serum total protein higher than 90 g/1.

Among patients of Group II, 7 had light chains myeloma, one had serum total protein above 90 g/l and five patients had hypercalcemia.

Serum creatinine ranged from 380 mol/l to 1550 µmol/l. Hemodialysis was necessary in 17 patients, 6 of whom were non oliguric (Table I). Among the dialysed patients only one improved its kidney function and one month later had serum creatinine 210 mol/l; the remaining required chronic hemodialysis until their death, including three patients with oliguric ARF.

Amont the 6 who did not require dialysis, only one had decrease of serum creatinine, 2 had stable serum creatinine of 400 and 800 µmol/l respectively for four months before they died.

Among the 23 patients the average survival after the acute renal failure was 9 months (from 15 days to 60 months).

After the onset of acute renal failure the actuarial survival was 55% at 3 months and 29% at 18 months. When considering the whole patients since the time of discovery of myeloma the average survival was 26.2 months (from 15 days to 121 months). In Group I, mean patient survival was 34.6 months (from 2 to 121 months) after the diagnosis of multiple myeloma and 2 months (range 4 days to 6 months) after the onset of acute renal failure. In patients of Group II, the average survival was of 16.8 months (from 15 days to 60 months).

Reasons of the death of the 16 patients were: three times a cerebral-hemorrhage, a digestive bleeding in 3 patients and s spesis in 3 others. The last seven patients died from the natural evolution of their disease.

III - COMMENTS

Mutliple myeloma is frequently (8 to 60%) complicated by progressive renal failure (1-6). Acute renal failure may occur in 7 to 8% of cases of myeloma (6,11) and it was the presenting clinical manifestation in 48% of our patients and in 46% of the patients reported by Cohen et al (11). Approximately 50% of our cases had non-oliguric ARF; this is similar to the findings by Cohen et al (11). These authors, however, found an association between the presence of non-oliguric ARF and hypercalcemia. On the contrary, we found a serum calcium greater than 2.75 mmol/l only in 2 out of 11 cases with non-oliguric ARF.

Two things of the patients with light chain myeloma presented with oliguric and volume depletion. 39% of patients with ARF in our series had light chain myeloma; which is not dissimilar from the incidence of 43-50% reported in the literature (8,11). Twenty-two percent of our patients had IgG myeloma, which is at variance with the incidence or 58% observed by others (6).

Most of our lyeloma patients with ARF and those reported in the literature displayed Bence Jones proteinuria (3,6,7,13). Several studies have demonstrated the nephrotoxicity of light chains. These proteins are easily filtered by the glomerulus, and most of them are reabsorbed and catabolized by the tubular cells, the remaining being excreted in the urine. Light chain can precipitate within the tubules and cause ARF. However, the recent studies have suggested the possibility of a direct toxic effect of light chains on the tubular cells as a cause for the ARF (9,16,). The nephrotoxicity seems to be related to the physicochemical properties of these proteins, rather than to their urinary concentration. Dehydration may promote light chain precipitation within the tubules or it may increase proximal tubular reabsorption of these potentially nephrotoxic proteins (8). It is of interest that 14 out of 23 of our patients displayed signs of volume depletion upon presentation.

Other factors, such as contrast agents, high serum calcium and spesis may be responsible for the onset of ARF in some patients with multiple myeloma.

Hypercalcemia, which is present in 30 to 70% of myeloma patients with ARF (6,8) can affect renal function in several ways; it may decrease renal blood flow and glomerular filtration rate through its hemodynamic effects, or through precipitation in the renal tubules and in the renal interstitium. Hypercalcemia can also affect water reabsorption in the distal tubule.

In 20 to 56% of the cases reported in the literature, renal function eventually improved (6,8,11). However, in our series only 2 patients displayed some improvement in renal function.

The survival rate among these patients is extremely poor (6,11,21). Among our patients the survival rate was only 2 months in patients of Group I and 34.6 months in patients of Group II. In the series of Cohen et al (11) the mean survival rate was 17.4 months.

CONCLUSION

Acute renal failure reveals the diagnosis of myeloma in approximately half of the patients.

Light chains myeloma, hypercalcemia, dehydration, sepsis and contrast studies appear to be predisposing factors.

Improvement of the renal function is rare.

After the onset of acute renal failure the mean survival is worse in these patients in whom the diagnosis of myeloma was already known than in those in whom the diagnosis was made after the onset of ARF.

REFERENCES

1 - D.A.G. Galton, R. Peto, : report on the first myelomatosis trail I. Analysis of presenting features of prognostic importance. Br. J. Haematol 24:123, (1973).

2 - R.A. Kyle, : Multiple myeloma - review of 869 cases. Mayo. Clin. Proc. 50:29, (1975).

3 - R. Alexanian, S. Balcerzak, J.D. Bonnet, et al. : Prognostic factors in multiple myeloma. Cancer 36:1192, (1975).

4 - M.J. Stone, E.P. Frenkel, : The clinical spectrum of light chain myeloma. Study of 35 patients with special reference to occurrence of amyloidosis, Amer. J. Med. 58:601, (1975).

5 - M. Martinez-Maldonado, J. Yium, W.N. Suki, G. Eknoyan, : Renal complications in multiple myeloma : pathophysiology and some aspects of clinical management. J. Chron. Dis 24:221, (1971).

6 - R.A. De Fronzo, R.L. Humphrey, J.R. Wright, C.R. Cook, : Acute renal failure in multiple myeloma. Medicine 54:209, (1975).

7 - C. Cauchie, Y. Kenis, P. Potuliege, J. Smulders, C.K. Compel, P. O. Lambert, : Les manifestations renales des dysglubulinemies. J. Urol. Nephro. 68:345, (1962).

8 - D. Ganeval, P. Jungers, L.H. Noel, D. Droz, : La nephropathie du myeloma : Acutalites Nephrologiques de l'Hopital Necker, 309, (1977).

9 - C.E. Bryan, J.K. Healy, : Acute renal failure in multiple myeloma. Am. J. Med. 44:128, (1968).

10 - C.R. Kjedsberg, R.E. Holman, : Acute renal failure in multiple myeloma, J. Urol. 105:21, (1971).

11 - D.J. Cohen, W.H. Sherman, E.F. Osserman, G.B. Appel, : Acute renal failure in patients with multiple myeloma. Am. J. Med. 76:247, (1984).

12 - F.G. Cosio, T.V. Pence, F.L. Shapiro, C.M. Kjellstrand, : Severe renal failure in multiple myeloma. Clin. Nephrology 15:206, (1981).

13 - J. Yium, M. Martinez-Maldonado, G. Eknoyan, W.N. Suki, : Peritoneal dialysis in the treatment of renal failure in multiple myeloma. South Med. J. 64:1403, (1971).

14 - A.N. Koss, C.L. Pirani, E.T. Osserman, : Experimental Bence Jones cast nephropathy. Lab. Invest. 34:579, (1976).

15 - J. Mc Geoch, J.F. Smith, J. Ledingham, J. Ross, : Inhibition of active-transport sodium-potassium ATP ase by myeloma protein. Lancet 2:17, (1978).

16 - D.H. Clyne, A.J. Pesce, R.E. Thompson, : Nephrotoxicity of Bence Jones proteins in the rat : Importance of protein isoelectric point. Kidney Int. 16:345, (1979).

17 - C.W. Bryan, K.R. Mc Intire, : Effect of substained diuresis on the renal lesions of mice with Bence Jones protein producing tumors. J. Lab. Clin. Med. 83:409, (1974).

18 - E.D. Rees, W.H. Waugh, L. Ky, : Factors in the renal failure of multiple myeloma. Arch. Intern. Med. 116:400, (1965).

19 - F.H. Epstein, : Calcium and the kidney. Am. J. Med. 45:700, (1968).

20 - L.S.T. Fang, : Light-chain nephropathy. Kidney International 27:582, (1985).

21 - H.M. Lazarus, D.J. Adelstein, R.H. Herzig, M.C. Smith, : Long-term survival of patients with multiple myeloma and acute renal failure at presentation. Am. J. Kidney Dis. 2:521, (1983).

ACUTE IMPAIRMENT OF RENAL FUNCTION

IN SYSTEMIC LUPUS ERYTHEMATOSUS

P. Coratelli, G. Pannarale, and R. Rizzi

Institute of Medical Nephrology
University of Bari
Bari, Italy

Acute impairment of renal function(AIRF)not infrequently complicates the course of patients with lupus nephritis.
Previous reports(1,2)indicated that renal failure in Systemic Lupus Erythematosus(SLE)was associated with a bad prognosis and was predictive of rapid and irreversible progression. However,in recent years,a few cases of acute anuric lupus nephritis,which recovered renal function after prolonged anuria,have been described(3,4). Moreover,not anuric acute renal failure and less severe degrees of AIRF are also frequent in SLE,but have not often been reported(5,6).
To further clarify the clinical and histological features so as the subsequent course of acute impairment of renal function in SLE,we report on 35 episodes occured in 26 patients.

PATIENTS AND METHODS

Between 1974 and 1985,35 episodes of AIRF in 26 patients with SLE were observed at the Institute of Medical Nephrology,University of Bari.
All patients fulfilled the preliminary (1971) and revised (1982) criteria of the American Rheumatism Association(7)for the diagnosis of SLE.
AIRF was defined as a rise in plasma creatinine concentration to 1.5 mg/dl or more and a change in serum creatinine of 33% or more over three months or less,a criterion commonly used to define "acute" impairment(6,-8)in SLE.
Twenty-two patients had a renal biopsy,16 of them during episodes of AIRF. Histological findings were categorized according to W.H.O. classification (9).
All patients received corticosteroid therapy. In 23 episodes treatment consisted of methylprednisolone(1-1.5 mg/Kg/day i.v.);in 8 of these im-

munosoppressive drugs(cyclophosphamide or azathioprine) were associated;- in a single episode plasmapheresis was also used. In more recent years 12 episodes were treated with three pulses of intravenous methylprednisolone(1 g. daily for three consecutive days)followed by intravenous metylprednisolone 0.8- 1 mg./Kg./day.

All patients had a follow-up period of at least one year after the onset of the first episode of AIRF,17 were followed for 5 years or longer.

On 16 patients a second renal biopsy was done 6-12 months after treatment was begun and comparison was made with the initial histological findings by pathological scoring system of activity and sclerosis,as described by Morel-Maroger(10).

Routine clinical and laboratory examinations,including renal function,- were done using standard hospital techniques.

Serum concentrations of C3 and C4 complement components were measured by radial immunodiffusion(Partigen plate,Behringwerke,West Germany). Normal values were established as 70 to 160 mg/dl for C3 and 20 to 70 for C4.

Antinuclear antibodies(ANA) were performed by standard techniques.

Anti-ds-DNA antibodies and complement-fixing anti-ds-DNA were determined by standard indirect immunofluorescence technique using Crithidia luciliae kinetoplast as substrate(Quantafluor n-DNA kit,Kallestad laboratories,U.S.A.). Serum specimen were considered positive for anti--ds-DNA if kinetoplast fluorescence was observed at minimum serum dilution of 1:10.

Kidney tissue specimens were obtained by percutaneous biopsy.

The removed tissue was fixed in Dubosq-Brazil and sections of 2-3 micron in tickness, cut from paraffin-embedded material,were stained routinely with Haematoxilin-eosin,periodic acid-Schiff,methenamine silver and Masson's trichrome.

Material was also frozen in liquid nitrogen and used for immunohistological studies. Cryostat sections 4 micron in tickness were incubated with fluorescein isothiocyanate coniugated rabbit antisera directed against human IgG,IgA,IgM,C3,Clq,Fibrinogen (Behringwerke,West Germany).

Statistical analysis was performed using standard Student's t-test,for comparison of mean value of tests for groups,and calculation of a correlation coefficent(r)by the method of least squares,for correlation of continous variables.

RESULTS

Of 26 patients,22 were female and 4 male,giving F:M ratio of 5.5:1. The mean age of the patients,at the time the first episode of AIRF occured, was 27 years,ranging from 14 to 60.

In 11 patients(42%)diagnosis of SLE was made during hospitalization for AIRF,in 15(58%)AIRF appeared 5 to 120 months (mean 35.4) after diagnosis of SLE.

Renal biopsy showed diffuse proliferative lupus nephritis in all examined specimens. Crescentic lupus nephritis(crescents $>$ 50%)was found in 12 biopsies;of these 6 had crescents $>$ 80%.

With regard to clinical findings,the majority of episodes of AIRF were accompained by nephrotic syndrome(74%);nephritic syndrome was present in 6 episodes(17%). Oliguria(/500 ml/day)characterized 16 episodes(46%),14 of these requiring dialysis. The mean serum creatinine peak during AIRF was 5.2 mg/dl, ranging from 1.5 to 13.4.

Extrarenal manifestations were present in 83% of episodes of AIRF; they consisted in haematological changes (29%), polyserositis (26%),polyarthritis and polyarthralgia (26%),nervous system disorders (11%).

Immunological features of AIRF included positive ANA in 33 episodes (95%),anti-ds-DNA antibodies ≥ 1/100 in 24 (68%),complement fixing anti--ds-DNA in 16(46%). Low C3 was present in 23 episodes(65%),low C4 in 19 (54%).

The above mentioned clinical immunological and histological findings and the presence of extrarenal symptoms confirmed the activity of SLE in all episodes of AIRF.

Active lupus nephritis was therefore considered the leading cause of AIRF, but in 7 episodes other factors were considered important in causing or precipiting renal failure. They were electrolyte disorders in 3 episodes, infections in 3 and drugs(Gentamicin for urinary tract infection)in another one.

The outcome of the 35 episodes of AIRF is shown in Tab.I. Treatment resulted in recovery of previous renal function in 21 episodes, in incomplete improvement of renal function in 7. Two patients developed end stage renal failure and required regular dialysis treatment and 5 other patients died, during episodes of AIRF. Two deaths occurred from sepsis and the three others respectively from cerebral lupus,acute cardiac failure and gastrointestinal hemorrage.

The outcome of the 16 episodes of oliguric renal failure was pooer than overall series. Treatment was effective in 11(68.5%):6 of these(37.5%)-resulted in recovery of previous renal function,5 (31%)in partial recovery. Moreover,2 patients(12.5%)remained on dialysis treatment which had been initiated for oliguric acute renal failure and 3 others (19%) died.

As complication of the treatment eleven patients suffered from infections, severe in 4 of them;two patients died from infection(Herpes zooster encephalitis, Staphilococcal septicaemia). A single patient developed psycosis during steroid therapy.

TAB. I OUTCOME OF ACUTE IMPAIRMENT OF RENAL FUNCTION IN SLE

		not oliguric	oliguric	overall series
Death during AIRF		2(10.5%)	3(19%)	5(14%)
End-stage renal disease		0	2(12.5%)	2(6%)
Recovery of previous renal				
function:	- partial	2(10.5%)	5(31%)	7(20%)
	- complete	15(79%)	6(37.5%)	21(60%)
		19(100%)	16(100%)	35(100%)

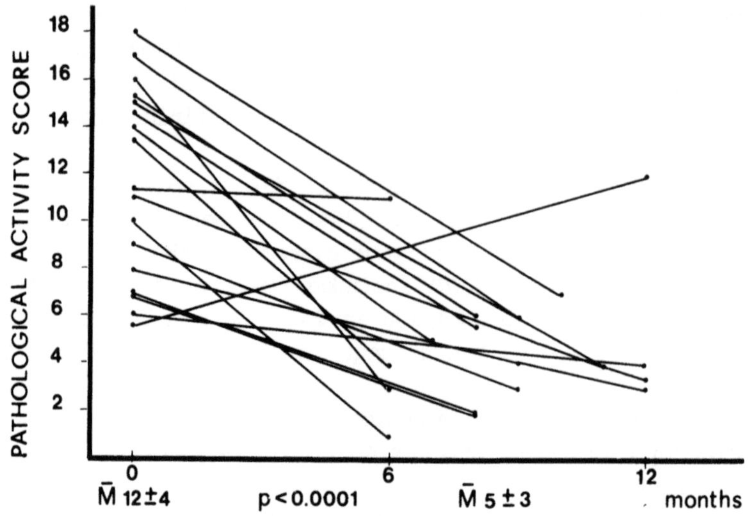

Fig. I Sequential changes in histological activity of the renal lesions.

During the first episode of AIRF,3 of the 26 patients died and another one developed end stage renal failure. Twenty-two patients(84.6%)were alive one year after the onset of AIRF, and 17 of them had a follow-up period of 5 years or more. During this follow-up period two patients died and 3 others developed end stage renal failure; twelve patients(71%)were alive at 5 years.

During follow-up period 9 episodes of recurrence of AIRF were observed in 8 patients;all patients who died and a single patient of three who lost renal function did so during recurrence of AIRF.

Figures 1 and 2 show sequential changes of histological activity and chronicity score in the 16 patients who had a second renal biopsy. Pathological activity score(fig.1)decreased from 12 ± 4 to 5 ± 3 ($p < 0.0001$), whereas chronicity score(fig.2)increased from 1 ± 1.15 to 3.5 ± 1.6 ($p < 0.0001$).

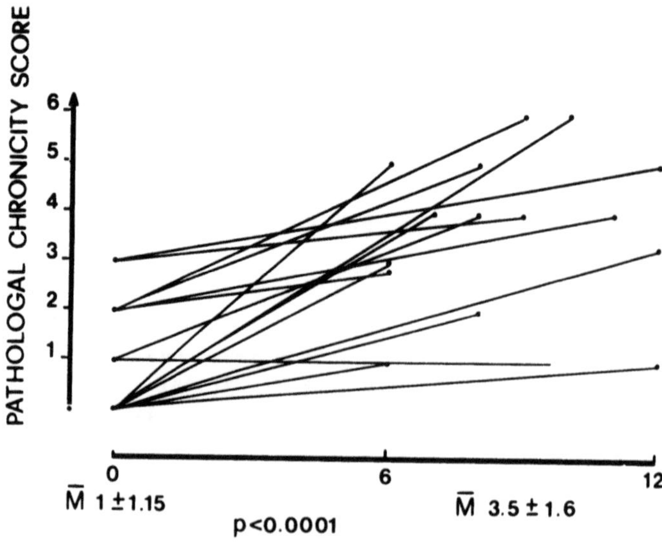

Fig. 2. Sequential changes in pathological chronicity score of the renal lesions

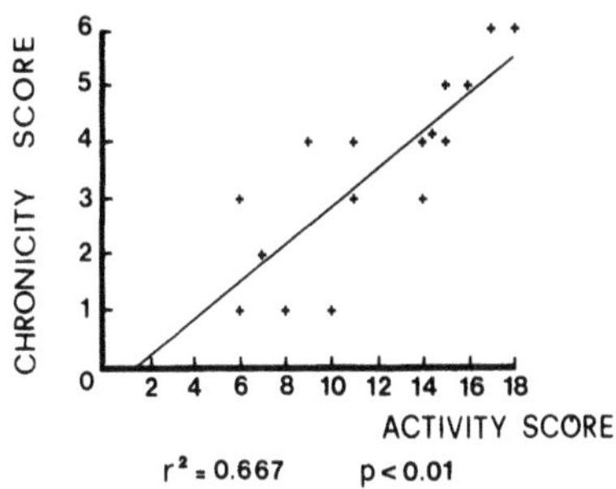

Fig. 3 Correlation betwenn activity score at first biopsy and chronicity score at second biopsy

Significant correlation was found between pathological activity score at first biopsy and chronicity score at second biopsy(r = 0.667, p/ 0.01),as shown in fig.3.

DISCUSSION

The results of this study confirm that active lupus nephritis is the most important cause of AIRF in SLE. In the majority of the examinated episodes,in fact,besides the symptoms of severe renal involvement,extrarenal manifestations,often severe,were also present: piastrinopenia and/or leucopenia,arthritis,central nervous system involvement as corea,-seizures,extrapiramidal manifestations. This is a clear evidence of generalized activity of SLE,which is also proven by immunological measurements. Moreover nephritis activity was demonstrated by renal biopsy: all biopsy specimens showed active lupus nephritis and more than 50% of these crescentic lupus glomerulonephritis. Although in a few episodes possible causes of AIRF other than active SLE have been also found these always occured in presence of active lupus nephritis,acting as aggravating or precipitating factors only.

Treatment was effective in the majority(80%)of AIRF episodes: complete recovery was obtained in 21(60%),partial in 7(20%). However, we are not able to attribute recovery to a specific form of therapy because this is a retrospective study on many years period and too many variables other than specific therapy can have conditioned the outcome.

Resolution of AIRF sometimes occured many months after episode was begun. By contrast,in anuric episodes,the average duration of anuria was relatively short,attaining maximum of 28 days; no patients were able to discontinue regular dialysis treatment after many months,as reported by others (11,12).

Oliguric patients,in our experience,have worse survival than the overall series,but not definitely bad prognosis,as in Yeung series (5).

Unlike previous reports(13,14)no patients in our series died from renal insufficiency,the deaths being in relation either to complications of therapy or to extrarenal manifestations of SLE,according to more recent series(15).

Steroid therapy,besides the improvement of renal function and extrarenal manifestations,allowed healing of histological lesions too. In all,but two,patients who underwent a second renal biopsy,treatment resulted in disappearance or decrease of the histologic signs of activity. However,in agreement with Pollak(16),complete suppression of active lesions,with little or no residual damage,occured only in the less severely involved cases. When active lesions had been suppressed in patients with the highest pathological activity score,chronic changes appeared,which resulted in high chronicity score at second biopsy.

Treatment results,therefore,in trasformation of active and rapidly progressive lupus nephritis in chronic and slowly progressive one, so delaying the renal failure for a long period of time,unless fresh active lesions develop in the future.

This is confirmed by the long term follow-up data of 17 patients. The highest survival rate (78%) of renal function was observed in the 9 patients who did not present further episodes of AIRF and,furthermore,-none of these died. However a few patients presented at the last observation some degree of renal failure,this in relation to the severity of clinical and histological involvement at the time of AIRF.

Of the 8 other patients 2 died and another one developed end stage renal failure,all during recurrence of AIRF;their survival rate was 62.5%. Developement of fresh active lesions in these patients precipitated the course of the disease. We emphasize,therefore,that patients,who have presented an episode of AIRF,are to be considered an high risk group. They need of careful clinical and immunological monitoring to detect initial development of recurrences,which are always life-threatening. In our experience, in fact,although a few episodes occured and progressed in spite of a prompt and adequate treatment,complete recovery of renal function was achieved in the majority of episodes in which aggressive therapy started in the initial phase, when renal function was not severly compromised.

In conclusion, our data suggest that AIRF in SLE is not rigidly predictive of rapid and irreversible progression,because prompt and adequate treatment often causes dramatic improvement of renal function and.of active histological lesions. Furthermore, in patients without recurrences of AIRF, long term prognosis is not significantly different from predicted survival for diffuse proliferative lupus nephritis.

REFERENCES

1) B. Zweiman,J. Kornblum,J Cornog,E.A. Hildreth.
The prognosis of lupus nephritis. Role of clinical-pathologic correlations. Ann. Intern.Med. 69:441 (1968)

2) D.S. Baldwin,J. Lowenstein,N.F. Rothfield,G. Gallo,R.T. McCluskey.
The clinical course of the proliferative and membranous forms of lupus nephritis. Ann. Intern. Med. 73:929(1970)

3) C. Ponticelli,E. Imbasciati,D. Brancaccio,A. Tarantino,E. Rivolta. Acute renal failure in systemic lupus erythematosus. Br. Med. J. 3:716 (1974)
4) M. Sugarman,A. Kamdar,B.H. Barbour,F.P. Quismorio,S. Massry, E.L. Dubois. Reversible renal insufficiency in systemic lupus erythematosus. Arthritis Rheum. 20:137(1977)
5) K.C. Yeung,W.L. NG,S.W. Wong,K.L. Wong,and K.M. Chan. Acute deterioration in renal function in systemic lupus erythematosus. Quarterly J. Med.,new series 56,393(1985)
6) R. Kimberly,M.D. Lockshin,R.L. Sherman,J.S. McDougal,R.D. Inman,C.L. Christian. High-dose intravenous methylprednisolone pulse therapy in systemic lupus erythematosus. Am. J. Med. 70:817(1981)
7) E..M. Tan,A.S. Cohen,I.F. Fries,A.J. Masi,D.J. Mcshane,N.F. Roth field,J.G. Schaller,N. Talel,J.R. Winchester. The 1982 revised criteria for the classification of systemic lupus erythematosus. Arthritis Rheum. 25. 1271(1982)
8) J.V. Donadio,K.E. Holley,R.H. Ferguson. Treatment of diffuse pro liferative lupus glomerulonephritis with prednisone and combined prednisone and ciclophosphamide. N. Engl. J. Med. 299:1151(1978)
9) G.B. Appel,F.G. Silva,C.L. Pirani,J. Meltzer,D. Estes. Renal involvement in SLE. A study of 56 patients emphasizing histologic classification. Medicine 57:371(1978).
10) L. Morel Maroger,J.P.H. Mery,D. Droz,M. Godin,P. Verroust,O. Kourilski,G. Richet: The course of lupus nephritis: contribution of serial renal biopsies. Adv Nephrol. 6:79(1976)
11) W.S. Moore,J.S.Guggenheim,I.R. Anderson. Diffuse proliferative lupus glomerulonephritis. Recovery from prolonged renal failure. JAMA 244:63(1980).
12) R.P.Kimberly,M.D. Lockshin,R.L. Sherman,J. Mouradian,S. Saal. Reversible end-stage lupus nephritis. Analisis of patients able to discontinue dialysis.AM.J. MED.74:361(1983)
13) E.L. Dubois,M. Wierzchowiecki,M.B. Cox,J.M. Weiner: Causes of death in 212 cases of SLE. Arthr. Rheum. 16:540(1973)
14) D. Estes,C.L. Cristian. The natural history of SLE by prospective an alysis. Medicine 50:8((1971).
15) P. Correia,J.S. Cameron,J.D. Lian,J. Hicks,C.S. Ogg;D.G. Williams,C. Chantler, D.G. Haycock. Why do patients with lupus nephritis die? Brit. Med. J. 290:126(1985).
16) V.E. Pollack,C.L. Pirani,R.M. Karw. Effect of large doses of prednisone on the renal lesions and life span of patients with lupus glomerulonephritis. J. Lab. Clin. Med. 57:495(1961).

ACUTE RENAL FAILURE AFTER SEPTIC SHOCK

Pasquale Coratelli, Giuseppe Passavanti,
Michele Giannattasio and Alberto Amerio

Institute of Nephrology
University of Bari
Bari,Italy

The problem of sepsis and acute renal failure(ARF)remains to date a major unsolved challenge to nephrologists. Despite the regular use of dialysis and other major improvements in the management of patients (pts) with ARF,mortality continues to be distressingly high(1,2).

Many factors,such as the age of pts (1,2,3,4),the severity of the underlying disease(5),multiple organ dysfunction,have been implicated for the persistence of high mortality,but the most widely recognized one is the role of sepsis(6,7). Infections are the leading cause of death in 30-70 % of pts with ARF.

Septic shock may be associated with gram positive infections (30 % of cases)although the most frequent etiology is due to gram negative bacteria(70 % of cases);the shock syndrome,however,is not due to bloodstream invasion with bacteria per se,but is related to release of bacterial toxins. The underlying diseases which may induce septic shock can be due to medical causes,and focused in the urinary tract,intestine,lung or skin. Often septic shock can be triggered by surgical maneuvers on the genito--urinary tract,gastroenteric apparatus or biliary tree;septic complications from urethral or vascular catheterism, tracheobronchial aspiration, etc may be included in this group. Lastly septic shock is the major precipitating factor in post-traumatic, post-partum and post-abortum ARF. In many pts sepsis appears to be the primary cause,or may develop during the episode,of renal failure.

HEMODYNAMIC PROFILE AND RENAL FUNCTION

Septic shock is a hemodynamic syndrome which consists of severe microcirculatory insufficiency and inadequate tissue perfusion. In gram negative sepsis,circulatory insufficiency is mainly due to cell injury initiated by endotoxin , and is the consequence of increased peripheral

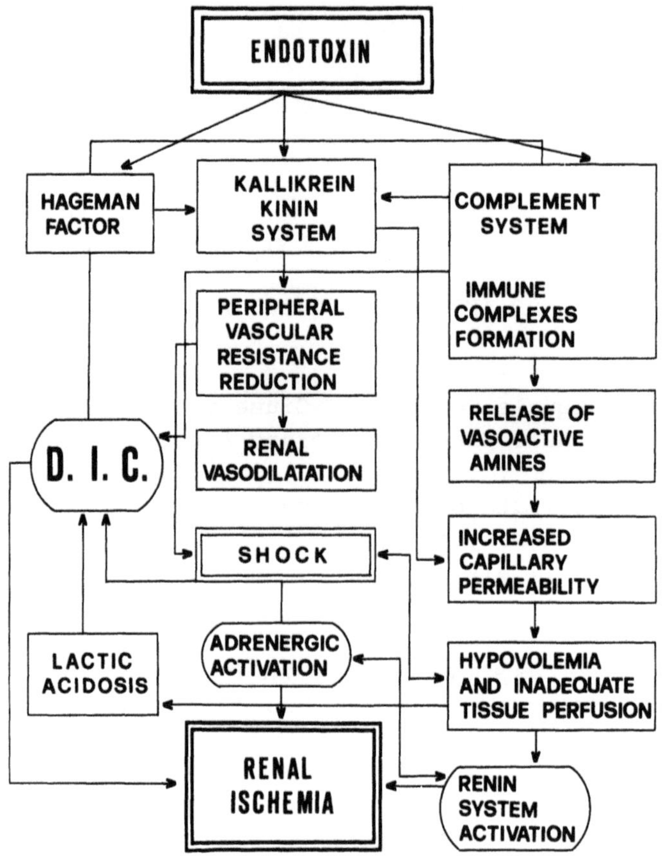

Figure 1. Pathogenesis of acute renal failure after septic shock

vascular resistance,blood pooling in microcirculation and reduced cardiac output as well as tissue anoxia(Figure 1).

Early in endotoxic shock,however,the clinical pattern is primarily one of vasodilatation with increased cardiac output,stroke volume and decreased central venous pressure and vascular peripheral resistance (8,9,10). Such hyperdynamic pattern is supported by the activation of the Hageman factor (11)by bacterial cell wall components(lypopolysaccharides) leading to an increased production of kallikrein from prekallikrein. The resulting bradykinin release may be responsible for peripheral vasodilatation,hypotension,pooling of blood in peripheral tissues,increased capillary permeability and,as a results,of a sharp decrease in effective circulating blood volume. Later in septic shock,the hemodynamic picture is therefore one of vasoconstriction;systemic vascular resistance increases,cardiac output and stroke volume decrease and so does the central venous pressure. Such hemodynamic pattern is supported by adrenergic activation caused by hypovolemia and shock,by the direct action of endotoxin on vascular alfa-receptors,by the renin system activation and by disorders in the coagulation mechanisms induced by activation of the Hageman factor.

The spectrum of renal damage ensuing from septic shock includes a reduction in renal perfusion with a sharp decrease of glomerular filtration volume,tubular necrosis,tubular obstruction due to the hemoglobin casts,vascular obstruction induced by coagulation system derangement and DIC secondary to endotoxemia,involvement(infiltration and edema)of interstitial tissue. Anuric syndrome after septic shock is the most frequent result of a potentially reversible acute tubular necrosis or the ominous result of a bilateral cortical necrosis.

It has been demonstrated that jaundice may be an aggravating and unfarovable prognostic factor in pts with ARF. It has also been shown that pts with liver and gall bladder diseases have an increased incidence of acute tubular necrosis(12,13). Jaundice in pts with ARF is an ominous sign,often reflecting liver ischemia(14). Gram negative bacterial sepsis is frequently associated with the development of a direct reacting hyperbilirubinemia(15);the syndrome of gram negative septicemia and jaundice involves a presumable defect in canalicular exscretion of conjugated bilirubin. In a previous study(16)in which we had evaluated the prognosis in ARF accompanied by jaundice, the mortality rate of 67 sequential cases of ARF with jaundice was compared with the mortality rate of 168 cases without jaundice. In jaundiced pts the mortality rate was 57 %,which was significantly higher than the 42 % mortality in pts without jaundice. The mortality rate correlated with serum bilirubin levels; pts with serum bilirubin higher than 20 mg% had an 85 % mortality rate,whereas pts with levels lower than 10 mg% had a mortality rate of only 33 %. Average blood pressures were significantly lower in pts with jaundice than in those without. The data indicate that ARF accompanied by jaundice carries a poorer prognosis ; the reduced blood pressure which accompanies this condition may be an aggravating factor,so that serum bilirubin levels may be used as a prognostic index. Many investigators have attempted to define the chemical components of icteric plasma causing ARF. In vitro studies have demonstrated that bilirubin and bile salt impair cell metabolism,-membrane integrity and membrane transport fuction. Bilirubin has been shown to decrease the respiratory quotient of tissue homogenates,to inhibit the oxidation of NADH in mammalian tissue culture and to uncouple oxidative phosphorilation by isolated mitochondria(17,18,19). Endotoxin exerts the same effects experimentally(20);the mutual potentiation of both factors can explain ominous prognosis when they act simultaneously.

THERAPEUTIC IMPLICATIONS

The goal of therapy in ARF after septic shock is to mantain the chemical composition of the body fluids as close to normal as possible until renal function returns. The major steps in therapy should include vigorous supportive care,immediate use of antibiotics,possibly a surgical approach to eradicate the septic focus,correction of pathogenetic factors(shock, hypovolemia, hemodynamic disorders, coagulation system activation),nutritional supply apt to preserve body protein stores,to prevent muscle wasting and to correct endogenous hypercatabolism and, chiefly,prevention of the uremic syndrome by intensive treatment with hemodialysis or peritoneal dialysis.

The weight of evidence supports the general concept that early initiation of dialytic treatment is useful in lessening the morbidity and mortality of pts with ARF. To day it is generally accepted that dialytic procedures must be employed prophylactically to prevent the occurrence of life threatening complications rather than as emergency treatment. The term "prophylactic dialysis" or "early dialysis", however, have been used to mean different schedules of dialysis in different studies.

We are now reporting on the results obtained in 85 pts affected with ARF after septic shock studied during the last 17 years. The aim of this retrospective study is to assess the efficacy of early dialysis in reducing mortality in those high risk pts. The diagnosis of estabilished ARF was based upon the combination of oliguria,progressive uremia,urinary sodium concentration above 30 mEq/l and failure to respond to intravenous infusion of mannitol or high doses of furosemide(400-1000 mg). Patients with a previous known history of renal disease or metabolic disordes or with non oliguric acute renal failure were excluded from the study. Only pts who got over the life threatening consequences of the shock through intensive care are included in the study. All pts underwent daily hemodialysis or continuous peritoneal dialysis until diuresis was restored and plasma creatinine levels dropped below 3-4 mg%.

Of the 85 pts,33 were males(mean age : 54.5 $\pm$ 17.6 yrs)and 52 were females(mean age : 36.7 $\pm$ 13 yrs). Dialyzing procedures consisted of hemodialysis in 33 cases and peritoneal dialysis in 52. The etiological factors,as well death rate,are listed in Table I.

Table I. Mortality in relation to etiology

Causes	Patients(n°)	Deaths(n°)	Percent mortality
post-abortum	29	9	31
post-partum	8	5	62.5
cholangitis	24	14	58.3
post-surgical, post-traumatic sepsis	11	7	63.6
others	13	11	84.6
total	85	46	54.1

Obstetric septic shock is the most frequent cause of ARF in our experience (29 cases of postabortum sepsis, 8 cases of septic post-partum complications). In 24 cases,ARF is a complication of a cholangitis,in 11 it is a septic surgical or post-traumatic complication. In 13 pts anuria was triggered by other septic conditions (pneumonia, peritonitis, etc.). Death rate is influenced by the clinical characteristics of the underlyng disease;indeed,in our experience,mortality fluctuates from 30 % surgical in post-abortum sepsis,to 58 % in cholangitis and ARF,to over 60 % in surgical and post-traumatic sepsis. Overall 39 of 85 pts survived and recovered fully while 46 (54 %) died.

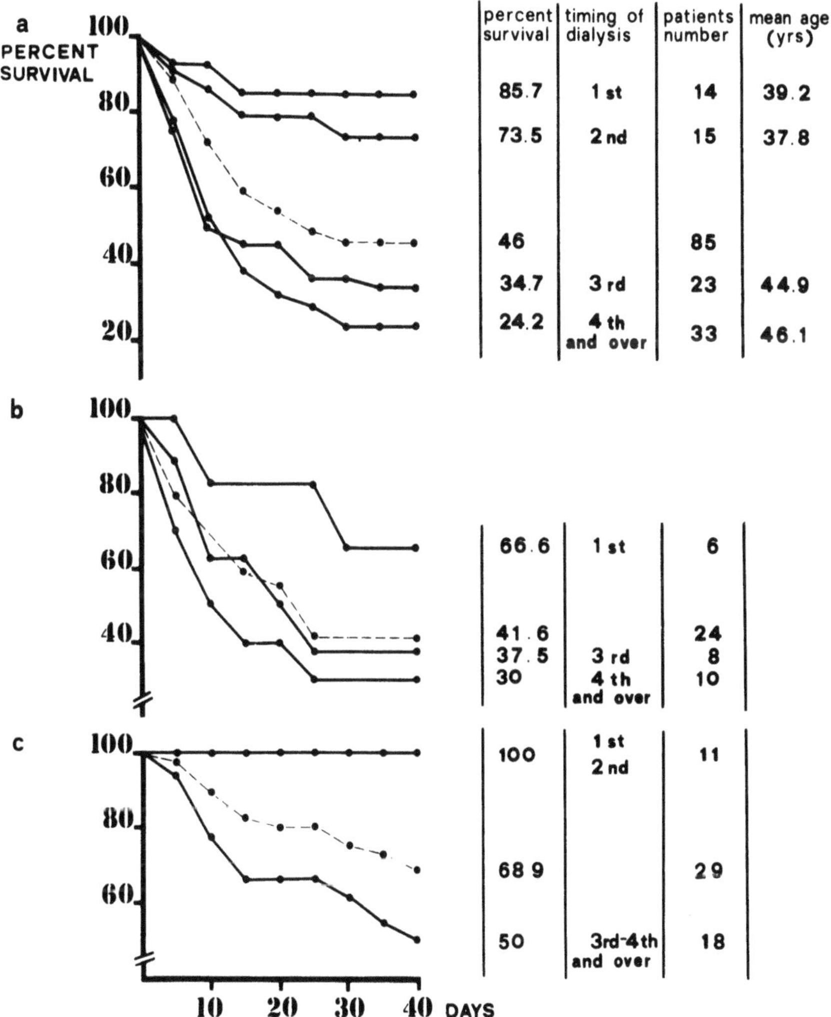

Figure 2. Actuarial survival referred to timing of dialysis (a = overall studied pts; b = ARF due to cholangitis; c = post-abortum ARF)

If the prognosis is compared with the starting day of dialysis during the anuric period,there appears to be a good correlation between survival rate and timing of dialysis(Figure 2). Actuarial survival curves after the onset of anuria show on the 40th day in all cases(Figure 2a)an 86 % survival rate the 14 pts dialyzed on the first day;73 % in pts treated on 2nd day(15 cases),35 % and 24 % in pts treated on the 3rd day(23 cases)and respectively,on the 4th day and over. The different survival rates in the 4 groups of pts cannot be related to age difference because the mean age of pts in the 4 groups does not show any significant difference. Similary, the survival curve calculated by the actuarial method in 24 cases of cholangitis and ARF shows a 67 % survival rate in the 6 pts treated on the first day of anuria,37.5 % in 8 pts dialyzed on the 3rd day and 30 % in 10 cases treated after the 4th day.(Figure 2 b). Actuarial survival curves evaluated in 29 post-abortum ARF causes show,on the 40th day,a 100 % survival rate for the 11 pts dialyzed during the first two days after the onset of anuria and 50 % for the 18 pts treated after the third day(Figure 2c).

Table 2 shows that the trend of survival curves related to the starting day of dialysis is comparable in pts treated either with hemodialysis or peritoneal dialysis. Peritoneal dialysis seems to provide better survival if compared with hemodialysis;differences,however,are not statistically significant.

The results of our retrospective study show a close correlation between early dialysis and survival rate; prophylactic dialysis , therefore, results in a dramatic improvement in prognosis of ARF after septic shock. In the past 30 years many studies (21,22,23,24,25,26) have shown prophylactic dialysis may significantly affect the survival rate in ARF. Kleinknecht et al (24),over a pool of 500 pts,showed that introduction of

Table II. Percent survival in relation to starting day of dialysis

Dialytic therapy	1st day	2nd day	3rd day	4th day +
Peritoneal dialysis(pts 52)	90 %	83 %	35.2 %	26.3 %
Intensive hemo-dialysis(pts 33)	75 %	66.6 %	33.3 %	21.4 %
Overall cases(pts 85)	85.7 %	73.5 %	34.7 %	24.2 %

prophylactic dialysis produced a drop in mortality from 42 %(in 173 cases treated prior to the institution of prophylactic dialysis) to 29 % (in 147 cases treated thereafter);the trend was confirmed in all etiological groups examined. The exact reason for this outstanding improvement is still not well understood,but it has been suggested that a more balanced correction of the biochemical abnormality is achieved if the dialysis is undertaken before the onset of clinical deterioration. The major therapeutic goal of prophylactic dialysis is to prevent uremic intoxication. A review of results of 20 series involving 1382 pts (25) shows that prophylactic dialysis,intended primarily to keep the BUN below 70-100 mg% decreased mortality from 54 to 32 %. A prospective study by Conger(26)intended to evaluate the importance of various dialytic schedules in the treatment of post-traumatic ARF showed that death rate decreased from 87 to 37 % whenever predialytic BUN decreased from 150 to 70 mg%. The improvement in survival was due primality to a decrease in the frequency of septic and bleeding episodes. The endogenous hypercatabolic rate is, therefore, the first and absolute indication for prophylactic dialysis in ARF. If the patient to be treated is hypercatabolic then, almost without exception,prophylactic dialysis means daily dialysis ; such treatment is mandatory for pts with tissue necrosis and sepsis(26).

Another goal of our study has been to evaluate the efficacity of early dialysis in correcting the etiopathogenetic factors of endotoxic ARF. In a group of 15 patients(Table III)affected by ARF after septic shock the presence of circulating endotoxins was documented by the positivity of Limulus Amebocyte lysate test (LAL test). All cases,except one, revealed systemic disorders of coagulation.

Table III. LAL test positive acute renal failure(cases 15)

PATIENTS SEX	AGE (yrs)	ETIOLOGY	DIC	DIALYSIS (STARTING DAY)	OUTCOME	CAUSE AND DAY OF DEATH
F	27	POST - PARTUM	+	1st	SURVIVED	
M	66	POST-SURGICAL	–		"	
M	77	"	+		"	
M	69	CHOLANGITIS	+		"	
F	37	POST-ABORTUM	+	2nd	SURVIVED	
F	18	"	+		"	
F	25	"	+		DIED	COMA (5)
F	23	"	+		SURVIVED	
F	53	POSTRAUMATIC	+		"	
F	44	CHOLANGITIS	+	3rd	DIED	RESP. INSUFF. (22)
M	72	POST-SURGICAL	+		"	HEART INSUFF. (38)
M	45	SEPSIS	+		"	SEPSIS (5)
M	65	SEPSIS (U.T.I.)	+		"	" (23)
M	62	PERITONITIS	+	4th	DIED	SEPSIS (15)
M	78	SEPSIS	+	6th	"	HEART INSUFF. (8)

The data reported in the table confirm the close relationship between the timing of dialysis and survival rate; interestingly, all the pts treated on the 1st day survived in spite of the life threatening underlyng diseases and, in 3 cases, of old age. In 8 pts (Figure. 3), the LAL test, evaluated daily before hemodialysis and immediately after it, showed a drop of positivity at the end of each dialytic session as well as a slow decrease of positivity with daily hemodialysis progression.

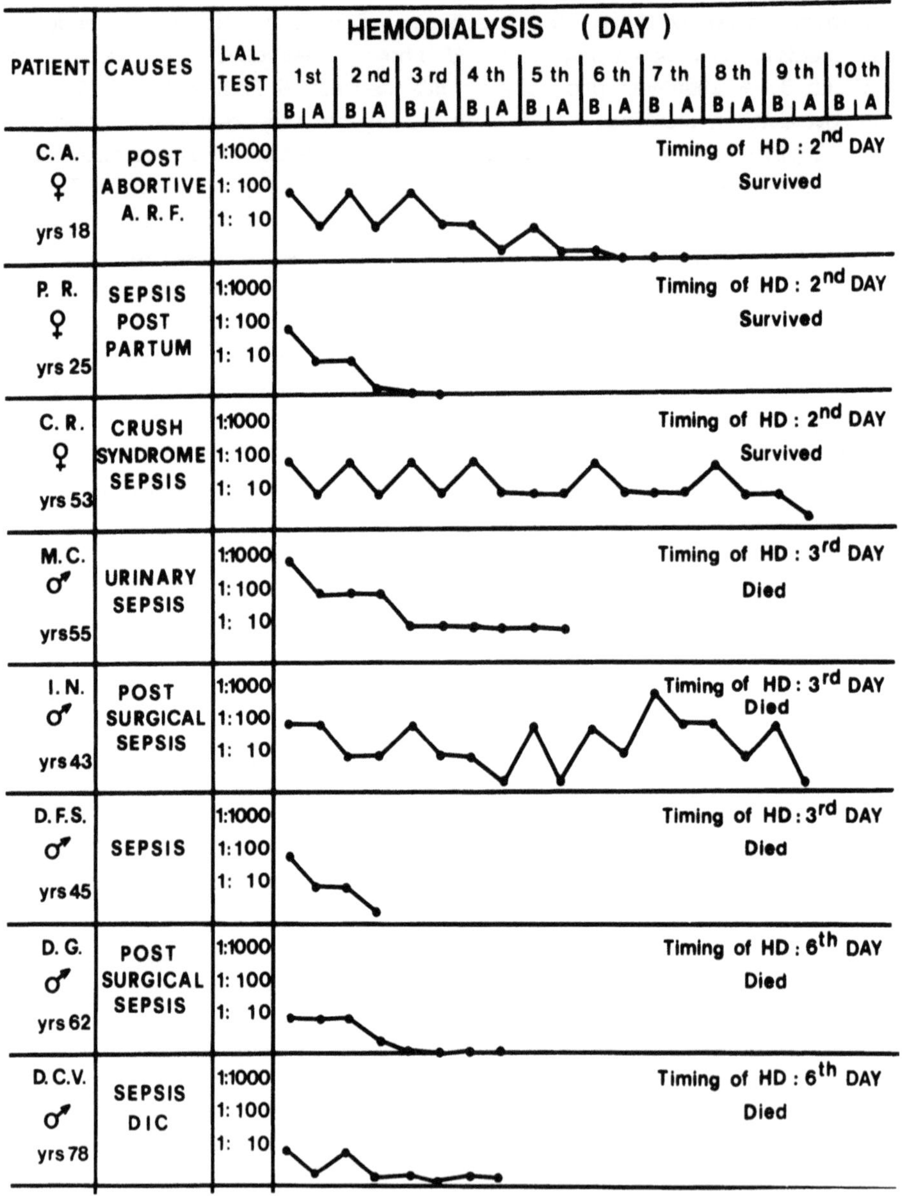

Figure 3. Limulus endotoxin assay in 8 septic ARF submitted to daily hemodialysis (B = before hemodialysis, A = after hemodialysis).

These results suggest that reactive LAL test substances may permeate the dialytic membrane. Raji et al(27)examined the permeability of dialyzing membranes to endotoxin and reported transfer in two of six trials with Kill hemodialyzer. On the other hand,negative results for endotoxin transfer were obtained by Bernick et al. (28,29). Theoretically, the dialyzing membranes should be an effective barrier to endotoxin(m.w.>100000 daltons). Endotoxins,however,could be fragmented into smaller molecules and thus cross the dialyzing membrane. It has been demonstrated that Lipid A is a fragment representing the biologically active endotoxin and this fragment is known to react with LAL. If such fragment is produced in the human body,naturally native lipid A would be easily dialyzed through highly permeable membranes since its molecular weight is as small as 2000 daltons. Clinical and experimental researches carried out by our group (30) have shown that dialyzing membranes are permeable to LAL reactive substances presumably related to small endotoxin fragments. Clinically, pts submitted to daily dialysis showed a progressive decrease to LAL reactive substances in the blood:in vitro experiments with polyacrylonitrile membrane demonstrated a decrease of lipid A concentration in the blood stream and the appearance of lipid A in the collected hemofiltrate.

These clinical and experimental results seem to suggest the hypothesis that early dialysis affords optimal chances of survival in ARF after septic shock not only through timely correction of biochemical abnormalities and prevention of the symptoms and complications of acute uremia,but also through timely removal of biologically active endotoxin fragments. The removal of the endotoxin from the blood stream,if done early in ARF,can either eliminate or depress the pathogenetic factors activated by the endotoxin itself and the consequent phenomenology (vascular injury,hemolysis,hyperbilirubinemia,DIC),if done late it is unable to prevent the cascade of events triggered by the endotoxin with obvious effects in prognostic implications.

ACKNOWELDGMENT

This research was supported by Ministero Pubblica Istruzione Grant 85/4478.

REFERENCES

1. R.B. Stott,J.S.Cameron,C.S. Oggs and M. Bewick, Why the persistently high mortality in acute renal failure?, Lancet 2:75 (1972)
2. D. Kleinknecht and D. Ganeval, Preventive hemodialysis in acute renal failure: its effects on mortality and morbidity, in : Proceedings of the conference on acute renal failure, E.A. Friedman and H.E.Eliahou, eds.,D.C. DHEW Publ. (NIH), Washington, (1973)
3. M. Lunding,I.B. Steiness and J.H. Thaysen, Acute renal failure due to tubular necrosis: immediate prognosis and complications, Acta Med.

Scand. 176:103 (1964)
4. R. Kumar, C.M. Hill and M.G. McGeown, Acute renal failure in the elderly, Lancet 1:90 (1973)
5. S.D. McMurray,F.C. Luft,D.R. Maxwell,R.J. Hamburger,D. Futty,J.J. Szwed,K.J. Lavelle and S.A. Kleit, Prevailing patterns and predictors variables in patients with acute tubular necrosis, Arch. Int. Med. 138:950 (1978)
6. J.L. Dawson, Jaundice,septic shock and acute renal failure, Am. J. Surg. 116: 516 (1968)
7. E.N. Wardle, Endotoxin and acute renal failure : a review, Nephron 14:321 (1975)
8. R.F. Wilson,A.P. Thal and P.H. Kindling, Hemodynamic measurements in septic shock, Arch. Surg. 91:121 (1965)
9. R.F. Wilson,E.J. Sarver and P.L. Leblanc, Factors affecting hemodynamics in clinical shock with sepsis, Ann. Surg. 174:939 (1971)
10. C.E. Lucas, The renal response to acute injury and sepsis, Surg. Clin. North Am. 56:953 (1976)
11. C.G. Cochrane,S.D. Revak,R. Ulevitch,A. Johnston and D. Morrison, Hageman factor:characterization and mechanism of activation, in : Chemistry and biology of the kallikrein-kinin system in health and disease, G. Pisano and S. Austen, eds., Fogarty Int. Center Proc. No 27. DHEW Publ. No (NIH) 76-791 (1977)
12. J.L. Dawson, Acute post-operative renal failure in obstructive jaundice, Ann. Roy. Coll. Surg. 42:163 (1968)
13. J.B. Andersen,F.H. Sorensen and H. Skjoldborg, Acute renal failure in association with choledocholithiasis, Acta Chir. Scand. 137:81 (1971)
14. O.S. Better, Acute renal failure complicating obstructive jaundice, in : Acute renal failure, B.M. Brenner and J.H. Stein, eds., Churchill Livingstone,New York, (1980)
15. D.J. Miller,G.R. Keeton and B.L. Weber, Jaundice and severe bacterial infection, Gastroenterology 71:94 (1976)
16. A. Amerio,V.M. Campese,P. Coratelli,F. Dagostino,M. Micelli,G. Passavanti and F. Petrarulo, Prognosis in acute renal failure accompanied by jaundice, Nephron 727:152 (1981)
17. R. Zetterstrom and L. Ernster, Bilirubin, an uncoupler of oxidative phosphorylation in isolated mitochondria, Nature 178:1335 (1956)
18. M.L. Cowger and R.F. Labbe, Bilirubin toxicity in cultured mammalian cells, Fed. Proc. 23:223 (1964)
19. R.Day, Inhibition of brain respiration in vitro by bilirubin. Reversal of inhibition by various means, Proc. Soc. Exp. Biol. and Med. 856:261 (1954)
20. W. Schumer,P. Erve,S.K. Kaika and G.S. Moss, Endotoxin effect on respiration of rat liver mitochondria, J. Surg. Res, 10:609 (1970)
21. P.E. Teschan,C.R. Baxter,T.F. O'Brien, J.N. Freyhof and W.H. Hall, Prophylactic hemodialysis in the treatment of acute renal failure, Ann. Int. Med. 53:992 (1960)
22. R.E. Easterling and M. Formand, A five years experience with prophylactic dialysis for acute renal failure, Trans. Am. Soc. Artif. Intern. Organs 10:200 (1964)
23. J.T. Baslov and H.E. Jorgensen, A survey of 499 patients with acute

anuric renal insufficiency. Causes,treatment,complications and mortality Am. J. Med. 34:754 (1963)

24. D. Kleinknecht,P. Jungers,J. Chanard,C. Barbanel and D. Ganeval, Uremic and non uremic complications in acute renal failure: evaluation of early and frequent dialysis on prognosis, Kidney Int. 1:190 (1972)
25. M. Brezis, S. Rosen and F.H. Epstein, Acute renal failure, in : The Kidney, B.M. Brenner and F.C. Rector, eds., W.B. Saunders Co., Philadelphia, (1986)
26. J.D. Conger, A controlled evaluation of prophylactic dialysis in post-traumatic acute renal failure, J. Trauma 15:1056 (1975)
27. L. Raji,F.L. Shapiro and A.F. Michael, Endotoxemia in febrile reaction during hemodialysis, Kidney Int. 4:57 (1973)
28 J.J. Bernick,F.K. Port,M.S. Favero and D.G. Brown, Bacterial and endotoxin permeability of hemodialysis membranes, Kidney Int. 16:491 (1979)
29. J.J. Bernick,F.K. Port and M.S. Favero, In vivo studies of dialysis related endotoxaemia and bacteriemia, Nephron 27:307 (1981)
30. P. Coratelli,G. Passavanti,D. Fumarola and A. Amerio, New trends in hepatorenal syndrome, Kidney Int. 28 Suppl. 17: S 143 (1985)

ACUTE RENAL FAILURE IN PREGNANCY

Jean-Pierre Grünfeld and Nathalie Pertuiset

Département de Néphrologie
Hôpital Necker
Paris, France

Acute renal failure (ARF) has become a very rare complication of pregnancy. In the 1960s, pregnancy-related ARF represented approximately 20 to 40 % of all cases of ARF. Since 1970, its incidence in industrialized countries has decreased dramatically because of the virtual disappearance of septic abortion and better prenatal care. At the National Maternity Hospital, Dublin, from 1961 to 1970, 20 cases of ARF occurred among 57,568 delivered women whereas from 1971 to 1980, only 4 cases were observed among 83,713 deliveries. At the same maternity hospital, during the same two periods, the number of cases of abruptio placentae and renal cortical necrosis went from 1,091 to 630 and from 6 to 1, respectively[1]. These data reflect the low incidence of pregnancy-related ARF. In other countries, however, the incidence of severe ARF in pregnancy is still high, for instance in northern India[2]. At the Mustapha Hospital, Algiers, pregnancy-related ARF represented approximately 20 % of all causes of ARF between 1979 and 1983, and this percentage is similar to that found from 1966 to 1978 (Drs. A.Merouani and M. Drif, personal communication).

The main causes of ARF in pregnancy are listed in Table 1.

Table 1. Main causes of pregnancy-related acute renal failure.

Septic abortion

Acute pyelonephritis

Preeclampsia-eclampsia

Volume contraction (hemorrhage, vomiting, etc.)

Idiopathic acute fatty liver

Bilateral renal cortical necrosis (complicating mainly abruptio placentae)

Idiopathic postpartum renal failure

Miscellaneous causes (obstructive uropathy due to enlarged uterus ; amniotic fluid embolism ; various causes unrelated to pregnancy, such as bacterial endocarditis, poststreptococcal glomerulonephritis, systemic disease, drug nephrotoxicity, or incompatible blood transfusion).

In industrialized countries, ARF due to septic abortion almost completely disappeared. The syndrome is characterized by severe sepsis due to Clostridia or gram-negative bacteria, shock, intravascular hemolysis, often anuric ARF, and in the most severe cases skin necrosis of the extremities and other features of significant disseminated intravascular coagulation[3].

Acute pyelonephritis is the most common infectious complication in pregnancy. Gravidas with acute pyelonephritis are more prone to develop ARF than are nonpregnant women. Acute renal failure may be precipitated or aggravated by the undue use of non-steroidal anti-inflammatory drugs or of potentially nephrotoxic antibiotics. Early antibiotic therapy, supportive management, and close supervision are mandatory for gravidas with acute pyelonephritis.

Severe preeclampsia-eclampsia may cause ARF, especially in older, usually multiparous gravidas. In our own series, which included cases collected from 1957 to 1979, severe preeclampsia-eclampsia was the apparent cause of ARF in 21 % of cases[5]. In subsequent studies dealing with eclampsia, the incidence of ARF was low. However, in the aforementioned Algerian series, eclampsia represented 56 % of the causes of pregnancy-related ARF in the 1979-1983 period vs. 18 % and 26 % in the 1966-1972 and 1973-1978 periods, respectively (Drs. A. Merouani and M. Drif, personal communication). In severe preeclampsia-eclampsia, ARF is most probably related to acute tubular necrosis. Disseminated intravascular coagulation (with microangiopathic hemolytic anemia) may contribute in rare cases.

Volume contraction is an important mechanism of ARF in pregnancy. In late pregnancy, the causal factor is often blood loss resulting from concealed or overt uterine hemorrhage. Hyperemesis gravidarum and late vomiting in pregnancy are less common causes[6]. The deleterious effects of blood loss are probably maximal in toxemic women whose intravascular volume is already contracted, who possibly have relative prostaglandin deficiency and who have increased reactivity to vasoconstrictive hormones, or in patients with abruptio placentae who show severe coagulation disturbances. Prerenal ARF and acute tubular necrosis or bilateral renal cortical necrosis may therefore result from volume contraction. Early and adequate restoration of blood volume should prevent renal failure. The attention paid to this preventive measure is probably the main factor involved in the decreased incidence of ARF in pregnancy.

Idiopathic acute fatty liver of pregnancy (AFLP) is characterized by microvesicular fatty metamorphosis in the centrilobular hepatocytes unaccompanied by inflammatory cell infiltration or hepatocellular necrosis. The first clinical manifestations usually appear suddenly during the last trimester of pregnancy and include nausea, vomiting and abdominal pain which are rapidly followed by jaundice, liver failure and encephalopathy. Hyperbilirubinemia, elevated serum aminotransferase and alkaline phosphatase levels, hypoglycemia, hyperamylasemia, elevated white-cell counts and thrombocytopenia are the most frequent biochemical and hematological abnormalities[7]. An association with preeclampsia has been noted in approximately 20 to 50 % of the cases[6]. The prevalence rate of AFLP has been estimated as approximately one in 13,000 to one in 1,000,000 pregnancies[8].

ARF develops in about 60 % of the patients. Shutdown in kidney function is due either to a prerenal mechanism or to acute tubular necrosis. Fibrin deposits in glomerular capillaries have occasionally been found. Renal failure is rarely severe enough to require dialysis.

"Liver disease presenting in the third trimester of pregnancy should be considered a medical emergency"[7]. The diagnosis is based on exclusion of other causes of hepatobiliary disease, and on liver biopsy if no other cause is detected and if coagulation tests are normal or correctable. Computed tomography may provide a noninvasive technique for demonstrating high liver fat content[6].

Maternal and fetal prognosis in AFLP has long been considered to be very poor. However, in the series reported after 1979, maternal and fetal mortality were 18 and 42 %, respectively[8]. Improved prognosis has been ascribed to earlier recognition and better supportive care leading to a decrease in deaths from extrahepatic causes, such as hemorrhage, hypoglycemia, or sepsis. Administration of blood products may reverse low antithrombin III levels found in cases of AFLP with disseminated intravascular coagulation[8]. Many authors advocate immediate delivery as soon as a diagnosis of AFLP is ascertained[7]. In survivors, no recurrence of AFLP has been observed in subsequent pregnancies[7].

Obstetric complications represent the most common causes of <u>acute bilateral renal cortical necrosis</u> (BRCN)[9,2]. In our study, BRCN was diagnosed in 21 % of cases of ARF in pregnancy (excluding ARF complicating septic abortion in which BRCN developed in only 1.5 % of cases)[9]. Abruptio placentae is the most common precipitating event, and prolonged intrauterine death, uterine hemorrhage, sepsis, or amniotic fluid embolism are much less frequent causes[9].

BRCN occurs more frequently in multigravidas 30 years of age or older, with ARF developing early in the third trimester of pregnancy, between the 26th and 30th gestational weeks[9]. The incidence of preeclampsia is lower in women with BRCN than in pregnant women with ARF due to acute tubular necrosis[9,2].

The clinical presentation of BRCN is characterized by anuria or severe oliguria of long duration, lasting 15 to 20 days or longer[9]. The diagnosis is based on renal biopsy and/or selective arteriography. Both techniques also provide information on the extent of cortical necrosis. The cortical nephrogram is absent on arteriogram (except in the subcapsular zone) in diffuse BRCN whereas it is heterogeneous in patchy cortical necrosis[9]. Cortical calcifications may develop in a few weeks and be seen on x-rays. In most patients who survive the acute phase, renal function resumes and more or less severe renal failure ensues. Recovery is probably related to patchy cortical involvement or to the frequent preservation of the juxtamedullary nephrons whose glomeruli lie in the deep cortex. Subsequent deterioration in renal function occurs frequently in the following months or years, depending on the preserved renal mass. This evolution may be related to hyperfiltration in the surviving nephrons[6]. However, some rare patients have stable renal function many years after the acute insult.

BRCN has been considered the clinical counterpart of the experimental Sanarelli-Shwartzman reaction. In pregnant animals, bilateral cortical necrosis is induced by a single endotoxin injection whereas two injections are required in non-pregnant animals. Coagulation disturbances, i.e., enhanced capacity to produce fibrin and depressed fibrinolytic activity, are found in pregnancy, and abruptio placentae is usually accompanied by severe coagulation abnormalities. These possibly contribute to the pathophysiology of BRCN. It is of interest, however, that the incidence of disseminated intravascular coagulation is not particularly high in women with BRCN (compared to women with ARF and acute tubular necrosis). Some experimental data also suggest that endothelial damage by endotoxin occurs first and that thrombi subsequently form in situ in a unilateral renal Shwartzman reaction (see ref. in 6).

The syndrome of idiopathic postpartum renal failure has been recognized since 1968 and occurs within days or weeks after an apparently normal pregnancy and delivery[6,10]. Respiratory or gastrointestinal symptoms frequently precede the appearance of rapidly progressive oligoanuric renal failure. Blood pressure is normal or slightly elevated at the onset, but severe hypertension may develop subsequently and be accompanied by seizures and heart failure. Microangiopathic hemolytic anemia and thrombocytopenia are found in 75 % of the cases, which can thus be termed "postpartum hemolytic and uremic syndrome" (HUS).

Prognosis of postpartum ARF is poor. Death occurred in approximately 60 % of reported cases and only 10 % of the women had complete renal recovery. In recent years, however, prognosis has improved although renal sequelae remain frequent. Recurrence of postpartum ARF has been reported. Renal transplantation may be successful although recurrence in kidney allografts has occasionally been observed[6].

Renal histopathological changes[6,10] involve interlobular arteries, afferent arterioles and glomeruli. Changes in arteries and arterioles are characterized by intimal swelling, subintimal deposits, concentric intimal fibrosis, and thrombosis in the lumen. Glomerular lesions may be similar to those found in HUS in children : i.e., enlarged tufts, endothelial swelling, subendothelial deposition of a pale granular fibrinlike material, leading to capillary obstruction and occasionally to thrombi. In other patients, however, the glomerular lesions are of ischemic type : i.e., with retracted tufts and wrinkled basement membranes, resembling those found in malignant nephrosclerosis or in scleroderma. The more severe the arterial involvement, the poorer the prognosis. Arterial changes are more frequent in adults than in children with HUS.

Various hypotheses and tentative classifications have been put forward concerning idiopathic postpartum ARF and HUS. These syndromes have been regarded as clinical counterparts of a generalized Shwartzman reaction. The lack of evidence for consumptive coagulopathy and for clear efficacy of anticoagulation therapy, however, does not support this hypothesis. In contrast, the primary lesion seems to be vascular endothelial damage. This mechanism may be involved in many cases, including the postinfectious form. Recently, the association between HUS and Escherichia coli that produces vero-cell cytotoxin (verotoxin) has been emphasized. A role of verotoxin-producing E.coli has been suggested in a woman with reversible postpartum HUS[11]. It should be kept in mind that the verotoxin elaborated by E.coli is probably similar to the toxin of Shigella dysenteriae 1[12].

Others have suggested that deposition of platelet thrombi in the microvessels may be the primary event in HUS. This may result from endothelial damage, from a circulating factor that causes agregation of normal platelets[13], or from a deficiency of prostacyclin (PGI_2) or of a plasma PGI_2-stimulating factor[14]. The latter hypotheses have lead to proposing plasma infusion, plasma exchange, PGI_2 infusion, PGI_2 synthesis stimulation[15], or platelet inhibitors for the therapy of HUS and related syndromes[14].

Additional pathogenetic mechanisms have been hypothetized in postpartum HUS. Oral contraceptives may provoke HUS whose manifestations are close to those observed in idiopathic postpartum ARF. Genetic predisposition to idiopathic, postpill or postpartum HUS has been found in some kindreds[6,12]. Immunologic abnormalities, including low plasma C_3, have been documented in some cases of HUS. The heterogeneous nature of HUS should be recognized. There is probably no single pathogenetic mechanism involved (as well as no single therapy)[12].

In postpartum HUS, as in idiopathic adult HUS, plasma infusion, plasma exchange and/or antiplatelet drugs are "currently in vogue"[12], and improvement has been ascribed to their use in uncontrolled studies[6,14]. Conservative management with dialysis and antihypertensive drugs (including converting enzyme inhibitors) is crucial[16].

REFERENCES

1. J.F. Donohoe, Acute bilateral cortical necrosis, in : "Acute Renal Failure", B.M. Brenner and J.M. Lazarus, eds., W.B. Saunders, Philadelphia (1983).

2. K.S. Chugh, P.C. Singhal, V.K. Kher,et al., Spectrum of acute cortical necrosis in Indian patients, Am. J. Med. Sci. 286 : 10 (1983).

3. M.D. Lindheimer, A.I. Katz, D. Ganeval, et al., in : "Acute Renal Failure", B.M. Brenner and J.M. Lazarus, eds., W.B. Saunders, Philadelphia (1983).

4. L.K. Atkinson, T.H.J. Goodship, and M.K. Ward, Acute renal failure associated with acute pyelonephritis and consumption of non-steroidal anti-inflammatory drugs, Brit. Med. J. 292 : 97 (1986).

5. J.P. Grünfeld, D. Ganeval, and F. Bournérias, Acute renal failure in pregnancy, Kidney Int. 18 : 179 (1980).

6. N. Pertuiset, D. Ganeval, and J.P. Grünfeld, Acute renal failure in pregnancy : an update, Sem. Nephrol. 4 : 232 (1984).

7. M.M. Kaplan, Current concepts : acute fatty liver or pregnancy. N. Engl. J. Med. 313 : 367 (1985).

8. P.J. Pockros, and T.B. Reynolds, Acute fatty liver of pregnancy, Dig. Dis. Sci. 30 : 601 (1985).

9. D. Kleinknecht, J.P. Grünfeld, P. Cia-Gomez, et al., Diagnostic procedures and long-term prognosis in bilateral renal cortical necrosis, Kidney Int. 4 : 390 (1973).

10. J.P. Hayslett, Current concepts : postpartum renal failure, N. Engl. J. Med. 312 : 1556 (1985).

11. B.T. Steele, J. Goldie, I. Alexopoulou, et al., Postpartum haemolytic uraemic syndrome and verotoxin-producing Escherichia coli, Lancet 1 : 511 (1984).

12. K.N. Drummond, Hemolytic uremic syndrome - then and now. N. Engl. J. Med. 312 : 116 (1985).

13. F.A. Siddiqui, and E.C.-Y. Lian, Novel platelet-agglutinating protein from a thrombotic thrombocytopenic purpura plasma, J. Clin. Invest. 76 : 1330 (1985).

14. G. Remuzzi, and E.C. Rossi, The hemolytic uremic syndrome. Intern. J. Artif. Organs 8 : 171 (1985).

15. S.T.S. Durrant, P. Joosten, and E.C. Gordon-Smith, Nafazatrom in treatment of thrombotic thrombocytopenic purpura, Lancet 2 : 842 (1985).

16. S. Rasmussen, M. Brahm, M. Damkjaer Nielsen, et al., Postpartum renal failure and malignant hypertension treated with captopril, Scand. J. Urol. Nephrol. 17 : 209 (1983).

ACUTE HANTAVIRUS NEPHROPATHY IN BELGIUM : PRELIMINARY RESULTS OF A SERO-EPIDEMIOLOGICAL STUDY

J. Clement * and G. van der Groen **

* Military Hospital Brussels, Belgium
** Institute of Tropical Medicine Antwerp, Belgium

INTRODUCTION

Hantavirus (HV) has recently been recognized as a cause of acute renal failure (ARF) in different countries of Europe, particularly in Belgium and France. This disease (HV-disease), hitherto unknown to the Western world, is marked by aspecific viral symptoms and minor thrombocytopenia at the onset, followed by a variable degree of ARF, most often with a self-limiting course of 2 to 6 weeks. This so-called HV-nephropathy is characterized by severe loin pain, oliguria, a heavy but transient proteinuria, and mostly a minor hematuria. On renal biopsy, acute interstitial nephritis with minimal glomerular hypercellurarity is found, whereas immunofluorescence shows no or very few and aspecific immuno-deposits. In the European patients, very faint or no hemorrhagic symptoms seem to appear, and the overall mortality is lower than 1 %. This is in contrast to the hemorrhagic forms with high mortality (up to 20 %) in the Far East, where the disease was known for a long time under various denominations and had been considered as a viral "hemorrhagic fever". Transmission of the virus occurs through exposure to infected rodents, probably by inhalation of contaminated aerosols (droplets of urine and/or saliva from apparently healthy rodents, who act as carriers). Diagnosis can only be ascertained by specific anti-HV serology. In this paper, we want to give an historical background of this "new" disease and illustrate it with 2 case-reports and the first preliminary results of a sero-epidemiological study in Belgium.

HISTORICAL BACKGROUND

A. Military History : " War nephritis"

HV-disease has an impressive military history, since many wars in the past have been plagued by epidemics ressembling in all parts the actual HV-syndrome: in 1862-1863, 14,000 of such cases were described among the Northern Armies of the Central Region in the American Civil War (1). On the other hand during the South African Boer War, the Japanese-Russian War, the Spanish-American War or the French-German War in 1870, no mention is found of a similar epidemic (1), proving at least that the responsible agent at those periods was not ubiquitous. The term "War nephritis" or "Trench nephritis" was coined for the first time in World War I, where from 1915 on, several thousand cases were reported among British soldiers in the trenches of Flanders' battlefields(1). A still worse epidemic however was rampant in the German lines where all the typical symptoms of the so-called "Kriegsnephritis" or "Feldnephritis" were lucidly analyzed (2). An annual variability and an almost exclusive occurrence in the trenches was noted.

When Japanese troops invaded Manchuria in World War II, they were confronted with the so-called Songo fever and suffered 12,600 cases. Japanese military doctors already suspected and later (1942) proved a viral etiology (3). On the European front, 16,000 cases of an epidemic clinically similar to nephropathia epidemica (NE) (see below) were noted among German troops in Lapland and in Yugoslavia (4).

At the outbreak of the Korean War (1951), the US military doctors were puzzled by a new and frightening disease consisting of fever, hemorrhages, shock and renal failure. The syndrome was called Korean hemorrhagic fever (KHF). In the United Nations Armed Forces, more than 3,000 cases were diagnozed with an overall mortality of 6 to 8 %, but in some small localized outbursts going up to 33 %, thus posing a major medical and military problem (5). Despite heavy research (see below) no etiological agent was found.

During military manoeuvres in Yugoslavia, 20 % of the soldiers stationed under tent near Fruška Gora fell suddenly ill from June 12th 1961 on. Since the overall mortality was 2.2 %, the cases were extensively, but without success, examined in the Military Medical Academy of Beograd (6). The only hint at that moment was that 1961 had been called "The mice year" and that nests of wild rodents (Apodemus, Microtus, etc) had been found under the tents.

B. Terminology of Viral Hemorrhagic Fevers in Relation to HV

Until recently, the nomenclature was an uncredible mess because all kinds of hemorrhagic fevers (all with RNA-viruses as etiologic agent) were mixed up and virtually each region in the Eurasian landmass had its own geographically labelled appellation (Crimean fever, Omsk fever, etc) resulting in a Babel of up to 60 synonyms for HV-disease alone ! This makes the extensive bibliography and classification by Gajdusek all the more valuable (6). In table 1 we list only the most important syndromes belonging to the HV-group, each time with the year of the first clinical description in literature, and the region affected.

TABLE 1 : TERMINOLOGY IN RELATION TO HV-DISEASE

1913 :	Hemorrhagic nephroso-nephritis (U.S.S.R).
1913 :	Epidemic hemorrhagic fever (EHF) or Songo Fever (China)
1930 :	Tula fever (Central Russia)
1934 :	Nephropathia epidemica (NE) (Scandinavia)
1934 :	Epidemic hemorrhagic fever (Eastern Europe)
1951 :	Korean hemorrhagic fever (KHF) (Korea)
1981 :	Hantaanvirus (Korea)
1982 :	Hemorrhagic fever with renal syndrome (HFRS)
1982 :	Muroïd virus nephropathy
1984 :	Hantavirus (HV) nephropathy

The working group on HFRS at a WHO-meeting in Tokyo, 1982, recommended that all the above mentioned diseases should be referred to as hemorrhagic fever with renal syndrome (HFRS), which is still the official denomination. Gajdusek proposed the term "Muroid virus nephropathy" because all these viruses are carried to man by rodents of the supra-family Muroidea, and belonging to the families Muridae (Apodemus and Rattus) and Cricetidae (Clethrionomys and Microtus) (7). He justly pointed out that the term "Hemorrhagic fever" is misleading to the clinician, since hemorrhagic symptoms do not always develop, the less so in the Eastern and Western European forms. At last, in 1984, J. Desmyter et al have proposed in a letter to the editor of The Lancet (8) the simple denomination "Hantavirus (HV) disease" which amongst others has the non negligible advantage of being the shortest and the most pronounceable version of them all...

C. Developments in HV-Research

Clinical and virological research was very long and extremely tortuous: see Table 2.

Rarely has an infectious disease been investigated as intensively as was HV-disease, particularly so since the Korean war. The oldest possible reference to HV-disease in the Far East is a suggestive description of a hemorrhagic fever associated with a renal syndrome in a Chinese Medicine Book written around A.D. 960 (9). Since 1934 a benign epidemic form of nephritis without hemorrhagic complication was described in Scandinavia under the name of nephropathia epidemica (NE) (10). In 1940 Russian, and in 1942 Japanese workers, independently established the first evidence for the infectious viral etiology, by producing typical HV-symptoms in human subjects after I.V. injection of bacterial-filtered blood and/or urine ultrafiltrate from acute phase HV-patients (3).

TABLE 2 : HV-DISEASE : Clinical and Virological Research

960 :	Chinese Medicine Book
1930 :	First description in Tula-region (U.S.S.R.)
1940 :	First evidence of viral etiology (U.S.S.R)
1951 :	Korean hemorrhagic fever (Korean War)
1976 :	Isolation of Hantaan virus (Korea)
1981 :	Culture in A 549 cells
1982 :	Culture in Vero E6 cells
1983 :	First European description of HV-laboratory outbreak (Belgium)
1984 :	Isolation of Puumala virus (Finland) and Hällnäs virus (Sweden)

HV-disease however did not attract great attention from the Western medicine until the Korean War, with its high fatality rate of Western KHF-cases (2,400 U.S. soldiers). The American Army Medical Service established an Hemorrhagic Fever Centre near Uijonbu in South Korea, and all suspected cases were evacuated by helicopter to the Centre's Hospital. Despite a careful investigative program, including inoculations into monkeys and animal and human continuous cell lines, no etiologic agent was found (11). The major breakthrough came only 25 years later in 1976, when H.W. Lee and co-workers found in the lungs of the Korean striped field mouse (Apodemus agrarius Coreae) an antigen which reacted in a virus-like pattern in an immunofluorescent (IF) test with convalescent, but not with early acute phase sera of patients (12). The rodent was wild-caught in an endemic area of Korea, and subsequent isolation of this infectious antigen resulted in the prototype strain 76-118. Lee named it in 1981 "Hantaanvirus" after the Hantaan river which runs near the famous 38th parallel between North and South Korea, where much of the battle had been fought out. So even the name of Hantaan (HTN) has a military consonance. It became clear that apparently healthy rodents acted as natural reservoirs for HV, excreeting the virus in their lungs, saliva and urine. The rat (or another rodent), that unliked but ever-present companion of the soldier at war, had been responsible for the War nephritis, and not the combination of cold and misery in the trenches, resulting in a renal vasospasm, as had been proposed by the great German physician Volhardt (2).

Still, the virus had to be cultured in continuous cell lines for allowing further characterization and taxonomic classification. French et al (13) were able to adapt HTN-strain 76-118 to A 549 (human lung carcinoma) in 1981, whereas Mc Cormick et al (14) used Vero E6 cells (a clone of African green monkey kidney-cells) in 1982 for isolation. Finally, in 1983 HV could be classified as a virus similar to viruses in the Bunyaviridae family (containing other hemorrhagic viruses e.g. Crimean fever virus), in that it possesses a tripartite single stranded RNA genome but with molecular differences, making it a new genus in that family.

At last, in 1984, exactly half a century after its first description as nephropathia epidemica (NE) in Scandinavia, the NE virus was successfuly adapted to Vero E6 cell culture. The virus was extracted from the lungs of the red bank vole (Clethrionomys glareolus), a common rodent in Europe, and collected in Finland (Puumala strain) and Sweden (Hällnäs strain) (15) respectively. Outside of Scandinavia, Ch. van Ypersele de Strihou was the first nephrologist in Europe to describe in 1983 acute HV-nephropathy in three laboratory technicians handling laboratory rats in a Belgian university campus (16), thus giving the clinical screening of this disease a much-needed stimulus.

MATERIALS AND METHODS

Serological Techniques (fig. 1)

We used an indirect immunofluorescent antibody technique (IFAT) as described by Mc Cormick et al (14), modified mainly by the use of HV-infected Vero E6 cells, inactivated by gamma irradiation and stored at - 80° in growth medium containing 10 % fetal calf serum (FCS) and 10 % dimethyl sulphoxide (DMSO) (17). Sera were screened at a dilution of 1-in-16 and all sera were also examined on uninfected E6 cells as a check for specificity. Sera giving the typical dotlike cytoplasmic fluorescence in Vero E6 cells infected with Hantaan strain 76-118, and no reaction on control cells, were considered positive. All of the military sera were also tested for another viral antigen, referred to as CG 18-20, from Clethrionomys glareolus (C.G.). This red bank vole, with a variant HV-strain in its lungs, was captured in the Western part

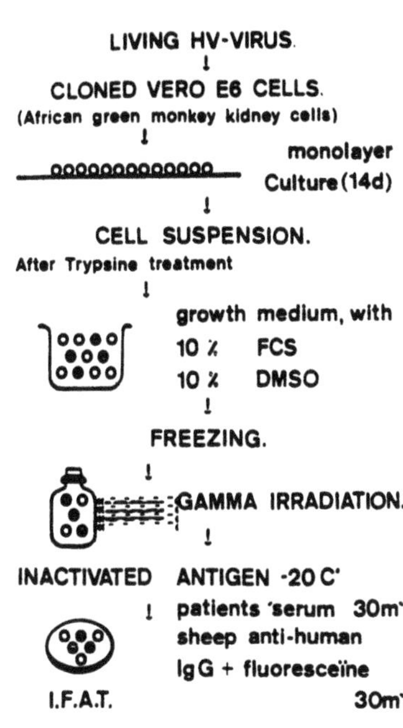

Figure 1

of the U.S.S.R. (Bashkiria region), in an area where a mild form of HV disease had been described, clinically similar to NE.
Military sera were first screened with the two above described IFA-techniques at the Military Hospital Brussels (HMB). Each positive military serum sample and 1 out of 10 negative samples, were controlled at least once in the Institute of Tropical Medicine (ITM) Antwerp, for further confirmation of the serological titre.

Sera :

Sera were stored at - 20° C. The vast majority of sera were provided by blood donors in the civilian as well as in the military study. Other sources are mentioned in the text.

CASE REPORTS

Case 1 : (see fig. 2)

Le. Ro., 20-years old male corporal of the Belgian Army.
4 weeks before the onset of symptoms (day 1), he participated in army manoeuvres in the surroundings of Spich (W. Germany), where he slept outside during 3 consecutive nights on his armoured vehicle. Later on, he made daily strolls with his dog in the forests around his natal town of Oostham, in the province of Limburg (N. Belgium). On day 1 (8 January 1984), he developed fever up to 40° C with viral symptoms, followed the next days by vomiting and diarrhoea. He was taken into the Military Hospital of Cologne on day 5, where a thrombocytopenia of 56,000/µl with some petechiae, oliguria with a total weight gain of 10 kg, 3-plus proteinuria and rapidly declining renal function was noted. On day 6 he was evacuated by helicopter to the Military Hospital Brussels for dialysis facilities. A top S. creatinine-level of 6.3 mg % was reached, whereas urinary output was remitting spontaneously at the end of the

same day.
The further evolution and all the other symptoms fitted remarkably well in the scheme as was given by P.Y. Lallement et al in 1984, presenting 4 French cases (18). From day 12 on, renal function was normalized. On day 11, a kidney biopsy was obtained, showing a discrete interstitial mononuclear infiltrate, but otherwise no abnormalities. Immunofluorescence was negative, as was an immunoperoxidase staining for HTN-antigen in the kidney tissue. The diagnosis was confirmed retrospectively by an unequivocal rise in the HV-antibodies, (strain 76-118) as demonstrated by IFAT: 1/64 and 1/128 in month 2, and 1/256 in month 3. The patient recovered completely.

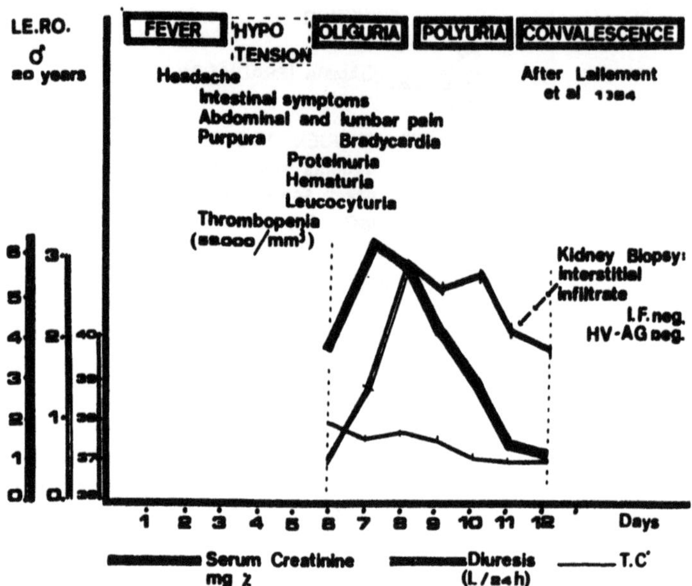

Figure 2

<u>Case 2 :</u> (not pictured)

Lo. Luc, 31-years old male, living in Couvin, a community in the South of Belgium, at the border of the forests of the Ardennes. Just before the onset of symptoms, he had done foundation works (digging) in his garden. On day 1 (9 February 1986), he presented a viral syndrome with headache, nausea and vomiting. On day 2 temperature went up to 39.9° C. He developed intractable abdominal colics and coercitive vomiting, together with repetitive bouts of epistaxis. On day 6, 3 plus-proteinuria, a thrombocytopenia (94,000/μl), and a reduction in renal function was noted, urging a hospitalization. Serum creatinine went up to 3 mg %, and proteinuria to 3.3 g/lit. Symptoms subsided under I.V. rehydratation, polyuria started from day 8 on, and on day 10 a normal platelet count and a S. creatinine of 1.4 mg % was recorded. Throughout, B.P. was normal, but there was a sinusal bradycardia of about 52/min. Hepatic tests where slightly disturbed. No kidney biopsy was performed, and the patient left hospital on day 12.
IFAT for Hantaan 76-118 antigen was positive on day 12 with a serum dilution of 1/128, whereas CG 18-10 antigen gave a 1/1024 positivity. The next month, the titres were 1/64 and 1/512 respectively. Table 3 shows the results of IFAT with a panel of different HV-antigens in the first serum sample of each case.

Table 3 : Indirect immunofluorescent antibody titres against different hantaviruses in sera of two sporadic Belgian cases of a mild form of hantavirus disease. (LR: case 1, 1984 - LL: Case 2, 1986)

	HTN	CG 18-20	NE	CG 13891	PH	TCH
LR V84-58	64*	512	512	64	128	64
LL V86-283	128	1024	512	1024	256	128

* Reciprocal of the highest dilution for which still characteristic fluorescence can be observed.

HTN: Hantaan strain 76-118 isolated from <u>Apodemus Coreae</u> in Korea;
CG 18-20: isolated from <u>Cl. Glareolus</u> (bank vole) in the Western part of the U.S.S.R.;
NE: Hällnäs strain isolated from <u>Cl. Glareolus</u> in Sweden;
CG 13891: isolated from <u>Cl. Glareolus</u> captured in Turnhout, Belgium;
PH: Prospect Hill isolated from <u>Microtus sp. in U.S.A.;</u>
TCH: Tchoupitoulas isolated from <u>Rattus-Rattus</u> in U.S.A.

Both patient sera showed a higher titre on HV-antigens (CG 18-20, NE) isolated from bank voles (<u>Cl. Glareolus)</u> captured in areas (Western part of U.S.S.R and Sweden), where an HV-disease has been described similar to the one reported here. Both sera reacted less well with the HTN antigen, etiologic agent of the more severe form of hantavirus disease in Korea, as well with <u>Rattus</u>-borne strain (TCH). L.R. serum (case 1) showed an equal affinity for the bank vole borne strains, the Belgian strain CG 13891 included.

EPIDEMIOLOGICAL STUDY
(preliminary results).

Civilian Study

From 1983 on, the IFAT using HTN-strain 76-118 as viral antigen, was used as a screening test in a prospective sero-epidemiological study of a cross-cut section (mainly blood donors) of the Belgian civilian population. Up to now (January 1986), a total N of 12,767 sera were examined, of which 205 (1.6 %) were found to be positive for the presence of indirect immunofluorescent anti-HTN-antibodies. So far we found antibodies in 124 (1.3 %) of 9413 blood donors, in 4 (0.7 %) of 596 chronic haemodialysis patients in Northern Belgium, in 16 (2 %) of 784 sera of veterinarians, farmers and foresters, in 44 (2.1 %) of 2055 sera submitted from all over Belgium to exclude leptospirosis, in none of all sera from personnel working at the institute of Tropical Medicine, and finally in 17 (6.3%) of 268 sera of which the clinician suspected a possible Hantavirus etiology.

With blood donors as a reference group, clinical suspected ($p < 0.001$ Fisher exact test), as well as leptospirosis ($X^2 = 10.52$ $p < 0.001$) suspected samples had a significant higher antibody prevalence.

On a total of 138 sera positive for antibodies against Hantaan virus, only two sera were also positive for leptospirosis, excluding a systematic crossreaction between the two. These data suggest that some Hantavirus infections in Belgium superficially mimic leptospirosis Chronic dialysis patients had a significant lower antibody prevalence. There is no straightforward explanation (humoral immunodepression ?) for this phenomenon, though this finding does suggest that HV-disease in Belgium rarely, and perhaps never, leads to severe permanent renal insufficiency.

A correlation has been observed between the prevalence of HTN-antibodies and the geographical origin of the human sera investigated (see fig. 3) (X^2 = 57.10 $p < 0.001$).

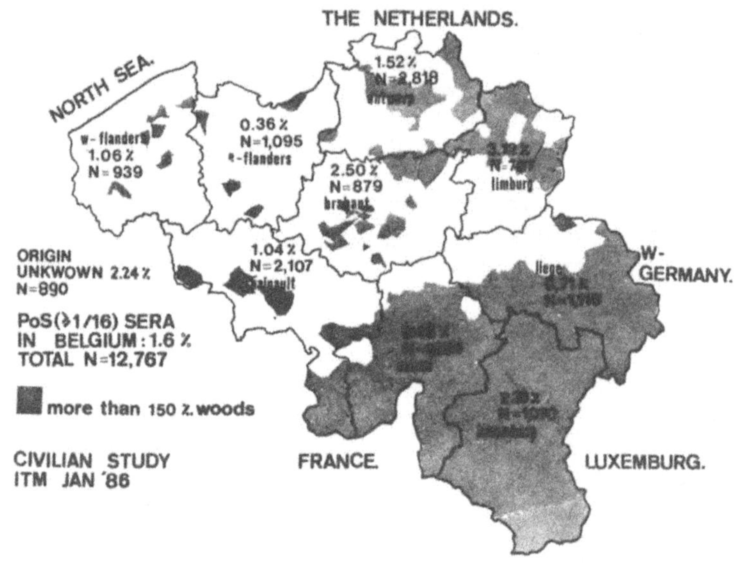

Figure 3

Fig. 3 is a map of Belgium, giving the total N of sera examined per province, each time accompanied by the total HTN-seropositivity (as percentage) per province. Densely forested areas (more than 150 ‰ of the surface) are shaded in grey.

A significant higher (X^2 = 23.3 $p < 0.001$) prevalence of HTN-antibody positive sera was observed in the South - Eastern part (2.2 %) (Luxemburg, Namur, Brabant, Liège, Limburg) than in the North - Western part (1 %) (Antwerp, E and W Flanders, Hainault) of Belgium. The highest prevalences were found in the Provinces Limburg (3.12 %) and Namur (2.48 %). The prevalences in these provinces were significant higher than in the remaining part of Belgium. (Limburg X^2 = 14.91 $p < 0.001$, Namur X^2 = 11.54 $p < 0.001$). East Flanders is the province with the lowest prevalence compaired to the rest of Belgium. (X^2 = 13.55

$p < 0.001$). It is also the least forested province in Belgium. The surprisingly low positive percentage in the province of Liège (0.71 %) can be explained by the fact that the vast majority of serum samples were harvested in the industrial city of Liège and/or its suburbs, where there are no woods at all.

The increased prevalence of Hantaan-antibodies in human sera of the S - E part of Belgium parallels the increased number of dense forest areas (see fig. 3). The majority of the clinical documented cases so far, were situated in the province of Namur, which is one of the most forested provinces in Belgium. To what extent a dense forest area reflects a difference in the occurrence of Hantavirus-positive free living animals as a potential source of infection for humans, must be evaluated further.
In order to study the groups at risk as well as the risk factors for HV-infection in Belgium, a case control study was set up.
For each seropositive person, three seronegative age- and sex-matched controls will be studied, using computer questionnaires with information about habitation(s), possible contacts with animals etc. The study is in progress.

B. Military Study

Military have been described to be at risk for the rodent-borne HV-disease (see military history above), probably due to open field activities (camping, digging, etc), carrying a higher risk of exposure to wild rodents.

To see if the same rule applies to the Belgian soldiers, an epidemiological case control study was worked out in the same way as the above mentioned civilian study, using 2,905 sera of an existing computerized sera bank of the Belgian Army, together with 4,218 sera of military blood donors of different garrisons. In this study, all sera were screened for antibodies against two different HV-antigens (HTN 76-118 and CG 18-20), and the computer questionnaire was completed with a special section asking information about recent camps, manoeuvres, bivouacs, etc.
Based on this individual data, all studied subjects were divided into two groups arbitrarly called "depot forces" (less than two open field activities in the past year) and "fighting forces" (two or more open field activities in the past year). On a total of 7,123 sera examined so far, only 65 or 0.91 % gave positive results with at least one of the two described IFA-tests. However, there was a statistically significant difference ($X^2 = 10.39$ $p < 0.005$) in the prevalence of positive sera between the so called fighting forces (49 positive sera out of 3,904 of 1.25 %) and the depot forces (16 positive sera out of 3,219 or only 0.49 %), suggesting a greater risk for HV-infection inherent to open field activities.
As in the civilian study however, valid conclusions can only be drawn after multiple regression analysis or equivalent statistical evaluation of the various data of this study, which is still going on. In addition, a prospective 3-years study comparing Para-Commando troops (intensive field activities) with Medical Service troops (fewer or no field activities) as a control group was started. Together with the questionnaire, blood samples will be taken at the beginning and at the end of the military service, in an effort to study risk factors, which could be important for a possible seroconversion.

CONCLUSIONS

HV-nephropathy should be added to the etiological list of ARF - at least in Europe- as a viral condition that often, in the more severe cases, is confounded with leptospirosis, and that in the milder cases, which are probably the vast majority, frequently can go unnoticed because of its self-limiting course. Symptoms are aspecific, but the clinician - and particularly the nephrologist - should grow suspicious if he is confronted with a clinical picture consisting of fever with abdominal symptoms, followed by oliguria, marked proteinuria and microhematuria. Pronounced *loin pain* before and during the oliguric phase (due to the interstitial edema) and initial but transient *thrombocytopenia* are the sole salient clinical features. This low platelet count (mostly between 30 and 70.000/µl) is in less than 10 % of the cases accompanied by hemorrhagic symptoms (petechiae, conjunctival hemorrhages, etc...), and seems to be in Europe the only common link with the more virulent hemorrhagic forms in the East, as they were recognized since the Korean War. In both Western and Eastern forms of HV-disease however, the main target organ is the kidney for reasons not yet understood. Careful questioning of the patient is (as always) very rewarding, particularly if a history of possible exposure to wild rodents 1 to 4 weeks prior to the onset of symptoms can be elicited. Besides of working in a barn (19) or stable, this contact can encompass all kinds of open air activities: camping, gardening (18), digging (18) around the (weekend)house, walking in the forest, and even jogging can be involved. The preliminary results of our sero-epidemiological study in Belgium seem to confirm the greater risk of seropositivity in densely wooded areas and among civilian and military professional groups with frequent open air activities. A special problem for scientific institutions is virus transmission to the staff by laboratory-bred white rats who act as healthy carriers: after Belgium (16), laboratory HV-outbreaks have been documented in France (20), the United Kingdom (21) and the Netherlands (22). So far, laboratory *mice* have not been implicated. It appears now that of all the hemorrhagic fever-viruses, HV is the only one that seems to be endemic and enzootic in Western Europe and in North America. HV is *not* arthropod-borne; neither is there any evidence for a person-to-person transmission.
Remission is almost always complete in 2 to 6 weeks, and HV-nephropathy has hitherto not been described as a cause of chronic renal failure, as was shown in Finland by Lähdevirta in 76 of his own patients with confirmed NE, and in 228 other patients followed in other Finnish institutions (23). One can only speculate about the possible implications of HV in the pathogenesis of unexplained "idiopathic" forms of interstitial fibrosis of the kidney. In such cases, this hypothesis could easily be ruled out by retrospective survey of specific anti-HV antibodies, because these markers of an ancient HV-infection have been detected as long as 34 years after the acute illness.

In a clinical setting suggestive for HV-nephropathy, the first serum sample should be taken as soon as possible during the first week after onset of fever, the second sample 2 to 3 weeks later, and the third preferentially 1 month later. The finding of immunofluorescent IgG anti-HV antibodies at a serum dilution of 1/16 or more(i.e. a positive IFAT-test) in the first sample is virtually diagnostic for acute HVdisease, since the prevalence of these antibodies is very low (1 to 2 %) in a standard population (mainly blood donors), as was shown in our and in a previous epidemiological study (24) in Belgium. Of course a subsequent rise in the titre is 100 % confirmative for the diagnosis. Titres can vary considerably depending on the virus strain that is used as antigenic substrate in the IFAT. The most widely used strain is still the prototype Hantaan virus (HTN) 76-118, isolated from the lungs of

a Korean striped field mouse.
More than 100 HV-strains have now been isolated. The genetic similarity between the original "native" Hantaanvirus (Korea), the Puumala strain (Finland) and the Hällnäs strain (Sweden), the latter both putative etiologic agents of the nephropathia epidemica (NE) in Scandinavia, has strengthened the clinical impression of the extension of HV-disease over the totality of the Eurasian continent. Moreover, HV-infected rodents and human serum samples containing anti-HV antibodies have also been found on the African and American continent: HV has probably a worldwide distribution. It is tempting to think that HV- *disease* also has,although until now no clinical reports of proven human HV-disease came in from the Americas or from the African continent. The question is if this curious situation stems only from the fact that outside Asia, HV-disease more than often has a benign and self-limiting course, and that as such the clinical diagnosis can easily be overlooked, the more so considering the complete aspecificity of the symptoms. It is noteworthy that even in the severe "classic" Korean Hemorrhagic Fever only 1/3 of the patients show hemorrhagic manifestations, whereas 2/3 have flu-like symptoms (25). Worldwide detection of HV-disease is further hampered by the fact that the final diagnosis can only be secured by a rather cumbersome indirect immunofluorescent antibody test (IFAT), demanding amongst others a cloned continuous cell line infected with HV. (see fig. 1). Variant serological techniques who were successfully used until now are hardly easier to perform: immune adherence hemagglutination assay (26), complement fixation (26), competitive inhibition with monoclonal fluoresceinated antibodies (27), variants of ELISA etc. An equally good alternative to immunofluorescent techniques has recently been developed, using immunoperoxydase-labelled protein A conjugate, and allowing examination by ordinary light microscope (28). The aim of all these tests is detection of specific anti-HV antibodies, which appear only at the end or after the illness (minimum 10 days from the onset of symptoms).
A very recent report from China (29) describes successful detection of the HV-antigen in white blood cells and in urinary sediment-cells of 138 patients with the Chinese form of HV-disease, scoring a positivity rate of 82,6 % and 71 % respectively. This technique would allow rapid diagnosis in the very first days of the illness. For antigen detection in white blood cells, blood should be taken on heparin in a sterile tube and immediately dispatched to a suitable laboratory.

The cases of acute HV-nephropathy that have been discovered by different European nephrologists in recent years, could well appear to be only the top of an iceberg.

REFERENCES

1. Brown: Royal Army Med. Corps 25 : 75 (1915).
2. F.R. Miller in "Lehrbuch des inneren Medizin" II p.85 J. von Mehring-Krehl, (1925).
3. S. Ishii, K. Ando, N. Watanabe et al: Studies on Songo Fever. Jap Army Med J 355 : 1755 - 1758 (1942).
4. Von Bergmann: "Lehrbuch der inneren Medizin" II p. 63, (1942).
5. D.P. Earle (Ed.) : Symposium on epidemic hemorrhagic fever. Am J Med 16 : 617-709 (1954).
6. D.C. Gajdusek, D. Goldgaber, E. Millard : Bibliography of Hemorrhagic fever with renal syndrome (Muroid virus nephropathy), U.S. dept. of health and human services, NIH Publication No. 83-2603, Maryland (1982).
7. D.C. Gajdusek: Muroid Virus nephropathies and muroid viruses of the Hantaan virus group. Scand J Infect Dis Suppl 36: 96-108 (1982).

8. J. Desmyter, Ch van Ypersele de Strihou and G. van der Groen: Hantavirus disease. Lancet ii: 158 (1984).
9. H.W. Lee: Korean Hemorrhagic fever. Prog Med Virol 28 : 96-113 (1982)
10. G. Myhrman : Nephropathia epidemica, a new infectious disease in Norther Scandinavia. Acta Med Scand 140: 52-56 (1951).
11. J. French, R.S. Foulke, J.W. Huggings et al: Korean Hemorrhagic Fever, Proceedings Symposium HFRS.
12. H.W. Lee and P.W. Lee: Korean hemorrhagic fever . Demonstration of causative antigen and antibodies. Korean J Intern Med 19: 371-384 (1976).
13. G.R. French, R.S. Foulke, O.A. Brand et al: Korean hemorrhagic fever: propagation of the etiologic agent in a cell line of human origin. Science 211: 1046-1048 (1981).
14. J.B. Mc Cormick, E.L. Palmer, D.R. Sasso et al: Morphological identification of the agent of Korean hemorrhagic fever (Hantaan virus) as a member of the Bunyaviridae. Lancet i: 765-68 (1982)
15. B. Niklasson, J. Le Duc: Isolation of the Nephropathia Epidemica Agent in Sweden. Lancet i: 1012-1013 (1984).
16. J. Desmyter, K.M. Johnson, C. Deckers et al: Laboratory rat outbreak of hemorrhagic fever with renal syndrome due to Hantaan-like virus in Belgium. Lancet ii: 1445-1448 (1983).
17. G. Van der Groen, T. Kurata, C. Mets: Modification to indirect immunofluorescence tests on Lassa, Marburg and Ebola material. Lancet i: 654 (1983).
18. P.Y.Lallement, B. Morinière, E. Kaloustian et al: Fièvre hémorrhagique avec syndrôme rénal: quatre cas autochtones. Med et Maladies inf 14: 425-430 (1984).
19. J.-Ph Mery, S. Dard, J.M. Chamouard et al: Muroid virus nephropathies Lancet ii: 845-846 (1983).
20. E. Dournon, B. Morinière, S. Matheron et al: HFRS after a wild rodent bite in Haute-Savoie and risk of exposure to Hantaan-like virus in a Paris laboratory. Lancet i: 676-677 (1984).
21. G. Lloyd, E. Bowen, M. Joes et al: HFRS outbreak associated with laboratory rats in UK. Lancet i: 1175-1176 (1984).
22. A. Osterhaus, J. Spijkers, B. Van Steenis and G. van der Groen: Hantavirusinfecties in Nederland. Nederl Tijdschr Geneesk 128: 2461-2462 (1984).
23. J. Lähdevirta: Nephropathia Epidemica in Finland. A clinical, histological and epidemiological study. Ann Clin Res 3 : suppl 8 1 - 154 (1971).
24. G. van der Groen, P. Piot, J. Desmyter et al: Seroepidemiology of Hantaan-related virus infections in Belgian populations. Lancet ii: 1493-1494 (1983)
25. H.W. Lee, M.C. Lee, K.S. Cho: Management of Korean hemorrhagic fever Med Prog 2: 15-21 (1980).
26. K. Sugiyama, Y. Matsuura, C. Movita et al: An immune adherence assay for discrimination between etiologic agents of hemorrhagic fever with renal syndrome. J Inf Dis 149: 67-73 (1984).
27. G. Song, C.S. Hang, H.X. Liao, J.L. Fu: Antigenic comparison of virus strains of mild and classical types of Epidemic Haemorrhagic fever isolated in China and adaptation of these two cultures of normal cells. Lancet i: 677-678 (1984).
28. G. van der Groen, G. Beelaert: Immunoperoxidase assay for the detection of specific IgG-antibodies to Hantaan virus. J of Virological Meth 10: 53-58 (1985).
29. Chen Bo-quan, Zhou Guo-fang, Liu Qing-zhi et al: Detection of the antigen of HFRSV by HFRS Mc Ab 25-1 in the cells of urine and white blood cells obtained from HFRS patients. Chinese J of Microbiology and Immunology 6:29-33 (1986).

Acknowledgements

We wish to thank Col. R. François M.C. and Maj. R. Van Hoof M.C. of the Medical Research Unit of the Belgian Army for their invaluable co-operation in this study.
We are indebted to Mrs. A. Midonnet and Miss F. Husson of the Laboratory Virology HBM, for their skillful assistance, and to Mrs. D. Du Bois of the Upjohn Co Belgium for the technical preparation of this manuscript.
Pat. Lo.Lu (case N° 2) was kindly referred to us by Dr. P. Colson, Centre de Santé des Fagnes, Chimay.
This study was made possible by a CCWO-grant (G46) of the Belgian Department of Defense, and by a FGWO-grant (3-0082-86).

Request for reprints of this paper should be sent to:

Dr. J. Clement, M.C. Lieut. Col.
Department of Nephrology
Military Hospital Brussels
Bruynstraat
B - 1120 Brussels, Belgium

ACUTE RENAL FAILURE IN LEPTOSPIROSIS-A 12-YEAR SURVEY

J. Drinovec, A. Kandus, AF. Bren, M. Šinigoj, I. Eržen
A. Ličina, R. Kveder, R. Ponokvar, M. Močivnik,
and M. Benedik

Department of Nephrology, Medical Centre, Ljubljana
General Hospital, Šempeter pri Novi Gorici
Institute for Public Health and Social Welfare
Ljublana, Yugoslavia

ABSTRACT

From the beginning of 1974 to the end of 1985 141 persons in Slovenia (population 1,9 million) contracted leptospirosis. 49 patients were 50 years old or more. All the patients have survived.8 male patients aged from 18 to 44 had more severe acute renal failure (ARF), 5 of whom were treated with hemodialysis. The authors found that this 100% survival rate did not agree with the findings of many other researches which quote a relatively high mortality rate among older patients. In all 8 patients kidney function was good 1 year or more after ARF. The authors consider that the survival of patients with ARF depends on early and appropriate supportive treatment, which also includes intensive hemodialysis.

INTRODUCTION

Leptospirosis is an acute infectious illness caused by different serotypes of one single species, L. interrogans.[1] When it is clinically manifested as Weil's syndrome, it is not infrequently fatal[1]. In Slovenia (surface area 20,000 km^2, 1,9 million inhabitants), the republic which comprises the north-western part of Yugoslavia, 141 persons contracted leptospirosis in the period from the beginning of 1974 to the end of 1985. The Icterohemorrhagiae serogroup (alone or together with other serogroups) was serologically established in 14 patients, while other serogroups were found in the remaining patients. All the patients survived. Table 1 shows the morbidity for leptospirosis in Slovenia from 1974 to 1985.

In a group of 92 patients, whose serogroup was not determined, 1 patient died. This group of patients was not taken into consideration in the analysis. All the patients with more severe ARF due to leptospirosis were treated in the Department of Nephrology at the Medical Centre in Ljubljana. This retrospective analysis shows the course of ARF in these patients.

Table 1. Morbidity with leptospirosis in Slovenia from 1974 to 1985.

Year	sex m	f	age in years <50	≥50	total no. of patients according to years
1974	21	11	26	6	32
1975	1	11	7	5	12
1976	19	24	31	12	43
1977	2	2	1	3	4
1978	2	3	1	4	5
1979	2	2	3	1	4
1980	2	4	4	2	6
1981	3	7	5	5	10
1982	0	4	1	3	4
1983	8	1	8	1	9
1984	4	5	4	5	9
1985	1	2	1	2	3
Total no. of patients	65	76	92	49	141

PATIENTS, METHODS AND RESULTS

8 patients (all male) aged from 18 to 44, with an average age of 34 years, had more severe ARF. Table 2 shows some clinical and laboratory findings in these patients. On admission 7 patients were poorly hydrated due to previous vomiting and/or diarrhea and/or severe sweating. Hyperbilirubinemia was predominantly conjugated. Only patient no. 4 had serious hemorrhagic complications (gastro-intestinal bleeding, more severe epistaxis), patient no. 2 and patient no.3 had a lighter form of epistaxis or petechial skin rash and conjunctival hemorrhages. The chest radiogram of patient no.7 taken in the first week of illness showed numerous small opacifications in both lungs. At the same time the patient had a nonproductive cough. After one week these symptoms and signs disappeared. Patient no. 4 had transitory signs of failure of the left heart with pulmonary congestion and pleural effusion in the chest radiogram. Patient no. 8 had paroxysmal atrial fibrillation together with clinical and echocardiographic signs of pericarditis when admitted. A kidney biopsy was made for patient no. 6 2 weeks after the onset of illness. By means of light microscopy we found changes congruent with acute interstitial nephritis (interstitial edema,moderate interstitial infiltration with neutrophilic leucocytes and mononuclear cells, slight dilatation of the tubules, thinning and polymorphism of the tubular epithelium and individual necroses and calcifications).By means of immunofluorescent microscopy we found fibrinogen diffusely present in the walls of the tubular capillaries.

The patients were given parenteral hydration and feeding. Antimicrobial drugs (penicillin G, ampicillin, amoxicillin, erythromycin, oxytetracycline)were administered to all the patients from the 4th.to the 8 th. day of the illness onwards. 5 patients with oliguric ARF were treated with hemodialysis. In all the patients a dialysis catheter placed in the femoral vein was used for vascular access. Table 3 presents the hemo-

Table 2. Some clinical and laboratory findings in our patients with ARF due to leptospirosis

Patient no.	patient	age (years)	serogroup	oliguria	max. creatinine (μmol/l)	max. urea (mmol/l)	max. total bilirubin (μmol/l)	max. SGOT (x upper limit of normal values)	max. SGPT (x upper limit of normal values)	minimal platelets ($x10^9/l$)	shock	hemorrhages	meningitis
1	MI	36	icterohem. and others	no	372	22	12	5	2	168	no	no	no
2	OJ	39	icterohem. and others	yes	1097	57	632	2	2	159		yes	yes
3	FI	40	icterohem.	yes	1708	75	450	3	2	56	no	yes	no
4	PM	31	icterohem. and others	yes	805	50	306	5	5	43	no	yes	no
5	ZE	28	icterohem.	yes	788	27	537	5	2	56	yes	no	no
6	KJ	34	australis	yes	1020	22	11	1	1	77	no	no	no
7	GJ	18	icterohem.	no	630	31	94	2	5	76	no	no	yes
8	ŽM	44	icterohem.	yes	980	44	288	3	3	36	no	no	yes

Table 3. Hemodialysis treatment of our patients with ARF due to leptospirosis

Patient no.	patient	predialysis days	no.of hemo-dialyses	no.of hemo-dialysis days	complica-tions
1	MI	-	-	-	-
2	OJ	7	5	6	no
3	FJ	12	5	7	hypo-tension
4	PM	9	1	1	hematoma with the catheter
5	ZE	-	-	-	-
6	KJ	8	2	3	no
7	GJ	-	-	-	-
8	ŽM	7	6	9	no

dialysis treatment of all the patients. During the period of restitution of kidney function 6 patients had polyuria from 4 to 8 litres per day. On discharge all the patients were free of the clinical abnormalities quoted in Table 2. Table 4 presents some laboratory findings in patients with ARF on discharge. The present serum concentrations of creatinine and urine findings in patients with ARF are shown in Table 5.

Table 4. Some laboratory data on our patients with ARF due to leptospirosis on discharge

Pa-tient no.	pa-tient	days from start of illness to discharge	serum crea-tinine (μmol/l)	total bili-rubin (μmol/l)	SGOT	SGPT
					(x upper limit of normal values)	
1	MI	29	124	normal	1	2
2	OJ	43	115	29	1	1
3	FI	47	177	normal	1	1
4	PM	42	97	37	1	2
5	ZE	42	88	42	1	1
6	KJ	27	90	normal	1	1
7	GJ	14	70	23	1	2
8	ŽM	38	139	normal	1	1

Table 5. Present serum concentrations of creatinine and urine findings in our patients with ARF due to leptospirosis

Patient no.	patient	years after ARF	creatinine (µmol/l)	urine
1	MI	8	95	normal
2	OJ	8	80	moderate proteinuria slight hematuria
3*	FI	1	97	normal
4	PM	6	78	normal
5	ZE	6	96	normal
6	KJ	5	92	normal
7	GJ	3	88	normal
8	ŽM	1	104	normal

*Data from 1980

DISCUSSION

During the last 12 years morbidity with leptospirosis in our country has been on average 11.7 cases per year, i.e. approximately 6 cases per year per 1 million inhabitants. It is very likely that the actual morbidity was greater, as our calculations did not take into account cases where the serogroup was not determined. We can conclude that leptospirosis is a relatively common illness in this country.[1-4] The illness here is mostly localized in two endemic regions. The 100% survival rate of our patients does not agree with the findings of some other researches which quote a relatively high mortality rate for older patients.[2-6] We do not have a reliable explanation for the good life prognosis of our patients, but we would concur with the opinion of certain other authors, who affirm that early and intensive hemodialysis treatment improves the prognosis for patients with Weil's syndrome.[3,5] Although clinical syndromes are not specifically linked to a serogroup, we - like other authors - have established the Icterohemorrhagiae serogroup in the majority of the most affected patients whom we have treated with hemodialysis.[2,4,7] The definitive diagnosis was confirmed serologically in agreement with acknowledged criteria [2]. Oliguric ARF was established in 6 patients, i.e. in 4.2% of the diagnozed cases of leptospirosis. 7 patients with ARF had clinical signs of dehydration on admission. We consider that dehydration in these patients was a significant contributory factor to causing ARF. Such a viewpoint is upheld by other authors as well.[8,9] A kidney biopsy was made for patient no.6 in the acute phase of his illness. By means of light microscopy we found changes congruent with acute tubulointerstitial nephritis, such as other authors have also

described.[10] Patient no. 7 , who had a nonproductive cough in the first week of illnes, also had numerous small opacifications in both lungs visible on the radiogram, which could be a sign of pneumonitis, which occurs rarely with leptospirosis[1]. The paroxysmal atrial fibrillation which we found in patient no. 8 and the transitory signs of failure of the left heart in patient no.4 were probably a sign of myocarditis due to leptospirosis.[1] All the 5 patients whom we treated with hemodialysis had oliguric ARF. Frequent hemodialyses allowed them adequate parenteral nutrition. Complications during hemodialysis (hypotension in patient no.3 and hematoma with the dialysis catheter in patients no. 4) were rare and clinically insignificant. In agreement with certain other authors we are of the opinion that bleeding diathesis in leptospirosis is not a contraindication for hemodialysis.[3,5] The majority concur that antimicrobial therapy started after the 4 th. day of illness is not beneficial.[2] We therefore assume that antimicrobial treatment, started with our patients only on the 4 th. to the 8 th. day of the illness, most probably did not influence the course of the basic illness. 7 our patients did not have signs of kidney illness even 1 year or more after ARF. This is in agreement with the observations of other authors and with observations in our patients with ARF due to leptospirosis prior to 1974.[10,11]
The moderate proteinuria and slight hematuria in patient no.2 8 years after ARF is probably a sign of chronic interstitial nephritis following leptospirosis,which some have described[10].

CONCLUSIONS

The 100% survival rate of patients with leptospirosis in our country during the last 12 years is not in harmony with the findings of many other researches. In our patients with ARF due to leptospirosis the prognosis regarding kidney function was good 1 year and more after the illness. Treatment with hemodialysis was safe and effective. We consider that early and intensive treatment with hemodialysis significantly improves the prognosis for patients with ARF due to leptospirosis.

REFERENCES

1. W.E. Farrar, 196. Leptospira species (leptospirosis), in: Principles and Practice of Infectious diseases, second edition, G.L. Mandell, R.G. Douglas, J.E. Bennett, eds. New York, John Wiley, 1985, 1338.
2. Centers for Disease Control: Leptospirosis Surveillance: Annual Summary 1978. August 1979.
3. N.D. Kennedy, D.J.Rainford, C.D. Pusey et.al, Leptospirosis and acute renal failure - clinical experiences and a review of the literature. Postgrad. Med. J. 55:176 (1979).
4. Leptospirosis Reference Laboratory and Communicable Disease Surveillance Centre (PHLS), Leptospirosis in man , British Isles, 1982, B.M.J., 287:1365(1983).

5. M. Borghi, G. Bertoli, U. Bodini et.al.,Leptospirosis Defeated? , in: Therapeutic Apheresis; A critical Look, edited by Y.Nose, P.S. Malchesky, and J.W. Smith, ISAO Press, Cleveland(1984),57.
6. C.W. Heath , A.D. Alexander, M.M. Galton, Leptospirosis in the United States: Analysis of 483 cases in man, N. Engl.J. Med. 273: 857, (1965).
7. M.L. Wong, S.Kaplan, L.M. Dunkle et al., Leptospirosis: A childhood disease. J.of Pediatrics, vol. 90:532 (1977).
8. V.Sitprija, Renal involvemend in human leptospirosis, Br. Med. J. 2: 656, (1968).
9. V.Sitprija, V. Pipatanagul, K. Mertowidjojo, et. al: Pathogenesis of renal disease in leptospirosis. Clinical and experimental studies, 17: 827, (198o).
10. M.Martinez-Maldonado, J.E. Benabe, J.M. Lopez-Novoa. Acute renal failure associated with tubulointerstitial disease including papillary necrosis, in: Acute Renal Failure, B.M. Brenner, J.M. Lazarus, eds. Philadelphia, Sounders Company,(1983) , 72.
11. S. Luzar, J. Drinovec, P. Jezeršek, Akutna bubrežna insuficijencija kod leptospiroze. in: IV Kongres internisa Yugoslavie sa međunarodnim učeščem, Zbornik radova, (1973), 553.

5. M. Bonati, G. Nicolini(?) [illegible] Fanelli(?), [illegible] In: Therapeutic apheresis, Critical Care, edited by Y. Nose, P.S. Malchesky, and J.W. Smith, ISAO Press, Cleveland(1983),67.
6. [illegible] Smith, [illegible] Alexander, M.J. Galton, [illegible] the method [illegible] analysis of [illegible] cases in [illegible] Res. 473-481, (1975).
7. [illegible]
[illegible] and response of [illegible], 141 [illegible] (1980).
9. [illegible]

PREVENTION AND TREATMENT

PROTECTION FROM ACUTE RENAL FAILURE

Michel Burnier and Robert W. Schrier

Department of Medicine
University of Colorado School of Medicine
Denver, CO

INTRODUCTION

The occurrence of acute renal failure (ARF), defined as an acute impairment of renal function resulting in the accumulation of nitrogenous waste which cannot be reversed by altering extrarenal factors, is frequent in contemporary medicine. In a recent prospective study, 4.9% of 2216 in-hospital patients developed some degree of ARF, and in some particular clinical situations, such as intensive care medicine or following cardiovascular surgery, the percentage of patients presenting with ARF may be as high as 50% (1,2). ARF is a major problem in clinical medicine not only because of its frequency but also because it represents a major cause of morbidity and mortality (1). Thus, the development of effective means to protect the kidneys against ischemic or nephrotoxic insults is very important in order to decrease the incidence of ARF and its related complications.

A decrease in renal perfusion due to, for example, shock, massive trauma or major surgery, and the administration of nephrotoxic or diagnostic agents are far the more common causes of ARF. Because the occurrence of ARF may sometimes be predicted, prevention of ARF may be possible. In many clinical situations, however, the occurrence of ARF cannot be prevented by general measures. In these cases, efforts have to be made to protect the kidneys or at least ameliorate the course of ARF using specific agents which can alter the degree of renal injury. In this regard, the understanding of the pathogenesis of ARF has led to significant advances in the use of pharmacologic agents to protect from ARF.

PATHOPHYSIOLOGIC BASIS FOR PROTECTION AGAINST ARF

ARF is characterized mainly by a decrease in glomerular filtration rate (GFR) and by the development of tubular dysfunction. The pathogenesis of the sudden decrease in GFR is multifactorial and involves both vascular and tubular factors, the relative contribution of these factors being dependent on the phase of ARF studied (initiating versus maintaining phase) and the animal model utilized (3).

The main vascular events involved in the decrease in GFR include a decrease in renal blood flow mediated by several possible factors such as the renin-angiotensin system, the sympathetic nervous system and/or endothelial cell swelling, and alterations in the permeability properties of the glomerular capillary wall. Tubular obstruction by necrotic tubular cells and non-selective backleak of filtrate across damaged tubules represent the main tubular events classically described in the pathogenesis of ARF.

The use of vasoactive drugs and diuretics to protect the kidneys from ARF has derived directly from these early pathophysiologic observations. However, more recently, considerable information has become available concerning the cellular events developing during an acute renal injury. These recent findings suggest that adenosine triphosphate depletion, the formation of oxygen-free radicals during reoxygenation and the increase in intracellular calcium are among the main cellular mechanisms inducing cell damage following an ischemic or a nephrotoxic injury. The understanding of these cellular events has not only contributed to explain the classic pathophysiologic processes discussed above, but has also led to interesting new alternatives in the pharmacologic protection from ARF such as the use of calcium channel blockers or the adminstration of adenosine triphosphate $MgCl_2$.

The list of pharmacologic agents that have been reported to be efficient in the protection of ARF either in clinical or in experimental situations is long and is constantly increasing (Table 1). We will not discuss each of these agents but instead will focus our attention on the use of diuretics, vasoactive agents and calcium channel blockers.

Table 1. Agents Used to Protect Against Acute Renal Failure

Diuretics	Nutritional Factors
Mannitol	Renal failure fluid
Polyethylene glycol	ATP-$MgCl_2$
Furosemide	
Vasodilators	**Miscellaneous**
Calcium channel blockers	Propranolol
Verapamil	Saralasin
Nifedipine	Clonidine
Diltiazem	Thyroxine
Dopamine	Theophylline
Prostaglandins E_1 and E_2	Chlorpromazine
Bradykinin	Methylprednisolone
Atrial natriuretic factor	

MANNITOL AND LOOP DIURETICS

Because oliguria is one of the most striking events when ARF occurs, it is not surprising that diuretics were among the first agents tested to protect the kidneys from ARF. However, although diuretics are widely used in clinical practice, a number of uncertainties remain regarding their mechanisms of protection and their clinical indication.

Diuretics can afford protection against ARF through several different mechanisms including: 1) increase renal blood flow and improve renal hemodynamics, 2) induce an osmotic diuresis and thus prevent cast formation and tubular obstruction, 3) prevent tubular cell swelling and therefore reduce the severity of tubular necrosis and intratubular obstruction, and 4) act as free radicals scavengers (4). Recent studies by Brezis et al have suggested that loop diuretics may also offer cellular protection by decreasing the energy expenditure of some nephron segments (5).

Early studies by Flores et al have suggested that the beneficial effects of mannitol in protecting from ischemic ARF were due to its ability to prevent endothelial cell swelling and therefore to prevent renal vasoconstriction (6). Later, micropuncture studies by Burke et al in the norepinephrine model of ARF have shown that the beneficial effect of mannitol is due both to decreased intratubular obstruction caused by the solute excretion and to improved renal hemodynamics (7). These observations were confirmed by Patak et al who also suggested that other agents that increase solute excretion but induce renal vasoconstriction, such as thiazides, may not be protective in the same circumstances (8). In addition, recent studies from our laboratory have shown that prophylactic mannitol prevented mitochondrial calcium accumulation and respiratory dysfunction during reflow following an ischemic injury, perhaps by preventing cell swelling (9).

The protective effect of mannitol was reported for the first time in 1945 by Selkurt in ischemic ARF (10). Since then, this original observation has frequently been confirmed and mannitol has been shown to afford significant protection in several experimental models. Mannitol improved renal function in the norepinephrine (7,8,11), and the renal artery clamping models of ischemic ARF (6,12) and in ARF caused by the administration of various nephotoxic agents such as glycerol (13), methemoglobin (14), cis-platinum (15) and amphotericin (16).

Clinically, the benefit of prophylactic administration of mannitol has been reported essentially in surgical situations including open heart surgery (17) and resection of aortic aneurysms (18). In a control study by Dawson, jaundiced patients undergoing surgery have been shown to benefit from prophylactic mannitol (19) and in renal transplantation, administration of mannitol immediately after completion of the vascular anastomosis was associated with a reduced incidence of acute tubular necrosis (20).

Medical indications to use mannitol as a protective agent are more limited. Two preliminary studies by Old et al (21) and Anto et al (22) have suggested that mannitol given prior to the administration of radiocontrast may protect against ARF in diabetic and non-diabetic patients. However, although these studies need to be confirmed by larger, controlled studies, mannitol is used frequently to prevent ARF induced by radiocontrast agents. In addition, there is also limited evidence that amphotericin B nephrotoxicity (23) and cis-platinum-induced ARF (24) may be prevented by the concurrent administration of mannitol.

Loop diuretics, such as furosemide, have also been studied extensively in both ischemic and nephrotoxic models of ARF, but the results are inconsistent and the efficacy of furosemide in protecting from ARF is still controversial. Furosemide significantly improved GFR in the norepinephrine model of ARF when injected before or immediately after the norepinephrine infusion (7,25) and prevented renal failure after renal occlusion in the rat when given both before and after release of the clamp (26).

Prophylactic administration of furosemide has been successful in few clinical situations. However, as for experimental models of ARF, the real efficacy of furosemide in protecting from ARF is still controversial, particularly when administered after ARF has occurred. Furosemide has been used in high risk surgical situations with some success (27), although there is less literature attesting to its efficacy than exists for mannitol. Cantarovich et al reported in two studies that patients with ARF treated with furosemide had a shorter duration of oliguria and needed less dialysis but mortality was unaffected (28,29). Recent studies have suggested an interesting synergism between furosemide and dopamine in oliguric patients. With this association 19 of 24 patients in the first study (30) and 6 out of 6 patients in the second study (31) were converted from oliguric to non-oliguric ARF. In view of the results of Anderson et al (32) showing that patients with non-oliguric ARF have a significant, lower morbidity and mortality than patients with oliguric ARF, the increase in urine output induced by furosemide alone or combined with dopamine may represent an important achievement to improve the outcome of patients with ARF.

VASOACTIVE AGENTS

Since renal vasoconstriction and diminished renal blood flow (RBF) were observed in animal models of ARF and in patients with established ARF, several groups of pharmacologic agents (Table 1) have been used to increase RBF and therefore potentially serve as therapeutic agents to protect from ARF. The effect of vasoactive drugs to attenuate ARF has been evaluated mainly in the norepinephrine and renal clamping model of ARF. Interestingly, although an increase in RBF was obtained following the administration of purely vasoactive agents such as acetylcholine (26) or secretin (8), GFR remained severely depressed and very little, if any, protection could be found in these conditions. Prostaglandins (PGE_1 and PGE_2) infused before or along with the infusion of norepinephrine provided significant renal protection (33) and the administration of either beta receptor blockers such as propranolol or beta receptor agonists such as dopamine also reduced the degree of azotemia in ischemic ARF due to renal artery clamping (34). However, Patak et al found that a better protection from ARF could be obtained when vasoactive agents were associated with drugs increasing renal solute excretion (8). As discussed above, a similar observation has been done clinically with the association of dopamine and furosemide (30,31). These results suggest that agents affecting both the vascular and the tubular determinants of ARF may be more effective in protecting the kidneys from ARF. In this context, calcium channel blockers which can increase renal blood and possibly prevent tubular damage by decreasing cellular calcium uptake may represent an important new pharmacologic development in the protection against ARF.

CALCIUM CHANNEL BLOCKERS

Animal studies by Farber et al in the liver (35) have suggested that cellular calcium accumulation represents a major pathophysiologic event in the development of ischemic and toxic cell injury. During the past several years, several studies performed in our laboratories have confirmed these important observations in the kidneys both in ischemic and nephrotoxic experimental models of ARF (36,37). Therefore, we examined the protective effect of calcium channel blockers in ischemic ARF.

In the norepinephrine model of ARF in the dog, verapamil infused in the renal artery either 30 minutes prior to the ischemic injury or for 2 hours after the ischemic insult afforded significant functional protection as assessed by the recovery of GFR (38). Following the ischemic injury, GFR recovered better when verapamil was administered before the injury. Protection against mitochondrial calcium accumulation and respiratory dysfunction was observed with both verapamil and nifedipine administered after the ischemic insult. A similar degree of protection was obtained with verapamil in the renal artery clamping model of ARF (39).

Additional studies from our laboratory, using the isolated perfused kidney, have shown that verapamil added to the perfusion media improved inulin clearance and sodium transport after 40 minutes of warm ischemia and in a cold model of ischemia. Addition of verapamil to the flushing solution also afforded significant protection against the ischemic injury (40). In addition to the protective vascular effects, a direct effect of calcium channel blockers on the tubular injury induced by anoxia has also been shown. In isolated rat proximal tubules subjected to 30 minutes of anoxia, verapamil and nifedipine decreased the ^{45}calcium uptake and the degree of cell damage (41) and in cultured proximal tubules verapamil increased cell survival following 45 minutes of anoxia (42).

Recently, calcium channel blockers have been shown to afford protection in a canine model of radiocontrast nephropathy (43) and preliminary results suggest that verapamil may protect against aminoglycoside nephropathy in the rat (44). Clinical studies demonstrating the beneficial effect of calcium channel blockers to protect from ARF are still few. In patients treated with cis-platinum, verapamil increased renal blood flow but did not affect the fall in GFR observed following four courses of cis-platinum (45). In renal transplant patients, results by Duggan et al (46) suggest that verapamil improves the early function of the graft when administered to the donors before harvesting the kidneys. Moreover, the patients who received the verapamil treated kidneys had a lower incidence of acute rejection episodes. A similar observation has been done by Wagner et al (47) using diltiazem, another calcium channel blocker, in transplant patients receiving cyclosporine and prednisone.

ATRIAL NATRIURETIC FACTOR

Because atrial natriuretic factor (ANF) possesses both vascular and tubular properties (48), it could be an important tool in protecting against ARF. For example, in the context of ischemic ARF, ANF could attenuate any decrease in RBF through its renal vasodilator properties and also decrease tubular obstruction and cast formation secondary to its diuretic and natriuretic properties. Although little attention has been given yet to this hypothesis, early results from our laboratory in the isolated perfused kidney showed that atriopeptin III given after 60 minutes of ischemia induced a significant functional protection from the ischemic injury as assessed by better recovery of GFR during reperfusion as shown in Figure 1 (49).

CONCLUSIONS

Thus, although the list of pharmacologic agents presently available to protect from ARF is long, the understanding of the pathophysiology of ARF has led to the appearance of new compounds that might improve our capacity to protect the kidneys against ischemic or nephrotoxic injuries. Clinical trials demonstrating the benefits of calcium channel blockers in the protection from ARF and additional experimental studies using ANF are awaited with extreme interest.

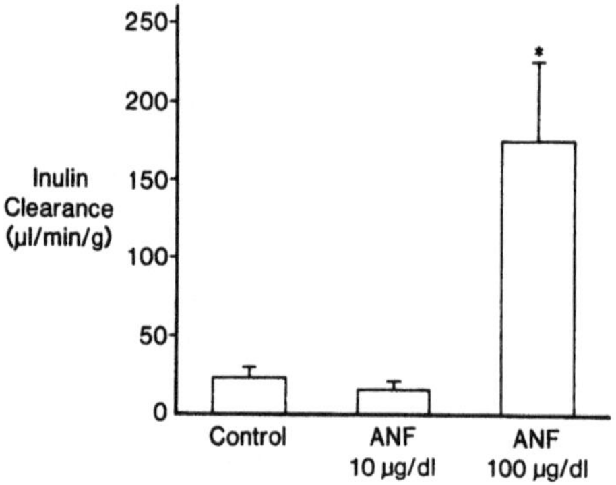

Figure 1. Effect of atriopeptin III (ANF) on the recovery of renal function in isolated perfused kidneys following 60 minutes of ischemia. Atriopeptin III, 10 μg/dl (n=4) or 100 μg/dl (n=6), was added after 30 minutes of reperfusion. *p<.05

ACKNOWLEDGEMENTS

Dr. Michel Burnier is a recipient of a grant from the Swiss Foundation for Medicine and Biology supported by the Swiss Academy of Medical Sciences.

REFERENCES

1. S. H. Hou, D. A. Bushinski, J. B. Wish, J. J. Cohen, and J. T. Harrington, Hospital-acquired renal insufficiency: A prospective study, Am. J. Med. 74:243 (1983).

2. R. J. Anderson, and P. A. Gross, Acute renal failure and toxic nephropathy, in: Contemporary Nephrology, Vol. 1, S. Klahr, and S. G. Massry, eds., Plenum, New York (1981).
3. N. G. Levinsky, Pathophysiology of acute renal failure, N. Engl. J. Med. 296:1453 (1977).
4. N. G. Levinsky, D. B. Bernard, and P. A. Johnston, Mannitol and loop diuretics in acute renal failure, in: Acute Renal Failure, B. M. Brenner, and J. M. Lazarus, eds., W. B. Saunders, Philadelphia (1983).
5. M. Brezis, S. Rosen, P. Silva, and F. H. Epstein, Renal ischemia: A new perspective, Kidney Int. 26:375 (1984).
6. J. Flores, D. R. Dibona, C. H. Beck, and A. Leaf, The role of cell swelling in ischemic renal damage and the protective effect of hypertonic solute, J. Clin. Invest. 51:118 (1972).
7. T. J. Burke, R. E. Cronin, K. L. Duchin, L. N. Peterson, and R. W. Schrier, Ischemia and tubule obstruction during acute renal failure in dogs: Mannitol in protection, Am. J. Physiol. 238:F305 (1980).
8. R. V. Patak, S. Z. Fadem, M. D. Lifschitz, and J. H. Stein, Study of factors which modify the development of norepinephrine-induced acute renal failure in the dog, Kidney Int. 15:227 (1979).
9. R. W. Schrier, P. E. Arnold, J. A. Gordon, and T. J. Burke, Protection of mitochondrial function by mannitol in ischemic acute renal failure, Am. J. Physiol. 247:F365 (1984).
10. E. E. Selkurt, The changes in renal clearance following complete ischemia of the kidney, Am. J. Physiol. 144:395 (1945).
11. T. J. Burke, P. E. Arnold, and R. W. Schrier, Prevention of ischemic acute renal failure with impermeant solutes, Am. J. Physiol. 244:F646 (1983).
12. M. J. Hanley, and K. Davidson, Prior mannitol infusion in a model of ischemic acute renal failure, Am. J. Physiol. 241:F556 (1981).
13. D. R. Wilson, G. Thiel, M. L. Arce, and D. E. Oken, Glycerol induced hemoglobinuric acute renal failure in the rat. III. Micropuncture study of the effects of mannitol and isotonic saline on individual nephron function. Nephron 4:337 (1967).
14. W. L. Parry, J. A. Schaeffer, and C. B. Mueller, Experimental studies of acute renal failure. I. The protective effect of mannitol, J. Urol. 89:1 (1963).
15. M. F. Pera, B. C. Zook, and H. C. Harder, Effects of mannitol or furosemide diuresis on the nephrotoxicity and physiologic disposition of cis-dichlorodiammineplatinum-(II) in rats, Cancer Res. 39:1269 (1979).
16. A. A. Hellebusch, F. Salama, and E. Eadie, The use of mannitol to reduce the nephrotoxicity of amphotericin B, Surg. Gynecol. Obstet. 134:241 (1973).
17. E. D. Yeboah, A. Petrie, and J. L. Pead, Acute renal failure and open heart surgery, Brit. Med. J. 1:415 (1972).
18. K. C. Barry, A. Cohen, J. P. Knochel, et al, Mannitol infusion. II. The prevention of acute functional renal failure following resection of an aneurysm of the abdominal aorta, N. Engl. J. Med. 264:967 (1961).
19. W. Weimar, W. Geerlings, A. B. Bijnen, et al, A controlled study on the effect of mannitol on immediate renal function after cadaver donor kidney transplantation, Transplantation 35:99 (1983).
20. J. L. Dawson, Post-operative renal function in obstructive jaundice. Effect of a mannitol diuresis, Brit. Med. J. 1:82 (1965).
21. C. W. Old, and L. M. Lehrener, Prevention of radiocontrast induced acute renal failure with mannitol, Lancet 1:885 (1980).
22. H. R. Anto, S. Y. Chou, J. G. Porush, and W. B. Shapiro, Mannitol prevention of acute renal failure associated with infusion pyelography (abstract), Clin. Res. 27:407A (1979).
23. J. J. Olivero, J. Lozano-Mendez, E. M. Ghafary, G. Eknoyan, and W.

N. Suki, Mitigation of amphotericin B nephrotoxicity by mannitol, Brit. Med. J. 1:550 (1975).
24. D. M. Hayes, E. Cvitkovic, R. B. Golbey, et al, High dose cis-platinum diammine dichloride. Amelioration of renal toxicity by mannitol diuresis, Cancer 39:1372 (1977).
25. A. De Torrente, P. D. Miller, R. E. Cronin, et al, Effects of furosemide and acetylcholine in norepinephrine-induced acute renal failure, Am. J. Physiol. 235:F131 (1978).
26. H. J. Kramer, J. Schuurmann, C. Wasserman, and R. Dusing, Prostaglandin-independent protection by furosemide from oliguric ischemic renal failure in conscious rats, Kidney Int. 17:455 (1980).
27. L. S. Nuutinen, M. Kairaluoma, S. Tuononen, and T. K. I. Larmi, The effect of furosemide on renal function in open heart surgery, J. Cardiovasc. Surg. 19:471 (1978).
28. F. Cantarovich, A. Locatelli, J. C. Fernandez, et al, Furosemide in high doses in the treatment of acute renal failure, Postgrad. Med. J. 47:13 (1971).
29. F. Cantarovich, C. Galli, L. Benedetti, et al, High dose furosemide in established acute renal failure, Brit. Med. J. 4:449 (1973).
30. A. Lindner, Synergism of dopamine and furosemide in diuretic-resistant, oliguric acute renal failure, Nephron 33:121 (1983).
31. G. Graziani, A. Cantaluppi, S. Casati, et al, Dopamine and furosemide in oliguric acute renal failure, Nephron 37:39 (1984).
32. R. J. Anderson, S. L. Linas, A. S. Berns, et al, Nonoliguric acute renal failure, N. Engl. J. Med. 296:1134 (1977).
33. R. H. Mauk, R. V. Patak, S. Z. Fadem, et al, Effect of prostaglandin E administration in nephrotoxic and vasoconstrictor model of acute renal failure, Kidney Int. 12:122 (1977).
34. K. Solez, R. J. D'Asostini, L. Stawowy, et al, Beneficial effect of propranolol in a histologically appropriate model of post-ischemic acute renal failure, Am. J. Physiol. 88:163 (1977).
35. J. L. Farber, Membrane injury and calcium homeostasis in the pathogenesis of coagulative necrosis, Lab. Invest. 47:114 (1982).
36. D. R. Wilson, P. E. Arnold, T. J. Burke, and R. W. Schrier, Mitochondrial calcium accumulation and respiration in ischemic acute renal failure in the rat, Kidney Int. 25:519 (1984).
37. T. J. Burke, M. Burnier, P. Shanley, and R. W. Schrier, Gentamicin (G) induces Ca abnormalities in renal proximal tubules (PT) before functional change (abstract), Kidney Int. 29:298 (1986).
38. T. J. Burke, P. E. Arnold, J. A. Gordon, et al, Protective effect of intrarenal calcium membrane blockers before or after renal ischemia, J. Clin. Invest. 74:1830 (1984).
39. D. Goldfarb, I. Iaina, S. Serbon, et al, Beneficial effect of verapamil in ischemic acute renal failure in the rat, Proc. Soc. Exp. Biol. Med. 172:389 (1983).
40. J. I. Shapiro, C. Cheung, A. Itabashi, L. Chan, and R. W. Schrier, The effect of verapamil on renal function after warm and cold ischemia in the isolated perfused kidney, Transplantation 40:596 (1985).
41. M. Burnier, V. Van Putten, P. Wilson, T. J. Burke, and R. W. Schrier, Beneficial effects of verapamil (V) and nifedipine (N) on Ca influx and cell viability in anoxic renal cortical proximal tubules (CPT) (abstract), Mineral Electrolyte Metab. 11:390 (1985).
42. U. Schwertschlag, R. W. Schrier, and P. Wilson, Beneficial effects of calcium channel blockers and calmodulin binding drugs on in vitro renal cell anoxia, Kidney Int., in press.
43. G. L. Bakris, and J. C. Burnett, A role for calcium in radiocontrast-induced reductions in renal hemodynamics, Kidney Int. 27:455 (1985).
44. H. Eliahou, A. Iaina, I. Serban, S. Gavendo, and S. Kapuler,

Verapamil's beneficial effect and cyclic nucleotides in gentamicin-induced acute renal failure (ARF) in rats (abstract), Proc. IX Int. Cong. Nephrol., p. 323A (1984).
45. J. J. G. Offerman, S. Meijer, D. T. Sliejfer, et al, The influence of verapamil on renal function in patients treated with cis-platin, Clin. Nephrol. 24:249 (1985).
46. K. A. Duggan, G. J. MacDonald, J. A. Charlesworth, and B. A. Pussel, Verapamil prevents post-transplant oliguric renal failure, Clin. Nephrol. 24:289 (1985).
47. K. Wagner, S. Albrecht, H. H. Neumayer, M. Molzahn, and G. Offermann, Prevention of delayed graft function by calcium-antagonism - a randomized trial in renal graft recipients on cyclosporin A, 2nd Int. Symposium on Organ Procurement (1985).
48. A. A. Seymour, E. H. Blaine, E. K. Mazack, et al, Renal and systemic effects of synthetic atrial natriuretic factor, Life Sci. 36:33 (1985).
49. M. Nakamoto, J. I. Shapiro, R. W. Schrier, and L. Chan, The protective effect of atriopeptin III on ischemic acute renal failure in the isolated perfused rat kidney, submitted.

ATRIAL NATRIURETIC FACTOR INCREASES GLOMERULAR FILTRATION RATE IN THE EXPERIMENTAL ACUTE RENAL FAILURE INDUCED BY CISPLATIN

Giovambattista Capasso, Pietro Anastasio, Dario Giordano
Loredano Albarano, Aldo Rufolo and Natale Gaspare De Santo

Chair of Pediatric Nephrology, 1st Faculty of Medicine
University of Naples, Naples, Italy

INTRODUCTION

Cis-diamminodicloroplatinum (CP) is a recently developed antineoplastic agent that has a remarkably broad spectrum of clinical activity in the treatment of solid tumors (1). Use of this drug has significantly improved the response rate in patients treated for metastatic testicular and ovarian carcinomas. Additionaly,cisplatin is an important component of many treatment programs for the management of bladder carcinoma,squamous cell carcinoma of the head and neck,bronchogenic carcinoma of the lung,cervical and endometrial cancer.However the clinical use of the drug is largely hampered by its nephrotoxicity. In fact the degree of renal toxicity rather than the therapeutic response often determines the dosage of this therapeutic agent. A chronic,repetitive low dosage of cisplatin in rats also leads to kidney failure creating a situation similar to kidney insufficiency clinically observed during the prolonged chemotherapeutic regimens used for various malignancies (2). An acute single dose of CP induces in rats a non oliguric acute renal failure (ARF) that is characterized by a reduction of whole animal glomerular filtration rate (GFR),with increase in serum creatinine concentration,diminished urine osmolality, decreased U/P creatinine concentration ratios,and a significant increase in the fractional excretion of sodium (3). Development of cisplatin to its present level of clinical usefulness was greatly facilitated by studies in which hydration-diuresis maneuvers were used in dogs (4) and subsequently in humans (5). Another promising approach to limit CP nephrotoxicity is pharmacologic inhibition of cisplatin tubular secretion. Administration of drugs such as probenecid may be effective in decreasing the intracellular concentration of drug by inhibiting its uptake by the contraluminal cell membrane (6). WR-2721,a radioprotective agent,and the enzyme,superoxide dismutase,also reduced nephrotoxicity in rats (7-8). However the research of new means to reduce CP adverse effects is still going on.Since one of the main feature of CP nephrotoxicity is a reduction of GFR,the use of substances able to prevent the decrease in GFR would be wellcome. In 1981 deBold et al. (9) reported that atrial but not ventricular extracts had marked natriuretic and diuretic effects. A family of peptides with natriuretic properties has since been isolated from atrial extractcs, sequenced and synthetized (10). The intravenous administration of these atrial natriuretic factors (ANF) leads to a brisk natriuresis,diuresis and kaliuresis of very rapid onset and relatively short duration. The peak sodium excretion reached as much as 30- to 40-fold basal levels,a magnitude of action which immediately situated ANF as the most powerful endogenous natriuretic substance described to date. The most striking renal hemodynamic action of ANF is its ability to markedly increase GFR in a sustained and reversible manner. This effect and the ANF-induced increase in filtration fraction was first described in the isolated perfused rat kidney (11) and thereafter in in vivo conditions (12). The ANF induced increase in GFR is not only remarkable in view of its magnitude,but also because it occurs with a decreased mean blood pressure and an unchanged or decreased renal plasma flow (RPF). It was therefore tempting to use ANF in the experimental model of ARF induced by CP in order to verify if also in this condition ANF was able to increase the reduced GFR.

METHODS

Experiments were performed on male wistar rats.They were anesthetized with inactine,placed on thermoregulated table,tracheostomized.Polyethylene catheters were placed in the carotid artery,in the jugular vein and in the bladder. Two groups of rats were studied: a) control rats b) rats treated with a single dose of CP (10 mg/kg) given intraperitoneally.The rats of group B were studied 72 and 96 hours after the CP administration. This treatment has been shown to induce non-oliguric ARF (3). The GFR was measured by ^{3}H-inulin.In group B after two thyrthy minutes control periods, synthetic rat aminoacid ANF (Ciba-Geigy,Basel) was given intravenously as prime,12 ug/kg,and then as costant infusion,1 ug/kg·min. ^{3}H-inulin concentration was measured by liquid scintillation counting; plasma and urine sodium and potassium concentration by flame photometry.

RESULTS AND DISCUSSION

In table 1 are reported the renal function of control rats and rats that have been injected with a single dose of 10 ug/kg of CP.The use

Table 1 : Renal function in control rats and after 72 hours intraperitoneal injection of 10 ug/kg cisplatin.

	Control (4)	CP (3)	p
GFR (ml/min/100 g)	1.01 ± 0.09	0.348 ± 0.057	<0.005
U/P Inulin	446 ± 88	86 ± 38	<0.005
FE_{Na} (%)	0.239 ± 0.081	2.63 ± 0.88	<0.05

Abbreviations: GFR,glomerular filtration rate; U/P,urine/plasma; FE_{Na} fractional excretion of sodium. In parenthesis the number of rats.

of the antineoplastic agent induces a non oliguric ARF characterized by a significant dicrease in GFR and in U/P inulin ratio,consinstent with an observed CP-induced concentrating defect,while there is a significant increase in fractional excretion of sodium. Micropuncture studies in rats have demonstrated that backleak of glomerular filtrate plays a major role in the pathophysiology of cisplatin induced ARF (3). Superficial single nephron GFR (SNGFR) was preserved relative to whole kidney GFR. However SNGFR could not be returned to control values by volume expansion,implying a distinct effect of cisplatin on GFR. Since there are no studies about the role of hydraulic permeability coefficient changes with or without renal hemodynamic alterations,the exact pathophysiologic mechanism resulting in the observed decrease in GFR is not clearly understood. However cisplatin induced acute renal failure is associated with declines in glomerular blood flow,intratubular obstruction and backleak of inulin. This pattern of nephron abnormalities is similar to other toxic and ischemic insults to the kidney and arises from the primary loss of renal cell viability and release of cellular debris into the tubule lumen with resulting obstruction,backleak and secondary hemodynamic consequences.

Table 2 : Effects of ANF administration on renal function of CP treated rats.

	CP (3)	ANF (3)	
GFR (ml/min/100 g)	0.330 ± 0.089	0.628 ± 0.121	<0.005
U/P Inulin	80 ± 25	52 ± 20	<0.05
FE_{Na} (%)	1.95 ± 0.90	3.99 ± 1.10	<0.05

The effects of ANF administration on the renal function of CP treated rats are reported in table 2. In the presence of no significant change in packed cell volumes,there was a significant increase in GFR and in the fractional excretion of sodium,while the concentrating defect was even more pronounced. Therefore ANF is able to partially restore the reduced GFR in the experimental model of ARF induced by cisplatin administration. The mechanism by which ANF increases GFR has not yet been elucitated. In functioning isolated perfused rat kidneys there is a major increase in filtration traction and a smaller but significant increase in renal vascular resistance (11). The combination of these effects strongly suggest that ANF is a preferential efferent vasoconstrictor and in this manner increases glomerular capillary pressure and hence GFR. Alternatively the increase in GFR might be mediated by a substantial alteration in the hydraulic permeability filtration area coefficient (K_f). An increase in K_f is an attractive possibility,but direct measurements of single nephron hemodynamics are necessary to elucidate the exact mechanism of the ANF induced increase in GFR. Whatever the case the increase in GFR is undoubtedly the central hemodynamic effect on the kidney. This is well illustrated in Fig. 1 and 2 where the time coarse of the effect of costant infusion of ANF on urine flow rate,GFR,Na and K urinary excretion are shown. The

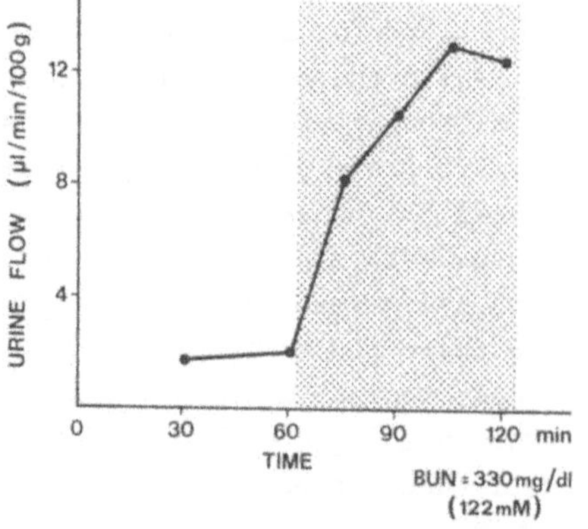

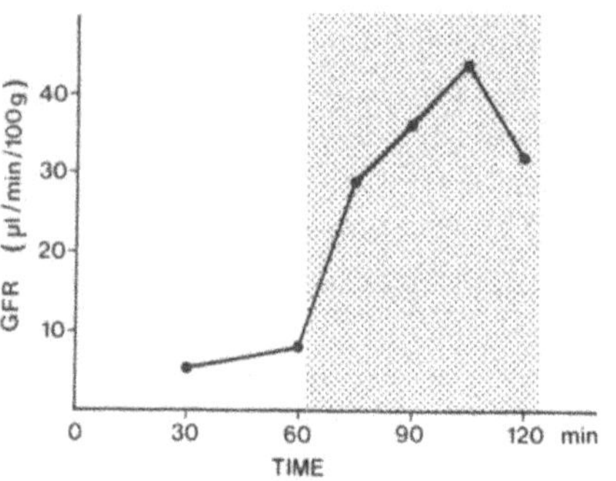

Figure 1. Effect of costant infusion of ANF on urine flow rate (upper pannel) and on glomerular filtration rate (lower pannel). Infusion period is represented by stippled area.

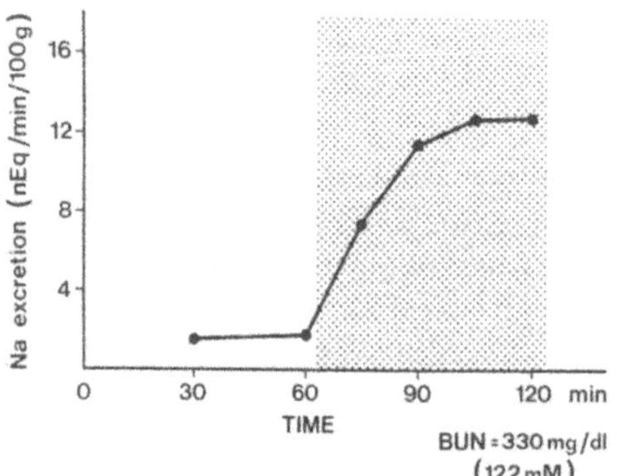

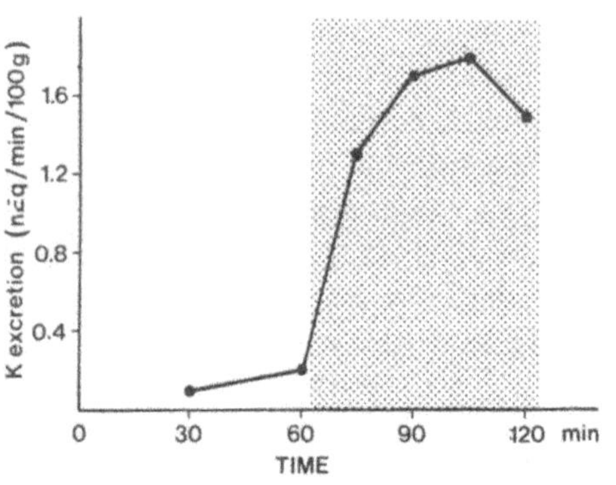

Figure 2. Effect of costant infusion of ANF on sodium (upper pannel) and potassium excretion (lower pannel). Infusion period is represented by stippled area.

natriuretic, kaliuretic, diuretic effect of ANF appears to be closely associated with the increase in GFR. It should be stressed that this rat was studied 96 hours after the CP administration,while the blood urea was as high as 60 mM.

Another possible explanation of ANF induced increase in GFR would be an action on the renin-aldosterone system. Since the work of Goormaghtigh (13) it has been suggested that the renin-angiotensin system may be involved in the pathogenesis of ARF. Indeed plasma renin activity has been repeatedly shown to be increased in the initial stages of both clinical and experimental forms of ARF. On the other hand intravenous infusion of ANF in anesthetized dogs markedly and reversibly decreased renin secretion rate,plasma renin activity and plasma aldosterone levels (14). This effect could be mediated by an increase in sodium load to the macula densa generated by the marked ANF induced increase in GFR. Finally a primary pathogenetic mediator of cellular injury has been identified in cytosolic free calcium levels. It has been proposed that calcium entry from the external medium increases intracellular free calcium to toxic levels thereby converting cellular injury from a potentially reversible to an irreversible state (15). It may be speculated that ANF protective effect on cisplatin induced ARF would have as a common denominator a decrease in cytosolic calcium ion activity brought about by an ANF-induced modulation of calcium uptake or release from intracellular stores.

REFERENCES

1. Einhorn L.H.,Williams S.D. : The role of cis-platinum in solid tumor therapy. N. Engl. J. Med. 300:289-291 (1979)
2. Ward J.M.,Fauvie K.A. : The nephrotoxic effect of cis-diammine-dicloro-platinum (II)(NSC-119875) in male F 344 rats. Toxicol. Appl. Pharmacol. 38:535-547 (1976)
3. Chopra S.,Kaufman J.S.,Jones T.W.,Hong W.K.,Gehr M.K.,Hamburger R.J., Flamenbaum W.,Trump B. : Cis-diamminodichloroplatinum-induced acute renal failure in the rat. Kidney Int. 21:54-64 (1982)
4. Cvitkovic E.,Spaulding J.,Bethune V.,Martin J.,Whitmore W.F. Improvement of cis-dichlorodiammineplatinum (NSC-119875) therapeutic index in an animal model. Cancer 39:1357-1361 (1977)
5. Hayes D.M.,Cvitkovic E.,Golbey R.B.,Schreiner E.,Helson L.,Krakoff I.H. High dose cis-platinum diammine dichloride: Amelioration of renal toxicity by mannitol diuresis. Cancer 39:1372-1381 (1977)
6. Ross D.A.,Gale G.R. : Reduction of renal toxicity of cis-dichlorodiammineplatinum (II) by probenecid. Cancer Treat. Rep. 63:781-787 (1969)
7. Yuhas J.M. and Culo F. : Selective inhibition of the nephrotoxicity of cis-dichlorodiammineplatinum (II) by WR-2721 without altering antitumors properties. Cancer Treat. Rep. 64:57-62 (1980)
8. McGinness J.E.,Proctor P.H.,Demopoulos H.B. : Amelioration of cis-platinum nephotoxicity by orgotein (superoxide dismutase). Physiol. Chem. and Physics 10:267-273 (1978)
9. DeBold A.J.,Borenstein H.B.,Veress A.T. and H. Sonnenberg : A rapid and potent natriuretic response to intravenous injection of atrial myocardial extracts in rats. Life Sci. 28:89-94 (1981)

10. Atlas S.A.,Kleinert H.D.,Camargo M.J.,Januszewich A.,Sealy J.E.,Laragh J.H.,Schilling J.W.,Lewisky J.A.,Johnson L.K.,Maack T. : Purification, sequencing and synthesis of natriuretic and vasoactive rat atrial peptide. Nature London 309:717-719 (1984)
11. Camargo M.J.F.,Kleinert H.D.,Atlas S.A.,Sealey J.E.,Laragh J.H.,Maack T. : Ca-dependent hemodynamic and natriuretic effects of atrial extract in isolated rat kidney. Am. J. Physiol. 246:F447-F456 (1984)
12. Beasley D.,Malvin R.L. : Atrial extracts increase glomerular filtration rate in vivo . Am. J. Physiol. 248:F24-F30 (1985)
13. Goormaghtigh H. : Vascular and circulatory changes in renal cortex in the anuric crush-syndrome. Proc. Soc. Expt. Biol. Med. 59:303-305 (1945)
14. Maack T.,Marion D.N.,Camargo M.J.F.,Kleinert H.D.,Laragh J.H.,Vaughan E.D.,Atlas S.A. : Effects of auriculin on blood pressure,renal function and the renin-aldosterone system in dogs. Am. J. Med. 77:1069-1075 (1984)
15. Farber J.L. : The role of calcium in cell death. Life Sci. 29:1289-1295 (1981)

AMELIORATION OF THE ISCHEMIC DAMAGE OF THE DOG KIDNEY SUBJECTED TO 90 MINUTES OF WARM ISCHEMIA BY LIDOCAINE PRETREATMENT AND LOW-DOSE DOPAMINE INFUSION ON REVASCULARIZATION

Wojciech Rowinski, Miroslaw Ruka, Frank Stuart,*
and Frank Buckingham*

Department of Transplantation Surgery, Medical Research
Center. Polish Academy of Sciences; Warsaw Medical School
Warsaw, Poland
Department of Surgery, The University of Chicago
Chicago, USA*

INTRODUCTION

Impaired renal function due to ischemic injury is still a common clinical problem in cadaveric renal transplantation. Profound high hypotension in the donor and the warm ischemia of the kidney are inevitable in this situations when nephrectomy can be performed only at the time of cardiac arrest. Ischemic damage due to these preagnoal events together with inadequate blood flow through the kidney after transplantation lead to development of oliguria in the recipient. The incidents of this complication is ranging from 15 to 70 %.

A number of protective regimens have been proposed including the donor pretreatment or the measures aiming to increase the renal blood flow in recipient after revascularization of the graft. In this report we are presenting the results of experimental studies on the effect of lidocaine pretreatment and constant low-dose dopamine infusion on the damage of the dog kidney subjected to 90 minutes of warm ischemia. We chose lidocaine hydrochloride, the local anesthetic agent which was described to protect the canine myocardium subjected to ischemia by preventing agregation of the platelets and vasodilatation. In addition this drug is also stabilizing the cell membrane.

MATERIAL AND METHODS

Experiments were performed in the mongrel dogs 14-26 kg of weight. Animals were fasted for 12-24 hours but were given water ad lib. before the experiment. After induction of anesthesia (nembutal, 15 mg/kg b.w.) dogs were hydrated by intravenous infusion of 0.9% saline and 5% dextrose (20 ml/kg b.w.) over 30 minutes. A polyvinyl tube was inserted to the right femoral artery for constant measurements of blood pressure.

The body temperature, 90 minutes, complete ischemia of the kidney was used as a model for the studies. The left kidney was used for experiment unless double renal arteries were found. After laparatomy renal artery and vein were dissected and the kidney was excised and left without perfusion within the abdominal cavity of the animal for 90 minutes. During that time the opposite kidney was removed. At the end of 90 minutes period the ischemic kidney was transplanted into the right illiac fossa using the standard technique. On revascularization of the kidney dogs were administered intravenously mannitol solution (0.5 g/kg b.w.) and furosemide (1 mg/kg b.w.). The abdomen was closed and then for six hours the animals were infused intravenously fluids (0.9% saline and 5% dextrose) in the total amount of 120 ml/kg. Furosemide was injected i.v. every hour in a dose of 1 mg/kg b.w. During that time arterial pressure and the urine output were monitored.

Animals were divided into four groups. Group I (Control-C) consisted of 6 dogs which underwent the transplantation of the ischemic kidney and besides fluids and furosemide received no other medications.

Group II (Dopamine after ischemia - D) comprised of 8 animals which were receiving continuous infusion of dopamine hydrochloride (INOTROPIN^{R} - Arnar Stone Laboratories) in a dose of 3 μ/kg/min for 6 hours from the time of revascularization of the ischemic kidney.

Group III (Lidocaine pretreatment - L) consisted of 8 dogs which before ischemia of the kidney received lidocaine hydrochloride (2 mg/kg as i.v. bolus followed by continuous infusion of 2 mg/min for 20 minutes). On termination of pretreatment the following part of the experiment was the same as in animals of group I.

Group IV (Lidocaine pretreatment. Dopamine after ischemia, L+D) included 8 dogs which received lidocaine infusion before ischemia as the animals in group II and the continuous infusion of Dopamine as dogs in Group II.

The serum creatinine was estimated postoperatively on days 1,3,5,7,14, 21 and in surviving animals 3 months after transplantation. Effective renal plasma flow (ERPF) was determined using 131-J Hippurane on termination of 6 hour observation period and than in surviving animals 3 months after transplantation. Microscopical examination of the kidney biopsy (taken 1 hour after revascularization) and of the kidneys removed at postmortem was performed.

RESULTS

Group I (Control). On revascularization the kidneys were mottled with a number of dark-blue spots indicating impairment of the microcirculation. Two out of six kidneys excreted some urine but the serum creatinine was rapidly rising after transplantation, all of the dogs became uremic and died 5-7 days post grafting (table 1). Microscopical examination showed very severe tubular necrosis and trombi in small vessels.

Group II (Dopamine after ischemia). On revascularization the kidneys at the beginning appeared similar to those in group I, but after 5-10 minutes the whole surface of the organ seemed to be well vascularized. There was no rise of arterial blood pressure or tachycardia during dopamine infusion. In all animals the serum creatinine level was rising after grafting. Six dogs died due to uremia between the 6th and the 10th day after transplantation. Microscopy revealed tubular necrosis. In two of these 6 animals however the postmortem revealed hydronephrosis. In the remaining two animals the serum creatinine after the initial rise decreased to near normal values on days 14 and 17 after transplantation (table 2).

Group III (Lidocaine pretreatment). The appearance of the kidney on revascularization was different from that observed in animals of groups I

Table 1. Early Results of the Experiments

Group	No of animals	Kidney on revascularization	ERPF ml/kg/min	Survival 9 days	Survival 3 months
I (C)	6	mottled	4 - 5	0	0
II (D)	8	mottled	5 - 6	2	2
III (L)	8	nearly normal	7 - 8	4	2
IV (L+D)	8	nearly normal	10 - 12	6	4

and II. Immediately after releasing the vascualr clamps the kidney became pink and the perfusion seemed to be perfectly normal. All but one kidney excreted urine soon after revascularization and 4 out of 8 animals survived beyond 7 days. Two animals then died on days 9 and 12 after transplantation due to uremia and in the remaining two the serum creatinine decreased to near normal level 3 weeks after transplantation (table 2). ERPF and the serum creatinine in two surviving animals 3 months after transplantation were close to normal (table 3).

Group IV (Lidocaine pretreatment, Dopamine after ischemia). The appearance of the kidney on revascularization was similiar to that observed in animals of group III. The surface of the kidney was pink and looked normal. Six out of 8 animals survived more than nine days after transplantation, two of them died on the tenth and 14th day due to uremia. Remaining 4 animals survived 3 months observation period. In the surviving animals there was an initial rise of the serum creatinine which decreased to normal 3 weeks after transplantation (table 2). Microscopy of the kidney biopsy showed the tubular necrosis but much less advanced than in the kidneys of dogs from group I. There were no thrombi in the lumen on the small vessels.

The follow-up renal function studies in the surviving animals (in 2 of D

Table 2. The serum creatinine level (mg/dl) in dogs after transplantation of autologous kidney subjected to 90 minutes of body temperature ischemia (min ± SD)*

Day post transpl.	Group I C	Group II D	Group III L	Group IV L+D
1	3.1 ± 1	1.8 ± 0.4	1.45 ± 0.4	2.2 ± 1
3	4.9 ± 1.6	2.9 ± 0.6	2.2 ± 0.0	2.6 ± 1.6
5	7.8 ± 1.8	3.6 ± 1.2	3.1 ± 2.0	2.8 ± 1.3
7	-	5.6 ± 2.5	3.7 ± 3	2.5 ± 1.4
14	-	1.7 ± 0.3	1.6 ± 0.2	1.5 ± 1.0
21	-	1.2 ± 0.5	1.5 ± 0.1	1.05 ± 0.2

* Up to the 5th day the mean values calculated from the estimated serum in all animals in each group. From the 7th day the serum creatinine estimated in the listed number of surviving animals:

	Day 7	14	21
Group II	6	2	2
Group III	6	2	2
Group IV	6	4	4

Table 3. Renal function in surviving animals after 3 months follow-up

Dog No	Urea nitrogen mg/dl	Serum creatinine mg/dl	ERPF ml/kg/min
D 60	22	1.9	8.5
D 61	12	1.14	12.2
L 77	25	1.1	11
L 88	40	1.4	8.2
L+D 102	43	1.02	15
L+D 105	23	1.32	12
L+D 106	28	1.2	9.5
L+D 109	21	1.6	9

group, 2 of L group and in 4 of 1*d group) were performed 3 months after transplantation. The results are shown in the table 3.

DISCUSSION

The preagonal events and the warm ischemia are the two important factos which limit the use of cadaveric kidneys for transplantation. A number of experimental studies have been published on the use of various pharmacological agents for protection against ischemia (phenoxybenzamine, chlorpromazine, mannitol, furosemid, calcium channel blocking agents, ATP-$MgCl_2$ and others). The results of these studies have often been contradictory and not always applicable to the clinical situation. One of the reasons for that being different models of ischemia used in studies. It should be remembered that in dogs the clamping of the whole renal pedicle (including ureter) still leaves approximately 6 % of the total renal blood flow through the perirenal capsule and fat. The excision and transplantation assures the reproducible model of total ischemia. There is no however experimental model of acute ischemic renal failure that would resemble the situation observed during the preagonal period in cadaveric donors before the cardiac arrest (Bell et al., 1974; Jablonsky et al., 1983).

In our studies we chose to use the body temperature complete ischemia of the dog kidney in order to investigate the possibility of pharmacological protection of the organ. According to a number of reports of our own experience ninty minutes of warm ischemia has been beyond the limits of the life supporting function of the dog kidney. Present results has proven this point. None of the animals from group I survived beyond the 7th day and all of them died of uremia.

In our studies we investigated the effect of lidocaine hydrochloride pretreatment and the low-dose dopamine infusion (acting only on the dopaminergic receptors in the vascular wall) after revascularization on the extent of damage of the dog kidney resulting from 90 minutes complete ischemia. The infusion of dopamine and furosemide (group II) to dogs which received the transplant of ischemicaly damaged kidney only slightly improved the outcome. Two of the eight animals survived for a period of 3 months after transient elevation of serum creatinien.

In recent years there have been a number of reports on the protective effect of combined dopamine and furosemide treatment in acute renal failure. Lindner et al. (1979) presented evidence that combined administration of dopamine (3 μg/kg/min) and furosemide (1 ml/kg/hour) ameliorates the course of the acute renal failure in dogs induced by intravenous uranyl nitrate injection. Treatment with both agents, dopamine and furosemide, produced renal vasodilatation, high urine flow rate and attenuation of the fall in GFR seen in the untreated animals. The data presented by these authors indicated that dopamine plus furosemide had a synergistic effect in preventing the early pathophysiological changes associated with acute renal failure in this animal model.

The mechanism of the synergistic effect of combined administration of dopamine and furosemide is not quite clear. The effect could be due to vasodilatation of the intrarenal vasculature with increased transport of the diuretic to the loop of Henle (in particular to its thick ascending part), natriuretic effect of dopamine itself and increased pO_2 within renal cortex due to furosemide (Docci, 1984; Graziani, 1980; Henderson, 1980).

Grundman et al. (1981) investigated the influence of the lenght and severity of hypotension on the results of the kidney preservation in dogs. They concluded that the level of hypotension was of more importance than its duration. Moreover, after 24 hours of cold ischemia the function of kidneys from hypotensive donors could be significantly improved if the dopamine was given in low doses to the recipient. The preservation injury itself however could not be counteracted by dopamine because the infusion od this drug did not improved the function of the kidneys which were removed from donors without hypotension.

Lidocaine pretreatment alone to some extend protected the dog kidney against ischemic damage. Half of the animals survived longer than 9 days, but only two of them for a long term observation period (group III). The best protection against ischemic kidney damage was observed in animals pretreated with lidocaine and receiving constant low-dose dopamine infusion on revascularization of the organ (group IV). Six of eight animals survived beyond 9 days and four of them fall the 3 months observation period.

One of the most striking observations made in lidocaine pretreated animals was the excellent blood flow through the kidney on revascularization despite the fact that the kidneys were not perfused before ischemia. This could have been due to antiagregatory effect of lidocaine which prevented formation of thrombi. The same was observed by Schaub et al. (1977) who used lidocaine in dogs subjected to myocardial ischemia. The lidocaine infusion in these animals decreased the extend of ischemic myocardial damage and the electromicroscopy revealed no sequestration of the platelets or other blood cells within the capillaries.

On the basis of the results of these experiments starting from January 1984 the same protocol was used in 131 patients undergoing cadaveric kidney transplantation in two centers - Warsaw Medical School and The University of Chicago. The analysis of this preliminary clinical trial showed in both centers a decreased incidence of ATN after transplantation of cadaveric kidneys from lidocaine pretreated donors (from 66% to 29% in Warsaw and from 52% to 26% in Chicago).

REFERENCES

Bell, P.R.F., Quin, R.Q., Calman, K.C., 1974, Donor pretreatment and organ preservation, Transpl.Proc. VI: 245.

Docci, D., 1984, Dopamine - furosemide in oliguric acute renal failure, Nephron, 36: 74.

Graziani, C. et al., 1980, Dopmaine and Furosemide in acute renal failure, Lancet, II: 1301.

Grundeman, R., Cammorer, B., Franke, E., Pichlmaier, H., 1981, Effect of hypotension on the results of kidney storage and the use of dopamine under these conditions, Transpl., 32:184.
Henderson, I.S., Beattie, T.J., Kennedy, A.C., 1980, Dopamine hydrochloride in oliguric states, Lancet, II:827.
Jablonsky, P., Howden, B., Leslie, E., Rae, D., Birrel, C., Marshall, V.C., Tange, J., 1983, Recovery of renal function after warm ischemia, Transpl., 35:535.
Lindner, A., Cutler, R., Goodman, W.G., 1979, Synergism of dopamine plus furosemide in preventing acute renal failure in the dog, Kidney Intern., 16:158.
Schaub, R.G., Stewart, G., Strong, M., Ruofolo, R., Lemole, G., 1977, Reduction of ischemic neocardial damage in the dog by lidocaine infusion, Am. J.Pathol., 87:400.

NUTRITION IN ACUTE RENAL FAILURE

Eben I. Feinstein

Associate Professor of Clinical Medicine
University of Southern California School of Medicine
Los Angeles, California

Malnutrition and loss of lean body mass are common occurrences in patients with acute renal failure. The degree of wasting is variable: it is likely that those patients who have the highest catabolic stress tend to be the sickest patients, the ones with the most number of co-morbid events, and those with the highest mortality rate. Indeed, a recent review of a large number of patients with acute renal failure listed hypercatabolism as one of the significant risk factors for poor outcome (1). Inadequate nutrition may affect outcome by impairing immune responses to infection and by slowing wound healing. This review will deal with several aspects of the nutritional therapy of patients with acute renal failure: the causes and mediators of the catabolic process in these patients, the role of amino acid infusions and caloric intake in nutritional therapy and finally the newer techniques for maintaining fluid balance during nutritional therapy in the oliguric patient.

In vitro observations point to the liver and muscle as key organs in the catabolic response to acute uremia. Frohlich et al. (2) demonstrated an increase in gluconeogenesis and ureagenesis when liver slices from uremic rats were perfused with amino acids. There is an increased release of certain amino acids, including alanine and glutamine, from the muscle of uremic rats (3,4). This increased release of amino acids may be accompanied by a decrease in muscle protein synthesis (5). Mitch and Clark have also demonstrated an impaired anabolic response to insulin in isolated muscle preparations from uremic rats (5).

The elevated rates of urea nitrogen appearance seen in patients with acute renal failure suggest that a similar catabolic process pertains in the clinical situation (6). The mediators of this catabolic response are currently under investigation. It is likely that circulating peptides with proteolytic activity and elevated circulating levels of certain hormones contribute in an important way to the catabolic response. A recent study in patients subjected to surgical stress and in patients with septicemia without acute renal failure indicated the presence of a circulating factor(s) with proteolytic properties (7). In patients with acute uremia, Horl and Heidland found increased concentrations of proteases in the circulation (8). Furthermore, acute uremia is characterized by elevated circulating levels of hormones such as glucagon and parathyroid hormone (9,10). The hormonal contribution to the protein breakdown has been investigated in an interesting experiment by Bessey and co-workers (11).

They infused normal subjects for 72 hours with epinephrine, glucagon and cortisol and obtained circulating levels of these hormones comparable to those seen in patients with surgical stress. They observed the development of negative nitrogen and potassium balance, glucose intolerance, insulin resistance, and sodium retention. There was a significant increase in both protein turnover and protein catabolism but no change in the rate of protein synthesis.

Among the other factors which may contribute to catabolism in patients with acute renal failure are the catabolic effects of hemodialysis. There is a loss of free amino acids (12). Furthermore, dialysis with glucose-free dialysate stimulates gluconeogenesis (13). Hemodialysis in patients with acute renal failure is associated with an increase in oxygen consumption (14). In chronically uremic patients, there is an increase in protein catabolic rate and negative nitrogen balance on days in which hemodialysis is performed (15). The negative nitrogen balance is in part dependent upon dietary protein intake.

Clinical Management of Patients with Acute Renal Failure

Patients with acute renal failure and marked catabolism present a challenge to the nephrologist and the nutritionist. Currently, there is no pharmacological means for reducing protein breakdown and stimulating protein synthesis. Most efforts to counter the catabolic stress have involved the provision of adequate nutrients. Many patients can receive adequate nutrition via the enteral tract alone or in association with peripheral intravenous supplementation, but the most catabolic patients usually require total parenteral nutrition (TPN) via a central catheter. A number of strategies have been advanced for the management of this group of patients. Abel et al reported that a regimen consisting of essential amino acids and dextrose was able to reduce the rate of rise in serum urea nitrogen potassium, magnesium and phosphorus in patients with acute renal failure (16). In a controlled double-blind study comparing this regimen with a glucose alone, they showed an improved recovery from acute renal failure in the group receiving essential amino acids and glucose but no improvement in overall hospital survival (17). They also noted that in patients with serious complications such as pneumonia and gastrointestinal hemorrage, the beneficial effects of nutritional therapy were most marked. These results were not confirmed by other investigators. Leonard et al, (18) found a marked negative nitrogen balance in patients receiving amino acids and glucose in a regiment similar to that of Abel et al.

Other lines of evidence suggested that essential amino acids alone might not be sufficient in treatment of the catabolic patients and that essential and nonessential amino acids should be administered. Toback and co-workers showed that in rats with acute renal failure, essential and nonessential amino acid infusions enhanced both renal protein synthetic activity and renal synthesis of phospholipids (19,20). There was a decrease in the rate of rise of serum creatinine in the animals treated with the essential and non-essential amino acids (21). In order to evaluate the relative benefits of three nutritional regiments (essential amino acids and dextrose, essential and nonessential amino acids and dextose, and dextrose alone) in the treatment of acute renal failure, a study was undertaken at the Los Angeles County-USC Medical Center and the VA Wadsworth Medical Center (6). There was no significant difference in recovery of renal function or survival among patients receiving no amino acids, 21 g of essential amino acids or 21 g of essential amino acids and 21 g of nonessential amino acids per day. Urea nitrogen appearance was markedly elevated (greater than 5 g nitrogen/day) in many patients in all three groups. There was a higher level of urea nitrogen appearance in the group receiving the greatest amount of amino acids. There was no significant improvement in the levels of serum albumin or total serum protein or transferrin among the three groups. In view of the persistent negative nitrogen balance even in patients receiving 42 g of amino acids, a subsequent study was performed comparing therapy with essential amino acids and glucose with a regimen of increased quantities of essential and nonessential amino acids (22). The amount of the latter regimen that was infused was varied in an attempt to approximate the urea nitrogen appearance and thus attain nitrogen balance. Patients in the essential amino acids alone group received a mean of 2.3 g of nitrogen per day, whereas those in the higher nitrogen intake group received an average of 11 g of nitrogen per day. Energy intake averaged about 25oo kcal per day in both groups. Patients in both groups exhibited a comparable level of catabolism as measured by the mean urea nitrogen appearance before the onset of the study. There was no difference in survival between the 2 groups. During the study, those patients receiving the higher nitrogen intake exhibited a mean urea nitrogen appearance of nearly twice that of the lower nitrogen intake group (14 g/day vs. 7.5 g nitrogen/day). There was no difference in nitrogen balance as estimated by the mean nitrogen intake minus the mean UNA. Thus, it would appear from these two studies that increasing the amount of nitrogen intake is not sufficient to produce nitrogen balance and furthermore contributes to an increased urea nitrogen appearance, without improving the survival rate.

Another important factor in the nutritional management of these patients is the administration of adequate caloric intake. In the two studies just described, caloric intake was approximately 30-35 kcal/kg/day. It is possible that for many of these patients, this level of caloric intake was inadequate. The importance of caloric intake in acute renal failure is underscored by the report of Mault et al. (23) in which the cumulative caloric balance of patients with acute renal failure in an intensive care unit was measured. Of twenty patients with negative cumulative caloric balances, eighteen died. However, of nine patients who were in positive cumulative caloric balance, only five patients died. That caloric balance is important in attaining nitrogen balance is suggested by the work of Spreiter et al. (24). In patients with catabolic acute renal failure, these investigators varied the amounts of amino acids and caloric intake and measured nitrogen balance. Nitrogen balance was attained when caloric intake reached a level of 50 Kcal/kg/day and amino acid nitrogen intake was approximately 200 mg nitrogen/kg/day. Both amino acids and glucose were varied at the same time in these patients, thus the relative contribution of each nutrient to attaining nitrogen balance is difficult to assess.

One of the major problems in providing acute renal failure patients with adequate caloric intake has been the large volumes of fluid that are ncessary to administer adequate calories. Recently, the use of continuous arteriovenous hemofiltration (CAVH) (25,26) or slow continuous ultrafiltration (SCUF) (27) has been advocated as a means of administering large volumes of parenteral nutrition fluid withou causing extracellular fluid volume overload. Kaplan and co-workers (26) were able to administer up to 15 g of nitrogen/day to patients with acute renal failure without inducing a rise in blood urea nitrogen and while maintaining fluid balance using the technique of CAVH. However, CAVH has the disadvantage of requiring close monitoring of fluid balance in order that replacement fluids match the losses via ultrafiltration.

One way of providing nutrition and continuous dialysis therapy without the need to scrupulous monitoring of replacement fluid is the technique of slow continuous hemodialysis or continuous arteriovenous hemodialysis with nutrients added to the dialysate. With this technique, which we have termed "nutrition hemodialysis" (28), the flow rate of dialysate is reduced significantly in order to allow adequate and efficient uptake of nutrients.

In vitro and in vivo studies have shown that the clearance of small molecules (urea and creatinine) at dialysate flow rates of less than 50 ml/min is equal to the to the dialysate flow rate. Such marked reductions in urea and creatinine clearances necessitate a prolongation of dialysis time in order to ensure adequate dialysis. In studies in chronically uremic patients receiving hemodialysis, a standard dialysate was modified so as to contain glucose, 5 g/dl, and essential and nonessential amino acids, 400 mg/dl. The patients were dialyzed for 3 to 5 hours at a blood flow rate of 200 ml/min and a dialysate flow rate of 20-30 ml/min. Urea clearance was 26 ml/min and creatinine clearance was 25 ml/min using this technique. Mean glucose absorbed by the patients was 49 g/hr or 78% of the administered glucose and mean amino acid absorption was 4 g/hr or 79% of the amino acids administered in the dialysate (28). This form of therapy is comparable to CAVH in that it is a slow and continuous treatment with low urea and creatinine clearances. However, unlike CAVH the patient receives nutrients via dialysis without the need for any fluid administration and therefore without the need for close monitoring of fluid balance. The high osmolality of the dialysate effects a slow ultrafiltration of fluid from the patient. Furthermore, since nutrients can be added to dialysate fluid, they need not be sterile and this may help reduce the cost of parenteral nutrition in such patients. To date there has been no clear evidence that either CAVH or slow continuous hemodialysis produces an improvement in the morbidity or mortality of renal failure. There is a need for controlled studies of standard hemodialysis and these newer forms of therapy in acute renal failure. However, it is reasonable to assume that in patients who are hemodynamically unstable and in whom hemodialysis is frequently difficult to do because of hypotension, these forms of therapy will have a role to play.

REFERENCES

1. M. L. Bullock, A. J. Umen, M. Finkelstein, W. F. Keane, The assessment of risk factors in 462 patients with acute renal failure, Am. J. Kid. Dis. 5:97-103 (1985).
2. J. Frohlich, J. Scholmerick, G. Hoppe-Selyer, K. P. Maier, H. Talke, P. Schollmeyer, W. Gerok, The effect of acute uremia on gluconeogenesis in isolated perfused rat livers, Europ. J. Clin. Invest. 4:453-458 (974).
3. W. E. Mitch, Amino acid release from the hindquarter and urea appearance in acute uremia, Am. J. Physiol. 241:E415-E419 (1981).
4. R. M. Flugel-Link, I. B. Salusky, M. R. Jones, J. D. Kopple, Protein and amino acid metabolism in the posterior hemicorpus of acutely uremic rats, Am. J. Physiol. 244:E615-E623 (1983).
5. A. S. Clark, W. E. Mitch, Muscle protein turnover and glucose uptake in rats with acute uremia, J. Clin. Invest. 72:836-845 (1983).
6. E. I. Feinstein, M. J. Blumenkrantz, M. Healy, A. Koffler, H. Silberman, S. G. Massry, J. D. Kopple, Clinical and metabolic responses to parenteral nutrition in acute renal failure - a controlled double blind study, Medicine 60:124-137 (1981).
7. G. H. A. Clowes, Jr. , B. C. George, C. A. Villee, Jr., C. A. Saravis, Muscle proteolysis induced by a circulating peptide in patients with sepsis or trauma, N. Engl. J. Med. 308:545-552 (1983).
8. W. H. Horl, A. Heidland, Enhanced proteolytic activity - Cause of protein catabolism in acute renal failure, Am. J. Clin. Nutr. 33:1423-1427 (1980).
9. F. Kokot, The endocrine systems in patients with acute renal failure, in: B. H. B. Robinson, J. B. Hawkins, A. M. Davison, eds., Proceedings of E.D.T.A., Vol. 18, Pitman, London, 617-619 (1981).
10. J. D. Kopple, B. Cianciaruso, S. G. Massry, Does parathyroid hormone cause protein wasting: Contr. Nephrol. 20:138-148 (1980).
11. P. Q. Bessey, J. M. Watters, T. T. Aoki, D. W. Wilmore, Combined hormonal infusion simulates the metabolic response to injury, Ann. Surg.

20:264-279 (1984).
12. J. D. Kopple, M. E. Swendseid, J. H. Shinaberger, C. Y. Umegawa, The free and bound amino acids removed by hemodialysis, Trans. Am. Soc. Artif. Int. Organs. 14:309-312 (1973).
13. R. Wathen, P. Keshaviah, P. Hommeyer, et al., The metabolic effects of hemodialysis with and without glucose in the dialysate, Am. J. Clin. Nutr. 31:1870 (1978).
14. J. R. Mault, R. E. Dechert, R. H. Bartlett, R. D. Schwartz, S. K. Fergeson, Oxygen consumption during hemodialysis for acute renal failure, Trans. Am. Soc. Artif. Intern. Organs. 28:510-513 (1982).
15. M. F. Borah, P. Y. Schoenfeld, F. A. Gotch, J. E. Sargent, M. Wolfson, M. H. Humphreys, Nitrogen balance during intermittent dialysis therapy of uremia, Kidney Int. 14:491-500 (1978).
16. R. M. Abel, W. M. Abbott, J. E. Fischer, Intravenous essential L-amino acids and hypertonic dextrose in patients with acute renal failure, Effects on serum potassium, phosphate, and magnesium, Am. J. Surg. 123:632-638 (1972).
17. R. M. Abel, C. H. Beck, Jr., W. M. Abbott, J. A. Ryan, Jr., G. O. Barnett, J. E. Fischer, Improved survival from acute renal failure after treatment with intravenous essential L-amino acids and glucose, Results of a prospective double-blid study, N. Engl. J. Med. 288: 695-699 (1973).
18. C. D. Leonard, R. G. Luke, R. R. Siegel, Parenteral essential amino acids in acute renal failure, Urology. 6:154-157 (1975).
19. F. G. Toback, R. C. Dodd, E. R. Maier, L. J. Havener, Amino acid administration enhances renal protein metabolism after acute tubular necrosis, Nephron. 33:238-243 (1983).
20. F. G. Toback, L. J. Havener, R. C. Dodd, B. H. Spargo, Phospholipid metabolism during renal regeneration after acute tubular necrosis, Am. J. Physiol. 232:E216-E222 (1977).
21. F. G. Toback, Amino acid enhancement of renal regeneration after acute tubular necrosis, Kidney Int. 12:193-198 (1977).
22. E. I. Feinstein, J. D. Kopple, H. Silberman, S. G. Massry, Total parenteral nutrition with high or low nitrogen intake in patients with acute renal failure, Kidney Int. 26:S319-S323 (1983).
23. J. R. Mault, R. H. Bartlett, R. E. Dechert, S. F. Clark, R. D. Swartz, Starvation: A major contribution to mortality in acute renal failure, Trans. Am. Soc. Aerif. Int. Organs. 29:390-394 (1983).
24. S. C. Spreiter, B. D. Myers, R. S. Swenson, Protein-energy requirements in subjects with acute renal failure receiving intermittent hemodialysis, Am. J. Clin. Nutr. 33:1433-1437 (1980).
25. A. A. Kaplan, R. E. Longnecker, V. W. Folkert, Continuous arteriovenous hemofiltration - a report of six months' experience, Ann. Int. Med. 100:358-367 (1984).
26. P. Kramer, J. Bohler, A. Kehr, H. J. Grone, J. Schrader, D. Mathaei, F. Scheler, Intensive care potential of continuous arteriovenous hemofiltration, Trans. Am. Soc. Artif. Int. Organs. 28:28-32 (1982).
27. E. P. Paganini, P. O'Hara, S. Nakamoto, Slow continuous ultrafiltration in hemodialysis-resistant oliguric acute renal failure patients, Trans. Am. Soc. Artif. Int. Organs. 30:173-177 (1984).
28. E. I. Feinstein, J. F. Collins, M. J. Blumenkrantz, M. Roberts, J. D. Kopple, S. G. Massry, Nutritional hemodialysis. in: "Progress in Artificial Organs," K. Atsumi, M. Maekawa, K. Ota, eds., ISAO Press, Cleveland, p. 421 (1984).

BAG-FILTER HEMODIAFILTRATION (BF-HDF): SIMPLE AND EFFECTIVE TREATMENT OF ACUTE RENAL FAILURE

Giorgio Bazzato, Ugo Coli, Silvano Landini, Agostino Fracasso, Paolo Morachiello, Flavio Righetto, and Flavio Scanferla

Nephrology and Dialysis Department
Umberto I Hospital
Venice-Mestre, Italy

INTRODUCTION

Many therapeutic approaches have been employed for treatment of patients with acute renal failure (ARF). Hemodialysis and peritoneal dialysis have been applied since the first attempts in uremia therapy with temporary blood or peritoneal access. In the last decades several other strategies have been experienced on the basis of the clinical status such continuous arterio -venous hemofiltration (CAVH)[1], intermittent hemofiltration[2], hemoperfusion[3], continuous peritoneal dialysis[4], hemodiafiltration[5], etc. Indeed the choice for appropriate treatment actually derives from the etiology of renal failure which may provide the best procedure for each patient. Hemofiltration with high volume exchange appears more indicated for septic hypotensive patients with ARF[6]; hemoperfusion associated with hemodialysis, on the other hand, seems more suitable for depuration of patients assuming different poisons or toxic substances[7]. More recently hemodiafiltration has demonstrated several advantages in the treatment of acute and severely ill uremic patients[8]. The rationale of hemodiafiltration as treatment of choice in such patients derives from the chance of removing water and uremic substances and simultaneous infusion of large volume as replacement fluids. In such a manner electrolytes and acid-base pattern can be adequately corrected by buffers and electrolyte solutions, in addition to the administration of calories by glucose, aminoacids and lipids.
On the basis of this therapeutic view our group has developed a new model of machineless artificial kidney* to be quickly set up in different medical and surgical wards for the therapy of ARF. We report the technical aspects, the feasibility and the effectiveness of this new apparatus for the treatment of patients with acute renal insufficiency hospitalized in non dialytic centers and assisted by not specialized paramedical personnel.

* Supplied by Bellco Spa - Mirandola, Italy.

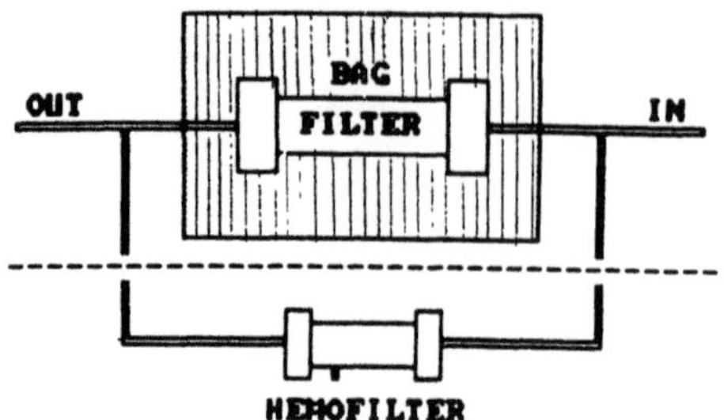

Fig. 1. Bag-Filter set for hemodiafiltration with (C-BF+HF) or without (P-BF) addition of a hemofilter.

METHODS

Our bag-filter apparatus for hemodiafiltration (BF-HDF) already employed for treatment of chronic uremic patients[9,10,11], consists in a decapsulated hollow fiber filter included in a plastic bag of 6 liters capacity which has to be filled by dialysate (Fig. 1). The first device was assembled with a cuprophane membrane which required to insert in parallel a hemofilter (Amicon 20) to obtain adequate fluid removal (C-BF+HF). In the last year we could unify the system by including into the bag a decapsulated

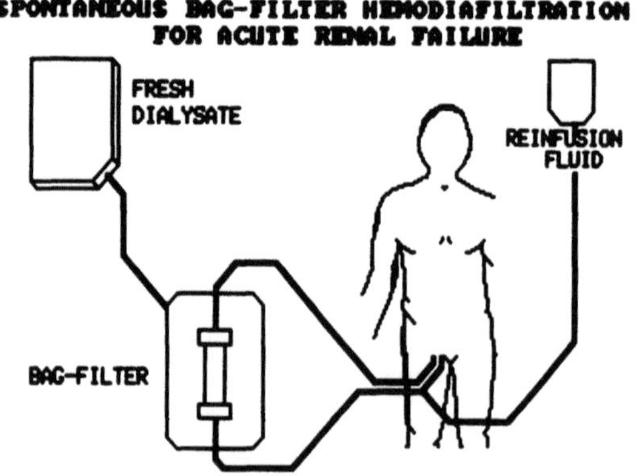

Fig. 2. Spontaneous BF-HD with blood flow obtained from femoral arterious and venous catheterization.

Tab. I. Patients with acute renal failure entered BF-HDF treatment and their outcome.

BAG-FILTER TREATMENT
FOR ACUTE RENAL FAILURE

PTS	SEX/AGE	CAUSE of ARF	BFmodel	# of SESSIONS	OUTCOME
1	M / 58	SURGERY	BF+HF	5	RECOVERY
2	M / 31	TRAUMA	BF+HF	4	DEAD
3	F / 65	SURGERY	BF+HF	10	CHRONIC
4	F / 77	NEPHROTOXIC	BF+HF	11	CHRONIC
5	F / 72	NEPHROTOXIC	BF+HF	3	RECOVERY
6	M / 64	THROMBOSIS	BF+HF	9	CHRONIC
7	M / 49	NEPHROTOXIC	BF+HF	4	RECOVERY
8	F / 61	SURGERY	P-BF	7	CHRONIC
9	F / 73	MYELOMA	P-BF	12	CHRONIC
10	F / 45	NEPHROTOXIC	P-BF	3	RECOVERY
11	M / 36	TRAUMA	P-BF	5	RECOVERY
12	F / 43	SURGERY	P-BF	3	DEAD
13	M / 54	NEPHROTOXIC	P-BF	6	RECOVERY

polysulfone filter (P-BF). The bag is filled with 5 liters of dialysis solution which is exchanged by gravity every 60-90 min for a total amount of 20-30 liters/session (Fig. 2). The dialysate composition employed is the following: sodium 150, potassium 1, chloride 110 mEq/L, calcium 12 mg/dl, magnesium 1.5 mEq/L, acetate 48 mEq/L. Blood flow of about 200 ml/min was obtained spontaneously by external A-V shunt (2 pts) or femoral arterious and venous catheterization (4 pts), or from large central vein by peristaltic pump (7 pts). The duration of the sessions were scheduled time after time according to the clinical conditions of the patients up to 10 hours. Similarly the amount of replacement fluid was monitored during the treatment. Since 1983, 13 patients, 6 males and 7 females aging 31-77 years, affected by ARF due to abdominal surgery or trauma with water-electrolyte diso-

BF HEMODIAFILTRATION
FOR TREATMENT OF ARF
TECHNICAL PROFILE

BLOOD FLOW	206±18 ml/min
DIALYSATE	20-30 L / session
SESSION TIME	4-10 hrs
ULTRAFILTRATION RATE	14±8 ml/min
REPLACEMENT FLUID (glucose,saline,buffer solution)	5-15 L / session

mean±SD

Fig. 3. Technical profile and fluid volume control of BF+HDF for treatment of acute renal failure.

rders, nephrotoxic or systemic disease, underwent BF-HDF treatment. Seven patients were treated with the combined C-BF+HF and 6 with the compact P-BF model. The patients underwent BF-HDF for a total of 82 sessions (3-12, mean 6.3/pts) (Tab. I).

RESULTS

Bag-Filter hemodiafiltration has resulted in effective and well tolerated therapy for our acute uremic population, either with the combined C-BF+HF either with the compact P-BF apparatus.
A blood flow of 206±18 ml/min, spontaneously derived or pump assisted, consented an ultrafiltration rate of 14±8 ml/min (Fig. 3). Such ultrafiltration capacity allowed in severe catabolic patients a fluid removal up to 15 liters during long dialytic sessions with simultaneous replacement by glucose, aminoacids or lipid solutions. On the other hand patients with water-electrolyte disorders or severe metabolic acidosis have been treated by BF-HDF with reinfusion of electrolyte or buffer solutions, which consented adequate correction of the altered parameters.
Concerning the depurative efficacy of the system, the mean clearances per session resulted 68.2±9.3 ml/min for urea nitrogen, 52.8±7.8 ml/min for creatinine, 44.0±8.5 ml/min for uric acid and 42.4±7.1 ml/min for phosphorus (Fig. 4). Of the 13 acute uremic patients entered our BF-HDF program 6 have had complete recovery of renal function, 5 remained on chronic hemodialysis and 2 died for sepsis and irreversible cardiac failure.

DISCUSSION

The therapeutic approach of acute renal failure currently deserves several options according to the clinical and logistic conditions. IPD has been applied not infrequently as treatment of ARF, with successful clinical outcome of the patients[12]. However this modality shows not adequate removal

BF HEMODIAFILTRATION FOR TREATMENT OF ARF

DEPURATIVE EFFICACY

	blood value (mg/dl)	clearance / session (ml/min)
UREA N	138±27	68.2±9.3
CREATININE	9.1±1.7	52.8±7.8
URIC ACID	8.5±2.4	44.0±8.5
PHOSPHORUS	5.6±1.2	42.4±7.1

mean±SD

Fig. 4. Depurative effectiveness of BF-HDF for treatment of acute renal failure.

of uremic toxins in very ill acute uremic subjects. In these cases the patients were managed by transfer to extracorporeal dialysis to achieve adequate depuration and fluid removal. CAVH represents the best procedure for severe ill patients with kidney failure treated in intensive care unit, because of easy set up and smooth continuous depuration[13]. In addition it consents better correction of metabolic acidosis or electrolyte imbalance and restoration of fluids volume. Indeed this therapy has several drawbacks in terms of adequate depuration because of implying only convective process and low volume of substitution fluids. Thus in particular conditions with accelerated metabolic catabolism this therapeutic procedure results in limited efficacy[14].

Our model employes the same technique by spontaneous heart-powered blood flow, throughout arterious-venous external or internal access, but increases the depurative effectiveness owing to the presence of dialysate in plastic bag which leads to a diffusive process with a dialysate/plasma equilibrium in about 90 minutes. This addictive dialysate compartment consents to remove about 30 g of urea each session by substituting 15 liters of plasma water for the convective process and 20 g of urea nitrogen for 75% D/P equilibrium, by exchanging 30 liters of dialysate. This theoretical calculation shows the feasibility of this procedure also for very ill patients with negative nitrogen balance such polytraumatized, post-surgery septic patients, etc. But the peculiarity of this technique is also due to the use of a new polysulphone membrane with a geometrical structure which includes high clearance rates in terms of filtration due to its high hydraulic permeability. This membrane resembles an ideal acqueous membrane close to cuprophane layer with the feature that there is not interaction between the diffusive solute transport and the convective process. This peculiarity makes this membrane able to provide high clearance either of small either of middle molecular weight substances.

The advantages of our BF-HDF system may also be split in technical and clinical. For the experience of our treated patients we may conclude that they have got an adequate depuration with the necessary administration of calories by glucose, aminoacids and lipid solutions. This technique allows no hemodynamic stress provided fluid monitoring is instituted.

The treatment was well tolerated by our patients even at high clinical risk. The 2 deaths were due to causes unrelated to the therapeutic procedure because of irreversible septic shock and multiple severe trauma.

This therapy infact is specifically indicated in acute renal failure from heart insufficiency, electrolytes disorders, and shocks of different origin. Besides these clinical indications we like to stress the technical advantages related to the semplicity in setting up and in monitoring the treatment. Infact we have treated patients with acute renal failure of different etiology in no nephrologic wards like intensive care units, traumatology, gastroenterology and surgery departments. Medical and paramedical assistance was limited and not specialized. The feasibility of the procedure, the semplicity of the technique, the absence of hemodynamic stress for its smooth treatment associated with efficacy in terms of adequate depuration also in hypercatabolic patients, makes this machineless artificial kidney a new deal in uremia therapy. The low costs and the abolition of the sophisticated machinery apparatus makes it a prêt à porter artificial kidney to be available in countries with low technical assistance, social and economical problems.

REFERENCES

1. P. Kramer, J. Böhler, A. Kehz, H. J. Gröne, J. Schrader, D. Matthaei and F. Scheler, Intensive care potential of continuous arterio-venous hemofiltration, Trans. ASAIO 28:28 (1982).
2. A. M. Pierides, B. Schniepp and W. J. Johnson, Hemofiltration in the treatment of acute and chronic renal failure, Proc. Clin. Dial. Transpl. Forum 9:50 (1979).
3. J. F. Winchester, Hemoperfusion in uremia, in: "Sorbents and their clinical applications" C. Giordano, ed., Academic Press, Inc., New York (1980).
4. K. D. Nolph, R. P. Popovich and J. W. Moncrief, Theoretical and pratical implications of CAPD, Nephron 21:117 (1978).
5. H. W. Leber, V. Wizemann, G. Gaubeaud, P. Rawer and G. Schütterle, Simultaneous hemofiltration/hemodialysis: an effective alternative to hemofiltration and conventional hemodialysis in the treatment of uremic patients, Clin. Nephrol. 9:150 (1978).
6. S. Shaldon, M. C. Bean, G. Deschodt, P. Ramperer and C. Mion, Vascular stability during hemofiltration, Trans. ASAIO 26:391 (1980).
7. J. F. Winchester, M. C. Gelfand, J. H. Kuepshield and G. E. Schreiner, Dialysis and hemoperfusion of poisons and drugs. Update, Trans. ASAIO 23:762 (1977).
8. G. Schütterle, V. Wizemann and G. Seyffart, Hemodiafiltration, Proc. 1 Symp. Giessen 1981 (Hygieneplan, Oberursel 1982).
9. G. Bazzato, U. Coli, S. Landini, S. Lucatello, A. Fracasso, P. Morachiello, F. Righetto, F. Scanferla, A bag-filter model as machineless artificial kidney, Trans. ASAIO 29:657 (1983).
10. G. Bazzato, U. Coli, S. Landini, F. Scanferla, A new model for spontaneous hemodialysis, Sem. Nephrol. 3:256 (1983).
11. G. Bazzato, U. Coli, S. Landini, S. Lucatello, A. Fracasso, P. Morachiello, F. Righetto, F. Scanferla, Combined hemofilter and bag-filter: an artificial nephron, Proc. ISAO Kyoto meeting 2:408 (1983).
12. T. W. Valk, R. D. Swartz and C. H. Hsu, Peritoneal dialysis in acute renal failure: analysis of outcome and complications, Dialysis and Transpl. 9:48 (1980).
13. P. Kramer, Arteriovenous hemofiltration. A kidney replacement therapy for intensive care unit, Springer-Verlag (1985).
14. C. Ronco, Arterio-venous hemodiafiltration (A-V HDF): a possible way to increase urea removal during CAVH, Int. J. Art. Org. 8:61 (1985)

DIALYTIC THERAPY OF ACUTE RENAL FAILURE

Albert Valek

Department of Medicine, Charles University
Medicine School, Prague, Czechoslovakia

INTRODUCTION

Acute renal failure is a serious illness from both the medical and social points of view. Its morality rate is high, it affects mostly young and healthy people and if patients survive the acute stage, the majority recover[1,2]. Modern methods of therapy are so effective that patients may die of an underlying disease or mortal injuries, but he should not die of renal failure and its complications. The treatment of patients with acute renal failure is a complex of diverse methods of therapy. Dialysis is only one of them.

HOW MANY PATIENTS WITH ACUTE RENAL FAILURE NEED DIALYTIC THERAPY?

The precise incidence of acute renal failure is not known. The number of patients per million population per year, found in individual countries differs substantially as well as incidence found by various authors in the same country /Table 1/. Also the number of patients per million population per year, dialysed in individual regions of one country differs /Table 2/.

The only explanation of this fact is that acute renal failure is not diagnosed and patients die without help. One of the duties of the specialized dialysis center is to teach physicians when to suspect and how to diagnose acute renal failure.

INDICATION FOR DIALYSIS

In 1960, Teschan et al.[9] and later others[10,11,12] have shown that "prophylactic" dialysis decrease mortality and morbidity. Also practice of regular dialysis treatment and good results of Bonomini's[13] "early dialysis" confirmed that the condition of patients is better, if blood urea concentration before dialysis is low.

Table 1. Incidence of acute renal failure.

Year	Author	Ref.	Country	Pat.pmp[a]
1958	Alwall	3	Sweden	30-40
1962	Sarre a Rothe	4	FRG	20
1963	Mackay a Dudley	5	Scotland	150
1964	Lundig et al.	6	Scandinavia	40
1979	Freiberg et al.	7	FRG	100
1984	Erben	8	Czechoslovakia	17

[a] Number of patients per million population

Dialysis treatment in acute renal failure should be initiated, if blood urea concentration is higher than 30 mmol/L and serum creatinine concentration higher than 800 μmol/L. Blood urea and creatinine levels should never exceed these values during the course of the disease. Other indications are hyperpotassemia over 6.5 mmol/L, if it is not treatable by cation exchange resins or by administration of hypertonic glucose infusions, and acidosis with pH lower than 7.2 and bicarbonate concentration lower than 10 mmol/L. Also hyperhydration, especially with manifestations of congestive heart failure, pulmonary and cerebral edema requires dialysis.

Frequency and duration of dialysis as well as protein catabolic rate may be ascertained by Sargent and Gotch urea kinetic modeling[14, 15, 16].

Who not to dialyse? Patients with hypovolemia due to blood and fluid losses in the initial stage. Its correction may improve renal failure and avoid dialysis. Patients with urinary tract obstruction. They will benefit more from relief of obstruction than from dialysis.

Table 2. Incidence of acute renal failure in individual regions of Czechoslovakia.

Region	Pat.pmp[a]	Region	Pat.pmp[a]
Prague	27	Northern Moravia	19
Central Bohemia	9	Southern Moravia	13
Eastern Bohemia	29	Western Slovakia	5
Northern Bohemia	3	Central Slovakia	5
Western Bohemia	12	Eastern Slovakia	7
Southern Bohemia	12		

[a] Number of patients per million population

CHOICE OF DIALYSIS TECHNIQUE

At present, peritoneal dialysis, hemodialysis and continuous arteriovenous hemofiltration /CAVH/ are available for treatment of acute renal failure. Which and when of these methods to use will be evident after comparing their effectivity, advantages and disadvantages.

Hemodialysis eliminates small molecular weight substances of protein catabolism including potassium five times more efficiently than peritoneal dialysis. Also resorption of bicarbonates or acetate from dialysate is five times more effective during hemodialysis. While more than 1000 ml water per hour and 140 mmol sodium per liter of filtrate is eliminated by hemodialysis, only 700 ml and 70 mmol is eliminated by peritoneal dialysis if hypertonic dialysate is used.

On the contrary, dialysis with a very effective dialyzer rapidly decreases the concentration of small molecular, osmotically active metabolites in the blood, which leads to disequilibrium syndrome. It also increases acetate flux from dialysate, which may cause so called acetate intolerance.

Peritoneal dialysis is indicated, if hemodialysis is not available, for children, in blood access problems, in patients with bleeding risk and with unstable cardiovascular status.

Peritoneal dialysis is unfavorable after abdomen trauma or operation, in patients with diaphragmatic defects, with peritoneal adhesions from previous abdominal surgery, with pulmonary complications and in hypercatabolic state.

Continous arteriovenous hemofiltration may be used, if long duration of anuria or oliguria is expected, if patients are confined to bed and if hyperalimentation and infusions will be necessary and if patients are hemodynamically unstable. CAVH operates without the use of a blood pump. The patient´s arterial pressure is a source of flow. Blood flow rate is 30-80 ml/min., ultrafiltration rate 500-1500 ml/hour. Low clearance due to spontaneous blood flow is inadequate to control the urea level in hypercatabolic patients in whom the support of haemodialysis is necessary. CAVH requires constant supervision and frequent readjustment of rate of substitutional fluid infusion because of variable filtration rates. Other drawbacks of CAVH include the high cost of substitution fluid and frequent filter clotting.

If acute renal failure is accompanied by exogeneous intoxication or hepatic failure, combination of hemodialysis and hemoperfusion is recommended.

BLOOD ACCESS

Catheterization of femoral or subclavian veins by Seldinger technique is the most advantageous method. It is safe in larger dialysis centers with experience gained, the catheter may remain in place for more than two weeks, patients can be dialysed also being hypotensive and in a state of shock. In between dialyses, the canula is kept from clotting by replacing the small dead space by heparin. The risk of thrombosis is lower than in arteriovenous shunt. Catheterization of veins also does not sacrifice blood access sites, which may become important, if acute renal failure is not resolved.

Catheterization of the femoral vein is, perhaps, the easier technique since the femoral artery is palpable. It is also in an area, in which no vital organ may be accidentally damaged. Catheters are withdrawn after dialysis and reinserted for each dialysis. The groin sites are alternated. The femoral catheter may also be left in place for repeated dialyses. However, a catheter restricts patients mobility and it is an area more prone to infection.

From this point of view, catheterisation of subclavian veins is more favourable. Mobility of patients is the best prevention of catabolism and pneumonia. Incidence of complications is low when cannulation is performed by trained personnel only.

Catheterization of the femoral artery for CAVH may be risky. Serious bleeding along the catheter between femoral muscles and into retroperitoneum during dialysis and especially after the catheter is withdrawn may happen. Inexplicable hypotension some hours after dialysis is the only sign. In one case, surgical intervention on the femoral artery was necessary. Arteriovenous shunt is safer for CAVH.

CLINICAL CONDITION MONITORING

Dialysis therapy should be as simple and safe as possible, so that personnel could take care of other aspects of the treatment. The same is true for monitoring parameters.

What is essential and what is complementary?

Essential is control of clinical manifestations, water and salt balance and protein catabolic rate. The rest is complementary. The extent of these parameters depends on the basic disease and complication, kind of therapeutic intervention, or on research. All essential features should be examined daily, or, if necessary, several times a day.

Clinical manifestations of uremia are not serious in patients with acute renal failure, properly treated in dialysis centers. Symptoms and signs of the basic disorder are specific and diverse. It is essential, however, to examine body teperature, pulse and respiratory rates, blood pressure, and to search for ankle, lumbar and eye-lid edemas, or for signs of dehydration. Also lung and heart percussion and auscultation are important.

Water and salt balance may be controlled by water and sodium intake and output, taking into account metabolic water and insensible perspiration, by serum sodium concentration and by body weight measurements, or plasma protein or hemoglobin concentrations. As patients with acute renal failure are catabolic, they should lose body weight between 0,2 and 0,4 kg daily. Hyperhydration is the cause of arterial hypertension, cardiac failure and pulmonary edema. Interstitial pulmonary edema is the first step. It is auscultatory silent, but typical on the x-ray picture: bilateral butterfly-like shadows originate from the lung hili and disappear into the periphery. Weekly chest x-ray pictures help to diagnose this manifestation. Sometimes central venous pressure measurement is necessary.

Protein catabolic rate may be checked by blood urea and serum creatinine and potassium concentrations. As hyperkalemia has a life-threatening effect on the cardiac conductive system, which is enhanced by hypocalcemia, hyponatremia and acidosis, electrocardiogram is more important than serum potassium concentration itself.

COMPLICATIONS

As complications of acute renal failure should be prevented or successfully treated, all physicians ought to be aware of them. They can be divided into two groups: not connected with dialysis and caused by dialysis.

Complications Not Connected with Dialysis

The most dangerous complications are infection, nonuremic bleeding from gastrointestinal tract and pancreatitis.

Infection affects lungs, urinary tract, wounds and operative sites. The exact reason for the high frequency of infective complications remains to be determined. However, disruption of anatomical barriers, impaired humoral and cellular immunity, and inappropriate use of antibiotics may all play a role.

Lung infections are common in critically ill patients. Pulmonary secretion is poorly cleared in bed-ridden patients, with subsequent development of atelectasis and pneumonia. Mortality is high in spite of antibiotics. Mobility of patients, physiotherapy or breathing excercise in bed-ridden patients is the only prevention. Urinary tract infection develops in anuric or oliguric patients easily as the stream of urine is lacking. Urinary bladder catheterization to obtain a sample of urine or to make sure that the patient is anuric or oliguric, or indwelling bladder catheter for measuring urine output is unacceptable because there is an unnecessary risk of infection. Wounds and operative sites as well as indwelling intravenous catheters must be treated by strictly aseptic technique. All necessary tubes and catheters should be removed.

Non-uremic gastrointestinal bleeding is usually caused by stress ulcers. Hypotension or shock of unknown origin may be the first manifestation. After one or two days, melena clarifies the reason. Presence of blood in the gut leads to urea and potassium loading, resulting in severe increase in blood urea and potassium levels. The investigation and therapy of gastrointestinal bleeding is similar to that in non uremic patients. Surgery has to be carried out between dialyses.

Pancreatitis is a rare complication, often not diagnosed. It occurs after prolonged hypotension and septicemia. Mortality is very high.

Complications Caused by the Dialysis Process

Hypotension may be brought about by several factors.

Depletion of extracelular volume is due to shifting blood into the extracorporeal circuit, to blood loss from a leak in the blood circuit or if the rate of ultrafiltration exceeds the rate of fluid mobilization from the interstitial and intracellular spaces in the vascular space. The larger volume of dialyzer and blood lines, the greater tendency for hypotension.

Acetate in dialysate has vasodilatory and cardiodepressant affects. Hypotension occurs more likely in patients, dialysed by large surface area dialyzer, in patients with liver disease or in diabetics, with nausea, vomiting and headache.

Also changes in osmolarity during dialysis play an important role in the pathogenesis of hypotension.

Antihypertensive medication contributes to the development of hypotension by blocking the compensatory response to intravascular depletion.

Hypotension during dialysis may be due to an underlying process such as myocardial disease or sepsis, to acute bleeding in the patient or to pericardial tamponade as well.

Prevention of hypotension by dialysis with small surface area dialyzer, with bicarbonate or high sodium dialysate, by withholding antihypertensive medication four to six hours prior to dialysis is possible.

Disequilibrium syndrome occurs the second or third hour after initiation of hemodialysis, particularly during the first or second dialysis. It appears as restlessness, headache, nausea, vomiting, and muscle twitching, confusion and generalized seizures. The pathophysiology is multifactorial. Urea concentration and osmolarity of the cerebrospinal fluid fall less rapidly than in plasma during dialysis, leading to inflow of water in the central nervous system and a rise in cerebrospinal fluid pressure. Subdural hematoma, intracerebral hemorrhage, hypertensive encephalopathy should be ruled out.

Measures to decrease the incidence of disequilibrium syndrome include deliberate decrease in clearance of uremic solutes by using small size dialyzers, decreasing the blood flow rate and limiting duration of first dialysis.

Excessive use of heparin, especially in patients with liver dysfunction, prolonged bleeding time due to platelet dysfunction or trombocytopenia prior to dialysis, may raise bleeding. Gastrointestinal bleeding, subdural or retroperitonal hematoma, hemopericardium are life-threatening bleeding diathesis.

Arrhythmias are produced by acute changes of serum electrolytes, particularly changes in potassium, calcium and bicarbonate cencentrations. They are potentiated in the digitalized patients.

Technical problems can be avoided by better technical care and nursing. There are air embolism during administration of intravenous fluid or during rinsing back of the blood at the end of dialysis; acute blood loss due to dialyzer leak; errors in dialysate composition, leading to hypo or hypernatremia; contamination of dialysate by disinfectants; overheated dialysate leading to acute hemolysis.

The most serious complications of peritoneal dialysis are peritonitis, hypotension, hyponatremia and hyperglycemia due to hypertonic dextrose dialysate; bowel and bladder perforations.

PROGNOSIS

In spite of dialysis and intensive care therapy improvement, mortality of patients with acute renal failure is still high and has not changed substantially during the past 30 years /Table 3/. The reason is that the proportion of patients with incurable underlying illness has increased as well as the age of patients /Table 4/.

Table 3. Mortality rates in patients with acute renal failure in Czechoslovakia between 1955-64 and in 1984

Year	Number of patients	Mortality %	Ref.
1955 - 1964	543	43	17
1984	180	37	8

Table 4. Influence of underlying illness and age on the mortality rate /18/

Period	1959-1967	1974-1976
Mortality rate /%/	38	67
Proportion of surgical patients /%/	54	75
Mean age /years/	43	58

WHEN TO TRANSPORT PATIENTS WITH ACUTE RENAL FAILURE TO SPECIALIZED DIALYSIS CENTERS

The number of patients with acute renal failure per million population per year, who require dialysis therapy is relatively low. Treatment of these patients is complicated and needs a trained and skilful personnel. The high standard and skill may be maintained only by constant activity. For this reason, it is better to concentrate patients with acute renal failure from an area of one million population or more to one center.

Whom, and when to transport patients to the specialized center?

1. Patients with anuric or oligurie phase of acute renal failure. Those in initial phase, in shock or with the urinary tract obstruction should be treated on the spot.
2. Uncomplicated cases, if anuria or oliguria persists for more than 3 days.
3. If blood urea concentration is higher than 30 mmol/L
4. If hyperkalemia is higher than 6.0 mmol/L in spite of conservative therapy.
5. Hyperhydrated patients, particularly with serious arterial hypertension, heart failure, lung and brain edema.
6. Patients older than 60 on the first day of the anuric or oliguric phase.

SUMMARY

1. On the basis of experience with dialysis therapy of 1000 patients with acute renal failure in the years from 1955 to 1985 the most important aspects of the treatment were discussed.

2. The precise incidence of acute renal failure is not known. It seems that a number of patients die without being diagnosed.

3. Dialysis therapy is indicated when blood urea concentration exceeds 30 mmol/L and/or serum potassium concentration is higher than 6.5 mmol/L, when patients are over-hydrated or show first signs of uremia. Hemodialysis remains the gold standard among all methods of blood purification.

4. Catheterization of subclavian veins is the most advantageous access to circulation for hemodialysis.

5. Majority of medical complications due to renal failure as well as technical ones may be avoided.

6. Mortality is still high and has not changed in 30 years in spite of medical and technical improvement of treatment because of higher proportion of patients with uncurable underlying disease and higher age.

7. Therapy of patients with acute renal failure should be centralized. No patient, should die of renal failure and its complications.

REFERENCES

1. A. Amerio, A. Vercellone, G. Benedictis, F. Linari, G. Picoli, P. Coratelli, G. Vacha, R. Ragni, F. Mastrangelo, G. Pastore, Long-term prognosis in acute renal failure of primarily tubular origin. Minerva Nefrol., 19:7/1972/.
2. V. Bonomini, A. Vangelista, G.M. Frasca, Value of renal biopsy for long-term prognosis in acute renal failure. In: Acute Renal Failure, D. Seybold, U. Gessler, eds., Karger, Basel, /1982/.
3. N. Alwall, Die Aktive Therapie der Niereninsuffizienz. Dtsch.med.Wschr., 83:950, 1008 /1958/.
4. H. Sarre, K. Rother, Akutes Nierenversagen. Thieme, Stuttgart /1962/.
5. W. D. Mackay, H. A. F. Dudley, An artificial kidney in a general hospital group. Scot.med.J., 8:109 /1963/.
6. M. Lundig, J. Steiness, J. H. Thaysen, Acute renal failure due to tubular necrosis. Immediate prognosis and complications. Acta med.Scand., 176:103 /1964/.
7. J. Freiberg, E. Schäfer, T. v. Lilien-Walden, J. Kindler, H. G. Sieberth, Prognose bei akuten Nierenversagen. Bericht über 1102 Fälle. In: Akutes Nierenversagen, H. G. Siebert, ed., Thieme Stuttgart /1979/.
8. J. Erben, E. Tschernoster, I. Skála, Hemodialysis activity in Czechoslovakia in 1984 /in Czech/, Transplant 4:21 /1985/.
9. P. E. Teschan, C. R. Baxter, T. F. O´Brien, J. N. Freyhof, W. H. Hall, Prophylactic hemodialysis in the treatment of acute renal failure. Ann.intern.Med. 53:922 /1960/.
10. F. M. Parsons, S. M. Hobson, C. R. Blagg, B. H. Mc Cracken, Optimum time for dialysis in acute reversible renal failure. Lancet, 1:129 /1961/.
11. D. Kleinknecht, P. Jungers, J. Chanard, C. Barbanel, D. Ganeval, Uremic and non-uremic complications in acute renal failure: evaluation of early and frequent dialysis on prognosis. Kidney Int., 1:190 /1972/.
12. J. D. Conger, A controlled evaluation of prophylactic dialysis in post-traumatic acute renal failure. J.Trauma, 15:1956 /1975/
13. V. Bonomini, Early dialysis stands the test of time. Life Support Systems, 3:1 /1985/.
14. M. F. Borah, P. Y. Schoenfeld, F. A. Gotch, J. A. Sargent, M. Wolfson, M. H. Humpreys, Nitrogen balance during intermittent dialysis therapy of uremia. Kidney, Int., 14:491 /1978/.
15. J. A. Sargent, F. A. Gotch, M. F. Borah, L. Piercy, N. Spinozzi, P. Schoenfeld, M. Humpreys, Urea kinetics: a guide to nutritional management of renal failure. Am.J.clin.Nutr., 31:1696 /1978/.
16. J. A. Sargent, F. A. Gotch, Nutrition and treatment of acutely ill patient using urea kinetics. Dial.Transpl., 10:314 /1981/.
17. A. Válek, Acute renal failure /in Czech/, SNZ, Praha, /1967/.
18. A. Linton, R. Lindsay, Why the continuing high mortality in acute renal failure? In: G. E. Schreiner, ed: Controversies in Nephrology, Vol. 1, /1979/.

INDEX

GPSR Compliance
The European Union's (EU) General Product Safety Regulation (GPSR) is a set of rules that requires consumer products to be safe and our obligations to ensure this.

If you have any concerns about our products, you can contact us on

ProductSafety@springernature.com

In case Publisher is established outside the EU, the EU authorized representative is:

Springer Nature Customer Service Center GmbH
Europaplatz 3
69115 Heidelberg, Germany

www.ingramcontent.com/pod-product-compliance
Ingram Content Group UK Ltd.
Pitfield, Milton Keynes, MK11 3LW, UK
UKHW051130260726
13967UKWH00010B/2969

* 9 7 8 1 4 6 8 4 8 2 4 1 6 *